Plastic Surgery Vivas for the FRCS(Plast)

This is the first Q&A-based revision book specifically aimed at candidates sitting the viva component of the FRCS(Plast) examination. It provides a selection of common clinical scenarios presented in a realistic way and presents a guide to answering the FRCS(Plast) questions, as well as advice on how to approach the revision process itself. Crucially, this will help to prepare candidates to organize their thoughts, demonstrate higher order thinking, and present a robust answer in the face of grey areas and controversies.

The text covers all topics from the syllabus, including Trauma, Burns, Facial and Soft Tissue Injuries, Acute Head and Neck Tumours, Cleft and Craniofacial, Congenital Anomalies, Facial Palsy, Vascular Anomalies, Trunk and Perineal, Skin Cancer, Basic Sciences, Aesthetic, Ethics and Medico-legal, and Consent. Candidates using this book will be able to realistically recreate the exam scenario either in private or in a group setting.

This book would be equally useful for candidates sitting plastic surgery post-graduate exams with equivalent syllabuses to that of the FRCS(Plast) such as the EBOPRAS exam, as well as others. In addition, it also makes an excellent companion for trainees throughout the course of their 6-year training rotation, allowing more junior plastic surgery trainees the opportunity to become acquainted with the format and content of the FRCS(Plast) exam. Lastly, it may be helpful to consultants who are interested in coaching their trainees in topics other than their subspeciality.

Plastic Surgery Vivas for the FRCS(Plast)

An Essential Guide

Monica Fawzy, MBChB,
MRCS, FRCS(Plast)

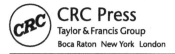

CRC Press
Taylor & Francis Group
Boca Raton New York London

CRC Press is an imprint of the
Taylor & Francis Group, an **informa** business

First edition published 2023
by CRC Press
6000 Broken Sound Parkway NW, Suite 300, Boca Raton, FL 33487-2742

and by CRC Press
4 Park Square, Milton Park, Abingdon, Oxon, OX14 4RN

CRC Press is an imprint of Taylor & Francis Group, LLC

© 2023 Taylor & Francis Group, LLC

ISBN: 9780367024888 (hbk)
ISBN: 9781138388215 (pbk)
ISBN: 9780429399268 (ebk)

DOI: 10.1201/9780429399268

Typeset in Times
by KnowledgeWorks Global Ltd.

*This book is dedicated to the loving memory of my mother,
Dr Seham Elrouby, and to my father, Professor M. E. Fawzy. A whole
book wouldn't be long enough to fit all my reasons why.*

Monica Fawzy

Contents

VIVA I

VIVA II

VIVA III

Foreword

I am honoured to have been asked to write the foreword for this addition to the Plastic Surgery literature.

I do this on the back of my experience in preparing trainees for the FRCS(Plast) over more than 15 years as a trainer and 8 years as a training programme director. I have been an examiner for the FRCS(Plast) for over ten years and during my time as chairman of the Specialty Advisory Committee (SAC) for plastic surgery sat on the intercollegiate exam board. This has afforded me an intimate knowledge of the examination process.

I am not surprised that Monica has embarked on this project as all my interactions with her have been in the field of surgical education. We first met when she assisted at national selection for plastic surgery training during my time as national selection lead for the SAC. Later, we met as co-faculty at various courses including a cadaveric programme she instituted in the East of England. I have always admired her commitment to training and to the specialty, which continues in her role as Communications Officer for BAPRAS.

In her quest for the correct tone and standard of this book, she has recruited some of the leading educators and sub-speciality experts in our field, many of whom are fellow examiners and up to date with any new changes in the curriculum and examination.

I have gone on record as saying that Plastic and Reconstructive Surgery is a very competitive specialty and our nationally appointed trainees are some of the brightest young minds in medicine. They present to the oral part of the FRCS(Plast) examination having been successful in a challenging multiple choice test which assures they have the required knowledge to be a day one consultant.

Unfortunately, some stumble at this hurdle, primarily due to a lack of examination technique. A few seem unaware of the structure of the examination process itself. Some are unprepared for the pace and precision required in the exam. Each question is only given five minutes and so Monica's two-minute rule is examination 'gold dust'. It also means that candidates may not leave themselves enough time to delve deeply into topics where the marks for higher order thinking are often awarded. Additionally, some believe that there must be a right or wrong answer to every question which is rarely the case in our specialty and this important issue is addressed here.

Trainees may also fall foul of the breadth of the specialty. If working in a region that does not offer subspecialty interests such as cleft, head and neck, genitourinary, or others, then the practical aspect of the exam may be more challenging. I believe this may be part of the aetiology for the struggles of some of the non-trainee candidates presenting to the examination, as they may be less likely to rotate through different firms or hospitals. I think that Monica's attempt to address this in the book is commendable.

I believe that reading this book will enlighten candidates not only on the breadth of content required for Section 2 of the FRCS(Plast) but also and perhaps more importantly on tips of technique regarding brevity and precision of answers.

Good luck to all.

Maniram Ragbir
President Elect BAPRAS 2022

Preface

I felt compelled to write this as I looked for a similar book when I prepared for the FRCS(Plast) exam just over 10 years ago. Most published materials, both then and now, are excellent in presenting and summarizing the theory required to pass but do not always address reasons why many good trainees fail the exam – such as a failure to demonstrate organization of one's thoughts under pressure, higher order thinking, and to present a robust answer when presented with grey areas and controversies.

The strength of this book is that I hope it presents a way of approaching the answers to demonstrate this.

Candidates have historically obtained this training from peers who have recently passed the exam, consultants who are willing and able to donate time from their own busy schedules, and formal exam courses that can be even more stress-inducing for some, as it is in effect practising 'in public'.

I hope this book will supplement these opportunities, allowing you to practise at your own pace, at a time that suits you, and in the comfort and privacy of your own home.

I wish you the best of luck.

About the Author

Ms Monica Fawzy, MBChB, MRCS, FRCS(Plast), is a Consultant Plastic Surgeon at the Norfolk and Norwich University Hospitals NHS Trust with a subspecialty interest in Head and Neck Reconstruction, Facial Palsy Reanimation, and Paediatric Plastic Surgery. She is co-lead of the Norwich Microsurgery Fellowship Program and Deputy Training Program Director of the East of England Plastic Surgery Training Program.

She graduated from Bristol Medical School and undertook her plastic surgery specialist training in the East of England, followed by fellowships in Paris and Cambridge.

She has always been passionate about medical education and spent a year teaching anatomy as a demonstrator first at the University of Oxford, then at GKT Medical School in London. She undertook a post-graduate certification in medical education, successfully coached many trainees to pass the FRCS(Plast) exam, and served as faculty on National FRCS Plast courses. She led the regional plastic surgery simulation programme in the East of England post-graduate deanery for 4 years. She was elected by her consultant colleagues as representative of the East of England on BAPRAS Council before being appointed as BAPRAS Communications Officer.

Acknowledgements

I am indebted to the NHS consultant colleagues and friends based around the United Kingdom, listed below, who have very generously donated their time to proofread the material relevant to their subspecialty, as well as lend their opinion with regard to grey areas and controversies.

Dhalia Masud, Peter Dziewulski, Chris Hill, Alex Crick, Patrick Gillespie, Wee Lam, Umraz Khan, Nora Nugent, Kalliroi Tzafetta, Juling Ong, Marc Moncrieff, Dean Boyce, Jonothan Clibbon, David Sainsbury, Walid Sabbagh, Fateh Ahmad, Martin Heaton, Richard Haywood, Ewan Wilson, Richard Sisson, Stuart Burrows, Helen Goddard, and Grainne Bourke.

I would strongly recommend that you seek the opportunity to spend time with these educators if you have the chance – both for exam purposes and to optimize your training in general.

I have included their NHS bases below.

They are masters of their subspecialities, passionate about education, and great company: I have enjoyed our many hours of discussion.

We are all so fortunate to be working within such an incredibly interesting and varied specialty.

Any remaining potential errors are entirely my own.

Ms Dhalia Masud
Consultant Plastic Surgeon
The Norfolk and Norwich University Hospital
Norwich

Professor Peter Dziewulski
Consultant Plastic and Burns surgeon
St Andrew's Centre for Plastic Surgery and Burns
Chelmsford

Mr Chris Hill
Consultant Plastic and Cleft Lip and Palate Surgeon
The Royal Belfast Hospital for Sick Children
Belfast

Ms Alex Crick
Consultant Plastic Surgeon
Salisbury District Hospital
Salisbury

Mr Patrick Gillespie
Consultant Plastic and Hand Surgeon
Royal Devon and Exeter Hospital
Exeter

Mr Wee Lam
Consultant Plastic and Hand Surgeon
Royal Hospital for Sick Children
Edinburgh

Mr Umraz Khan
Consultant Plastic Surgeon and Orthoplastic
    Lead for Lower Limb Trauma Services
North Bristol NHS Trust
Bristol

Ms Nora Nugent
Consultant Plastic and Burns Surgeon
Queen Victoria Hospital
East Grinstead

Ms Kalliroi Tzafetta
Consultant Plastic Surgeon
St Andrew's Centre for Plastic Surgery and Burns
Chelmsford

Mr Juling Ong
Consultant Plastic and Craniofacial Surgeon
Great Ormond Street Hospital
London

Professor Marc Moncrieff
Consultant Plastic Surgeon
The Norfolk and Norwich University Hospital
Norwich

Mr Dean Boyce
Consultant Plastic and Hand Surgeon
Swansea NHS Trust
Swansea

Mr Jonothan Clibbon
Consultant Plastic Surgeon
The Norfolk and Norwich University Hospital
Norwich

Mr David Sainsbury
Consultant Cleft and Plastic Surgeon
Newcastle upon Tyne Hospitals
Newcastle

Mr Walid Sabbagh
Consultant Plastic Surgeon
The Royal Free Hospital
London

Mr Fateh Ahmad
Consultant Plastic Surgeon
St Andrew's Centre for Plastic Surgery and Burns
Chelmsford

Mr Martin Heaton
Consultant Plastic Surgeon
The Norfolk and Norwich University Hospital
Norwich

Mr Richard Haywood
Consultant Plastic Surgeon
The Norfolk and Norwich University Hospital
Norwich

Mr Ewan Wilson
Consultant Plastic Surgeon
North Bristol NHS Trust
Bristol

Mr Richard Sisson
Consultant Oral and Maxillofacial Surgeon
The Norfolk and Norwich University Hospital
Norwich

Mr Stuart Burrows
Consultant ENT Surgeon
The Norfolk and Norwich University Hospital
Norwich

Dr Helen Goddard
Consultant Head and Neck Anaesthetist
The Norfolk and Norwich University Hospital
Norwich

Ms Grainne Bourke
Consultant Plastic and Hand Surgeon
Leeds Teaching Hospitals
Leeds

Introduction

This book is designed to be a revision guide for those preparing for the UK FRCS(Plast) Viva plastic surgery exam, and equivalent examinations, to help you practise applying your knowledge in an exam format with complex scenarios.

It provides a flavour of common questions and how one answer may lead to the next, with a realistic style of questioning and interruptions by the examiner.

Hand drawings are also included as examples of what you may be expected to produce on the day. They are not annotated, as you won't have time to do that in the exam. You will just be expected to talk through them, as included in the model answers.

However, it is almost guaranteed that you will never be asked so many questions about one scenario: it will more commonly be three to four questions before they move you on to the next topic, but many more have been included here to help prepare you for more potential questions depending on which path you are taken down.

Also, the questions are purposefully set at the level of a very comfortable pass, so please do not panic if you find some of them difficult!

In addition, there are several 'heart-sink' scenarios such as those covering ethical, legal, and duty of candour issues to prepare you for some very difficult decisions that you may need to make on the day.

Lastly, management algorithms may differ between units and even between consultants in the same unit. If you have seen a patient managed differently from what is described in the book, then that is perfectly acceptable to describe that on the day, but please be prepared to justify it. The book describes an accepted way of management, including controversial grey areas (that has been fact-checked and approved by an NHS consultant of the relevant subspecialty).

How to use this book and approach the revision process:

This can be used as a starting point for your revision to know what to aim for before starting your revision, or to test yourself when you are ready to practise.

- The three viva tables cover the range of subjects as listed in the Guide to the Scope of the Examination. The scope of the exam is covered in the curriculum published by the Specialist Advisory Committee on the websites of the Intercollegiate Surgical Curriculum Programme and Joint Committee on Intercollegiate Examinations.
- Most of the exam is about breadth, as a 'day-one consultant', more than depth.
  It is important to understand that the examiner wants to know your opinion and why you will manage a patient in a certain way, rather than just what you know about the topic. Regurgitating theory alone is not enough to pass.
- Many of the very complex scenarios won't have a right or wrong answer. They are being asked to test how you apply your knowledge, in addition to your own personal approach. You will score well if you:
  - are organized,
  - justify your decisions and pre-empt the opposing view,
  - are able to 'look ahead' and avoid burning bridges, and
  - are patient-focused, ethical, and reasonable,
  - even if the examiner would personally manage the scenario differently.
- I would suggest you take the time to explore the many excellent summary books available. They not only summarize information but also provide a skeleton on which to hang more detail/ evidence/your prepared opinion regarding controversies in the topic.
- After completing the revision of a particular topic:
  1. I would suggest that you organize your thoughts in order to give a potential two-minute uninterrupted monologue about the topic in general, e.g., 'Tell me about Dupuytren's disease'.

Unless you are interrupted, this should include the relevant:
- definition – if appropriate,
- epidemiology,
- pathophysiology,
- clinical presentation,
- your management, and
- your treatment algorithm.

2. Next, be prepared for all the different subsections of the topic, as they will be likely follow-on questions, including how to manage any complications.
3. Then list any possible related basic sciences questions/drawings that may be asked within that topic, so you are not caught off-guard on the day.

In this way, you will have compiled a potential list of questions for each topic.
- After completing this process, I would suggest you ensure that you are comfortable with the following:
  - Be able to describe five free-flaps in detail, which should cover most reconstructive management questions (even if you would use something else in reality), such as:
    - LD for a very large muscle flap with a long pedicle – possible to offer chimeric options
    - Free fibula for a bony flap
    - Radial forearm – for a thin fasciocutaneous flap, with a long pedicle
    - ALT – large fasciocutaneous flap with a long pedicle. Also, possible to raise a chimeric option with muscle for bulk
    - DIEP for breast reconstruction
- Local flaps – know how to draw and talk through in detail:
  - A bilobed flap
  - A rotation flap (scalp/buttock)
  - A transposition flap
  - A rhomboid flap
  - A Z-plasty
- Draw planning incisions on a photograph/illustration presented to you:
  - A cleft lip repair
  - A cleft palate repair
  - Syndactyly release planning incisions
  - Cleft lip planning incisions
  - Hypospadias incisions
  - Fasciotomy incisions
  - Escharotomy releases
  - Dupuytren's access incisions
- Talk through emergency procedures in detail such as:
  - Tracheostomy
  - Fasciotomies
  - Escharotomies
  - Lateral canthotomy
  - Debridement of necrotizing fasciitis
- Anatomy – please draw:
  - Cross-section of lower limb
  - Cross-section of penis
  - Cleft lip repair
  - Brachial plexus
  - Extensor tendon mechanism
  - Proximal interphalangeal joint
  - Cruciate pulley system
  - Skin layers
  - Neck levels (including cross-section)
  - Eyelid (including cross-section)

- Ear
- Nose, including sagittal cross-section
- Craniofacial bony anatomy and LeFort fractures
- Wrist ligaments
- Basic science questions:

Embryology of:
- the face including cleft lip and palate/facial clefts,
- the ear,
- the hand,
- external genitalia
- the breast.

Pathophysiology:
- wound healing – acute, chronic, and foetal
- skin graft healing
- scars
- nerve healing
- bone healing
- distraction osteogenesis
- fat grafts
- tendon healing
- cartilage healing
- LASERS
- coagulation cascade
- complement cascade
- tissue expansion
- delay phenomenon
- microcirculation of the skin
- classification of flaps
- topical negative pressure therapy
- radiotherapy, and sequelae
- imaging: MRI, CT, PET
- local anaesthesia
- dressings
- Glascow Coma Scale
- MRC grading for muscle function
- dermoscopy
- osteomyelitis

Guidelines to be aware of:
- Lower limb trauma guidelines (most up-to-date),
- Melanoma – including the most up-to-date AJCC guidelines,
- BCC – the most up-to-date BAD guidelines, and
- SCC – the most up-to-date BAD guidelines.
- In the last few days prior to the Viva, I would go through the 'list of potential questions' for your topics (without the answers), just to re-organize your thoughts and prepare yourself for potential 'tangential' questions so you are not caught off guard.

On a good day, you will pre-empt most, if not all the questions that are asked.

Recommendation 1: I would suggest you pay attention to the basic sciences topics/and diagrams.

This is frequently forgotten by candidates, or left until the very end, and it can help you get out of trouble and impress examiners again if you have been struggling. It is not impressive for a candidate, who is in effect a potential future day-one consultant plastic surgeon – if they are unable to give a clear succinct answer on how a wound heals, or how a nerve heals, or how a LASER works. Lastly, you will also find that the same basic science questions can be asked in so many different scenarios, so they are worth the extra effort.

Recommendation 2: I would suggest you pay particular attention to ensure you are able to confidently describe the common emergency surgical procedures that all plastic surgeons should be comfortable with.

As you won't have time to 'phone a friend' as a day-one consultant when managing these life- or limb-threatening scenarios, examiners will take a particularly dim view if you are not confident about describing them in the exam (such as a tracheostomy, fasciotomy, escharotomy, lateral canthotomy, and debridement of necrotizing fasciitis).

How to answer questions:

- Posture and non-verbal body language:
    - Sit up straight with a clear, confident, and audible voice. Many speak too quickly or mumble.
    - Think of it as an interview – maintain eye contact and smile. Examiners are human beings and will relax if you behave like a pleasant one!
    - Take 2–3 seconds after the question to collect your thoughts before beginning to answer.
- If you are asked to manage a patient in a scenario with very little information – such as a clinical photograph with little clinical history, then I would suggest answering with an opening statement that qualifies your answer with a potential contraindication such as: 'In a patient who is otherwise fit for a general anaesthetic, I would', or 'In a patient who has been assessed as per ATLS principles, I would manage this hand injury by', etc. If they want you to focus on the contraindication or opening remark, they will.
- Many candidates have trouble approaching very open questions and answer with 'it depends', or worse still – they start asking the examiner specific questions regarding the history or examination findings such as: 'Are they diabetic/How old are they/Are they fit for a general anaesthetic'? Please avoid that. You will waste time and potentially irritate the examiner. If they wanted to ask your management plan for a specific case, they would have presented you with more information for that scenario.

    If you have the urge to say 'it depends on whether they have X or Y', then I would convert that answer to 'I will manage a patient with X by performing the following', or 'In a patient who has Y, then I will' and list all eventualities and their management that way.

    I would also suggest that you offer a bullet-point-style overview in the first instance, to allow the examiner to know you have a good broad understanding of the topic, before expanding each point, if they have not interrupted you.

    Here, they are initially testing your ability to see the bigger picture, such as the complete management algorithm of a complex topic.

    This allows the examiner to move you on if they want to, and for you to cover more topics and higher marks. The alternative would be for you to go into minute detail about points that they may not be interested in and waste time with little points gained.
- Listen to the question – e.g., there is a difference between 'How would you manage this condition' versus 'How would you manage this patient'.
- I suggest you use I 'will' as much as possible rather than I 'would' – especially for emergency scenarios. This will make you sound more confident and believable, as this is all about convincing the examiner that you are ready to be their colleague.
- I would also ensure you recognize and pre-empt any essential points (such as the need to exclude malignancy, e.g., or any important contraindications to what you are suggesting) and mention them without requiring any prompts.

    (If you find yourself giving one-worded answers, something is wrong.)
- If the scenario demands an MDT approach, please say: 'I will suggest the following management option to the MDT' or 'I will manage this within the MDT and suggest X', rather than 'I will refer this to the MDT'. The latter implies that the candidate is delegating complete responsibility to the MDT, which will worry the examiner greatly.
- Similarly, if this is clearly to be managed in a specialist centre, please let the examiner know that you are aware of that, but ready to demonstrate your understanding of the subject by saying – 'I would manage this within a Craniofacial centre', etc. – rather than saying 'I would refer this to the Craniofacial centre', etc.

What to do if you don't know

If you prepare correctly for this exam, then I anticipate that you will sail through.

However, no one can prepare for absolutely everything, so it is important to prepare for a very small risk that you are caught out.

- If you do not understand the question, then politely state that, rather than risk wasting time and irritating the examiner with an answer that doesn't address their question.

    I would suggest saying something like: 'I am not sure I completely understand the question – would you like me to describe X or discuss Y'? This will give them the opportunity to rephrase it for you.

- If you are really struggling with a management question, then just think – 'what would you do in reality?' Now is the time to buy time with:

    'This is a challenging situation, I would
    – discuss this with my senior consultant colleagues/within the MDT and
    – obtain further imaging/biopsy'.

    This will at least demonstrate that you are reasonable/collegiate/safe, even if you may have a gap in your knowledge (which will hopefully prompt them to give you clues and try and help you to work it out yourself).

    This may be helpful to get you out of the odd tight spot.

- Lastly, if you are asked to describe an emergency procedure that you have failed to cover in your revision, rather than just saying 'I don't know', I suggest you add that you would call for support (e.g., your ENT consultant colleague for a tracheostomy/orthopaedic consultant colleague for a fasciotomy/ophthalmology colleague for a canthotomy, etc.).

    Whilst I do believe this is essential knowledge to pass – and more importantly – will help you to become a safe consultant surgeon, this will at least dampen the examiners' ire by showing that you recognize your limitations and that you would save the patient by asking for help, even if it won't improve your marks.

VIVA I

Case 1.1

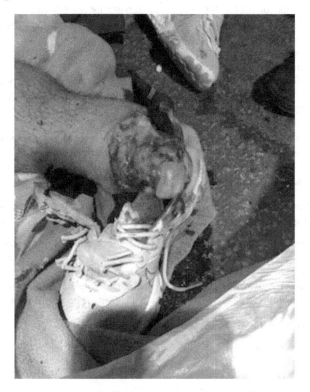

This patient drove his car into a wall whilst intoxicated. Please describe this image.

This is the photograph of a patient's dislocated right ankle with an off-ended midfoot, with possible associated fracture – taken in what appears to be the prehospital environment. I would be particularly concerned about the vascularity of his foot.

You are called to assess him in the emergency room. How would you proceed?

- I will manage him according to ATLS guidelines and the updated UK Standards for the management of open fractures.
- With regard to the foot injury, my primary concern is its vascularity.
  - I will first document the neurovascular status of the limb prior to administering any analgesia and then reduce the fracture and reassess the neurovascular status.
  - Looking at the photo, I don't anticipate the need to remove any gross contaminants.
  - Next, I will ensure IV antibiotics are given in the emergency room – as NICE guidelines suggest this should be given within 1 hour of injury and continued for 24 hours following wound excision, as the first of the two-phase antibiotic protocol for open lower limb fractures.
  - I will administer tetanus prophylaxis if required.
  - I will complete my primary management by obtaining a CTA of the limb as part of the head-to-toe trauma CT scan.
- Throughout my assessment, I will have a high degree of suspicion for established and evolving limb-threatening situations, such as limb ischaemia and compartment syndrome.

DOI: 10.1201/9780429399268-2

You have mentioned the neurovascular examination; please describe the examination you would perform.

- This consists of palpation for the dorsalis pedis and posterior tibial pulses.
- If these are not palpable, then I will exclude hypovolaemia and swelling and use the other limb as a comparative reference point – if uninjured.
- If there is no Doppler pulse in a swollen limb, then I will proceed with urgent exploration and management of an acutely ischaemic limb.
- If pulses are present, then I will proceed with motor nerve examination by confirming common peroneal nerve function with dorsiflexion, and that of posterior tibial nerve function with plantarflexion. This also helps to exclude a compartment syndrome if pain-free.
- With regard to sensory examination, I will examine:
  - the sole of the foot supplied by the medial and lateral plantar nerves and the medial calcaneal branch of the tibial nerve, which are all branches of the tibial nerve, and
  - the dorsum of the foot supplied by the superficial peroneal nerve, except for the first dorsal web space that is supplied by the deep peroneal nerve.

You mentioned antibiotics: what is the evidence for this? And what is the antibiotic protocol for the rest of this patient's inpatient stay?

The guidance from both the latest UK guidelines and NICE for open lower limb fractures suggests a two-phase antibiotic protocol – with co-amoxiclav given in the first hour post injury aimed at environmental flora, and continued for 24 hours post wound excision. The second phase is aimed at nosocomial organisms, which are the most common cause of subsequent deep infections, with teicoplanin and gentamicin given on induction at the time of definitive skeletal stabilization and soft tissue cover.

Will you take this patient to theatre in the middle of the night?

No, I won't unless there is evidence for a specific indication for this, such as:

1. acute limb ischaemia,
2. gross contamination of the wound-with marine, agricultural, or sewage sources,
3. compartment syndrome, or
4. a multiply injured patient that requires stabilization.

What about other patients who do not fulfil those indications? When would you take them to theatre?

I will arrange for the first debridement to occur during a scheduled orthoplastic operating list in normal working hours – ideally within 12 hours of the injury as this is a high-energy injury, as opposed to 24 hours for low-energy injuries.

What about the 6-hour rule that was mentioned in the previous guidelines – surely the sooner the primary excision, the better?

- There is no evidence for the previous 6-hour rule. The strongest predictor of deep infection is the grade of the fracture and administration of broad-spectrum antibiotics.
- There is evidence that delays of up to 24 hours have no effect on outcomes such as infection, union potential, and time to return to work, amongst many others.

What would you do if neither pulse is palpable, and the foot appears pale?

- As this is not a child, where the time reference may be longer, this is an emergency where circulation needs to be re-established within 3–4 hours of the injury to prevent irreversible muscle damage, after which revascularization may result in systemic problems such as myoglobinuria, renal failure, and possible death.
  - I will first confirm the absence of pulses with a handheld Doppler if one is readily available.
  - If the limb is not straightened already, I will do so and check the pulses again to exclude simple kinking of the vessels.

- If the problem persists, I will ensure adequate resuscitation as part of the secondary ATLS survey and take the patient to theatre urgently along with my orthopaedic colleague (and/or vascular surgery colleague depending on the protocol of my unit) with the following order of play:
  1. insertion of vascular shunts,
  2. temporary skeletal fixation, followed by
  3. definitive vascular reconstruction using autologous vein grafts
- Once circulation is restored, I will alert the anaesthetist as ischaemic products may result in hypotension.
- My orthopaedic colleague will then proceed with external fixation.
- Next, I will reassess the patient an hour after shunting. If the patient responds favourably and is systemically stable, then I will perform prophylactic fasciotomies. If the muscle is viable, then I will proceed with a vein graft.
- There is some controversy regarding the optimal vein graft donor site. I prefer the saphenous vein as it saves injuring the upper limbs in the situation of potential lower limb loss. However, I am aware that others may prefer the cephalic vein as it is less prone to spasm.
- Lastly, I will reconstruct any deep venous injury that is proximal to the level of the trifurcation, as this has been shown to reduce swelling and improve long-term functionality.

Your orthopaedic colleague would like to fix the fracture first as they are worried about the possibility of dislodging the shunt. What would you do?

- Re-establishing circulation should be our common primary goal. I will insist that revascularization occurs first as there is evidence to suggest increased morbidity in those who are fixed first rather than revascularized.
- I will also suggest that external fixation is less likely to dislodge the shunt.
- Lastly, I will reassure them that a dislodged shunt, although unlikely to occur, can be easily re-inserted.

You mention that you would only reconstruct venous injuries above the level of the trifurcation – why not also reconstruct more distal injuries?

There is evidence that infra-popliteal repairs thrombose soon afterwards, so they are not recommended.

What would you do if you take the patient to theatre with your orthopaedic colleague and the anaesthetist informs you that the patient is hypotensive, possibly due to other injuries, and is becoming coagulopathic?

This demands a 'damage control strategy' to avoid tipping the patient's inflammatory response in a physiologically unstable patient, into a SIRS picture with possible consequent ARDS, DIC, and multiple organ failure.

1. I will make a joint decision to shunt and ex-fix the fracture with removal of gross contamination from the wounds as efficiently as possible, then
2. transfer the patient to intensive care, with a plan to either:
   - bring the patient back to theatre for definitive vascular repair once their condition improves, with the agreement of the intensivists and orthopaedic surgeon, or
   - a joint decision to amputate is made at that point.

You've mentioned SIRS, ARDS, and DIC. What is the pathophysiology of these?

- Systemic inflammatory response syndrome is the clinical manifestation of dysregulated immune responses to infectious and non-infectious stimuli. It involves activation of the inflammatory cascade – with its humoral and cellular responses and complement and cytokine cascades. This may culminate in multi-organ failure, if left untreated.
- Acute respiratory distress syndrome is a non-cardiogenic pulmonary oedema where an inflammatory or mechanical insult causes endothelial cell dysfunction with leakage of cells and inflammatory exudate into the alveoli. This affects lung function with consequent hypoxia, increased work of breathing, atelectasis, and lung fibrosis.

- Disseminated intravascular coagulation is a disorder characterized by generalized widespread activation of coagulation, with thrombotic complications and diffuse haemorrhage due to consumption of platelets and coagulation factors.

You mentioned assessing the limb for the potential for salvage: what are your general indications for primary amputation of the limb?

- My absolute indications are:
  1. damage control for either uncontrollable haemorrhage or a crush injury exceeding a 6-hour period of warm ischaemia,
  2. an avascular limb with a period of warm ischaemia between 4 and 6 hours,
  3. incomplete traumatic amputations, where the distal remnant is significantly injured, and
  4. extensive crush injury, particularly of the foot.
- In addition, there are several grey areas, which would lead me to consider an amputation, such as:
  1. absent plantar sensation in the context of an ischaemic limb,
  2. segmental muscle loss affecting more than two compartments, especially if the posterior compartment is involved, and
  3. a severe open foot injury.
- In addition to the anatomical and functional deficits, I will consider the patient's:
  – general physiological reserve, as well as
  – psychological,
  – socio-economic, and
  – cultural factors.
- For example, a patient with a 'grey area' scenario with continued haemodynamic instability, or with concomitant comorbidities and who is self-employed, may shift the decision towards amputation.
- I will make the decision in agreement with another consultant surgeon and – if possible – patient and family involvement. If any disagreement occurs, then I would discuss the case with another specialist centre.

You mentioned absent plantar sensation as a grey area for a possible amputation. Why is that and how would you manage such a patient?

- This is not an indication for amputation on its own, as there is evidence that half of the patients with initial absent plantar sensation have neurapraxias that eventually recover completely.
- However, the outcome is less certain if the nerve is divided – even if it is repaired, as long-term outcomes for patients with permanent absent plantar sensation are unknown.
  Despite analogies having been made with other neuropathic conditions; both groups are not exactly comparable as pain and functional outcome may be influenced by muscle loss and scarring in the traumatic group.
- So given that evidence, I would explore the tibial nerve: an intact nerve would lead me to take an expectant approach. However, if the nerve is divided in addition to a 'grey area' scenario I have mentioned before, then I would consider an amputation.

You mentioned a neurapraxia. What is that, and what is its pathophysiology?

This is a type of nerve injury that involves local ion-induced conduction block and segmental demyelination, without loss of axonal continuity. A complete recovery is expected within 3 months.

What other types of nerve injury are you aware of?

- Other nerve injuries may involve:
  – localized structural injury of the axon, endoneurium, perineurium, or epineurium, orcomplete transection of the nerve, with or without segmental loss.
- These were originally classified by Seddon into neurapraxia, axonotmesis, and neurotmesis.
  – Axonotmesis involves direct damage to the axons with preservation of the endoneurium, perineurium, and epineurium. Wallerian degeneration, axonal regeneration, and target reinnervation occur because the remaining uninjured mesenchymal latticework provides a path for subsequent sprouting axons.

- Neurotmesis is complete transection of the nerve and requires surgical repair to potentially regain any function.
- This was further classified by Sunderland into five grades with:
  - neurapraxia equivalent to grade I;
  - axonotmesis equivalent to grade II;
  - additional grades III and IV specific to endoneurium and perineurium injury, respectively;
  - grade V is equivalent to Seddon's neurotmesis; and
  - MacKinnon further added a Grade VI to refer to mixed levels of injury and/or segmental loss.

You mentioned segmental muscle loss affecting more than two compartments as a possible indication for an amputation – especially if the posterior compartment is affected. Why is that?

- This is because the functional loss of more than two compartments increases the likelihood of dependence on orthotics to support the foot and ankle, whereas the loss of one compartment can be offset with a tendon transfer, such as a tibialis posterior transfer through the interosseous membrane, to compensate for the loss of the anterior compartment or the lateral compartment.
- Whilst this alone is not an indication for an amputation, it may sway the decision in that direction if considered with other factors.

You mentioned bone loss. Please describe the different treatment options that you know of to manage this.

- The various management options are dependent on the size of the bone gap and include:
  1. primary bone shortening,
  2. bone grafting – with or without membrane induction,
  3. primary bone shortening and subsequent distraction lengthening, and
  4. reconstruction with vascularized bone.
- Primary bone shortening is an option for segmental defects up to 5 cm long, to prevent potential kinking of the neurovascular bundles with attempted shortening of gaps of more than 5 cm.
- Bone grafting is usually performed in non-articular small gaps of up to 6 cm. It may be performed immediately with free-flap reconstruction of the soft tissues or delayed until after the soft tissues have healed.
- Primary bone shortening and subsequent distraction lengthening is an option in gaps of up to 8 cm.
- Reconstruction with bony free flaps is possible in gaps up to 25 cm, with a free fibula or DCIA flap. The patient must be informed that vascularized bone takes a considerable amount of time to hypertrophy and strengthen.

You mentioned membrane induction. What is that?

- This is a two-stage technique that creates a membrane around the bone graft, which has been shown to decrease graft resorption and improve its vascularity and corticalization:
  - The first stage involves insertion of a cement spacer that forms a pseudo-synovial membrane, followed by
  - the replacement of the spacer with a cancellous bone graft in the second stage.

You've mentioned distraction osteogenesis. Please tell me more about that. What is its pathophysiology?

- This is a technique developed by Ilizarov and consists of intramembranous formation of new bone after the creation of an osteotomy, by controlled gradual distraction of the fracture ends. This results in a tension stress effect leading to:
  1. increased cell activity,
  2. increased vascularity, and
  3. increased type 1 collagen production.
- Within one week, a fibrous interzone is formed – consisting of a bridge of dense longitudinally aligned collagen.

- In the subsequent week, a primary mineralization front is formed – with bony spicules at the edges of the osteotomy extending into the fibrous interzone.
- This progressively extends to close the gap – with remodelling and maturation of the bone it leaves behind as it progresses, with the formation of lamellar bone.

Which factors affect new bone formation?

- These include those that will affect tissue healing in general and those specific to bone formation.
- Factors affecting wound healing in general are local and systemic which may be congenital and acquired.
  - Local factors include:
    - infection,
    - radiation, and
    - local blood supply.
  - Congenital factors include conditions that will affect collagen and elastin, such as Pseudoxanthoma elasticum, Ehlers-Danlos and Cutis Laxa syndromes, amongst others
  - Acquired systemic factors include:
    - malnutrition – such as deficiencies in vitamin A, C, E, and Zinc – amongst others,
    - medication – such as steroids, NSAIDs, and colchicine – amongst others,
    - Diabetes mellitus, and
    - smoking.
- Factors specific to bone formation include:
  1. fixation stability,
  2. the osteotomy type,
  3. the latency period, and
  4. the distraction rate and rhythm.
- With regard to fixation stability – the more the better, as it encourages more intramembranous healing via Haversian remodelling, as opposed to secondary bone healing via inflammation, callus formation, and remodelling.
- With regard to the osteotomy, better results are achieved with techniques that:
  - preserve blood supply – such as a subperiosteal corticotomy, and
  - decrease energy transfer – such as the use of osteotomes rather than a saw.
- With regard to the latency period, the optimal period is 5–7 days. This avoids the acute inflammatory phase, although shorter periods may be possible in children. Premature consolidation occurs from two weeks onwards so it's best to start before then.
- A distraction rate of 1 mm/day is optimal. The rhythm refers to the frequency: the more frequent the better, with a regular rhythm better than a random one.

You have just described the management options for bone loss – including reconstruction of 25-cm gaps. So why would severe bone loss be a possible indication for an amputation?

- The goal of lower limb reconstruction is to return the patient to as close to their pre-injury functional state as possible, rather than to simply achieve an anatomical restoration of soft and bony tissues. So, it is important to consider the scale and time needed to recover from salvage surgery versus that following an amputation, especially as their outcomes have been shown to be functionally equivalent.
- An adult transtibial amputee will take approximately 5–6 months to rehabilitate to independent walking if there are no other injuries. This is equal to the time taken for consolidation of a bone-grafted segmental defect of less than 2 cm (provided the site is well vascularized and the patient is a non-smoker).
- However, an adult who undergoes distraction osteogenesis for a 5-cm gap will take about 7.5 months to consolidate (at 45 days/cm), which only well-motivated patients with appropriate domestic and financial support will be suitable for.
- Worse still, the time to achieve hypertrophy of free bony transfer, and allow safe loading, is in the region of 18–24 months. So, this is a significant undertaking for the patient from a personal and financial point of view.

Why are open foot injuries a 'grey area'?

These injuries commonly have a poor outcome, so an early recommendation for an amputation may provide a functionally equivalent outcome with a shorter rehabilitation period. This is because of the following:

- Joint stiffness and chronic pain are common, due to the ligamentous and bony injury altering the mechanics of the foot.
- In addition, the loss of plantar skin is very difficult to reconstruct.
- Salvage of early post-traumatic degeneration of joints will need arthrodesis, leaving the patient with the functional equivalent of a below-knee amputation.

Both you and another surgical consultant colleague have agreed with the patient that a below-knee amputation is the best plan. How would you perform this?

- As this is not an emergency amputation, I will plan the exact length and shape of the amputation stump in conjunction with my consultant colleague in rehabilitation medicine, as well as the patient – to best optimize the planned prosthesis for that specific patient.
- This is because the metabolic cost of gait after amputation is inversely proportional to the length of the residual stump.
- However, an overly long stump is also more difficult to fit with a prosthesis and allows a more mobile fibula which may become symptomatic.
- In emergency situations, my preference is for a bony tibial level of 13 cm distal to the tibial tubercle if the injury allows this.
- Before I start the procedure, I will ensure that the patient is supine with an inflated high tourniquet and an epidural for pre-emptive pain control:
  1. I will plan for an extended posterior flap as opposed to a classic fish mouth incision to ensure the scar is positioned off the weight-bearing aspect of the stump.
  2. Unless otherwise recommended by the rehabilitation consultant, I mark the anterior skin incision 10 cm distal to the tibial tubercle, and plan the posterior skin flap to allow tension-free closure – ensuring it is distal to the musculotendinous junction of gastrocnemius.
  3. I then control and divide the saphenous vein and nerve. All nerves are divided at the level of the anterior skin incision so that they are proximal to the stump level.
  4. Next, I divide the lateral compartment and superficial peroneal nerve, followed by the lateral interosseous membrane, to gain access and divide the anterior compartment and anterior tibial neurovascular pedicle.
  5. I then osteotomize the tibia at 13 cm distal to the tibial tubercle, unless we have a preoperative decision otherwise – bevelling at 45 degrees, and rasping the sharp edges, followed by the fibula osteotomy – 1 cm proximal to this.
  6. I then divide the posterior compartments and posterior tibial neurovascular bundle at the tibial level except for gastrocnemius, followed by haemostasis and release of the tourniquet.
  7. I then perform a myodesis through the gastrocnemius aponeurosis by drilling holes anterior to the tibial bony level.
  8. This is followed by placement of a submuscular drain, and securing the borders of gastrocnemius to the proximal anterior fascia.
  9. I then close the skin in layers: I may need to trim the posterior flap to length if required. In addition, I will consider a negative pressure incision vacuum dressing if the skin and soft tissues are swollen.
  10. Lastly, I will start prophylactic neuropathic and phantom limb pain management with gabapentin as my first-line option, unless the rehabilitation or pain team suggests otherwise.

You see the patient a few months down the line in clinic and they report a 'troublesome stump'. What might be the cause for this?

Stump complaints are commonly due to infection of the soft tissues or bone, mechanical problems and nerve-based problems:

- mechanical problems include:
  - an ill-fitting socket – with a stump that is too bulky or too loose,

–   incorrect alignment and pressure distribution – with resultant unstable scars or ulceration, and
    –   bony spurs or heterotopic ossification,
*   Nerve-based problems include:
    –   neuromas, and
    –   pain syndromes with a central component, such as phantom limb pain or CRPS.

FURTHER READING

1. Eccles S, Handley B, Khan U, McFadyen I, Nanchalal J, Nayagam S. Standards for the management of open fractures. Oxford Medicine Online. 2020. doi:10.1093/med/9780198849360.001.0001. https://oxfordmedicine.com/view/10.1093/med/9780198849360.001.0001/med-9780198849360
2. Higgins TF, Klatt JB, Beals TC. Lower extremity assessment project (LEAP) – the best available evidence on limb-threatening lower extremity trauma. Orthop Clin North Am. 2010 Apr;41(2):233–239.
3. Menorca RM, Fussell TS, Elfar JC. Nerve physiology: mechanisms of injury and recovery. Hand Clin. 2013;29(3):317–330.
4. Masquelet AC, Fitoussi F, Begue T, Muller GP. Reconstruction des os longs par membrane induite et autogreffe spongieuse [Reconstruction of the long bones by the induced membrane and spongy autograft]. Ann Chir Plast Esthet. 2000 Jun;45(3):346–353.

Case 1.2

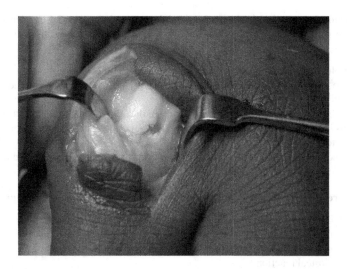

Please describe this photograph.

This is an intraoperative photograph of the dorsum of a patient's left hand, with an open metacarpophalangeal joint of the left index finger.

How would you manage this patient? The patient admits that he was involved in a fight.

- After excluding any other injuries according to ATLS principles, if appropriate, I will ensure tetanus prophylaxis is administered if needed.
- I will obtain a radiograph of the hand to exclude a foreign body such as a tooth, or any associated fractures.
- If he is of African or Afro-Caribbean heritage, then I will confirm his sickle cell status pre-operatively, although I am aware that the importance of this is debated in the anaesthetic community regarding procedures under tourniquet.
- An open joint, such as in this case, requires both IV antibiotics and an intra-operative washout:
  - Intravenous co-amoxiclav is my first-line therapy as it provides broad cover. This can be modified later as per the intraoperative microbiology results.
  - With regard to the intra-operative management, I will:
    - obtain a sample for Gram stain and culture of the wound or any purulent fluid,
    - wash the joint with copious normal saline, then
    - pack the wound for a relook in 24–48 hours if pus was found.
    - If not, I will repair any structural injuries, then
    - splint the hand in the position of function and start hand therapy as appropriate for any of the repairs.

Why do you need broad antibiotic cover?

Human saliva contains a mixture of aerobic and anaerobic bacteria.

- Aerobic bacteria include *Staphylococcus aureus, Staphylococcus epidermidis*, and *Streptococcus viridans*.
- Anaerobic pathogens include *Eikenella corrodens, Peptostreptococcus*, as well as *Corynebacterium* and *Bacteroides*.

DOI: 10.1201/9780429399268-3

The patient self-discharges before he is taken to theatre, as he was frustrated with the wait on the emergency list. He then returns sometime later with a protracted history of multiple episodes of a swollen and painful metacarpophalangeal joint, with 'intermittent discharge from the scar', despite numerous courses of antibiotics in the community.

What do you suspect? And what is the pathophysiology of this process? I am concerned regarding osteomyelitis in this patient. The pathophysiology of direct inoculation osteomyelitis, which is a likely cause of the infection here, includes:

- Bacterial proliferation within the bone inducing an acute suppurative response.
- This leads to raised intramedullary pressure, lower pH and oxygen tension, and formation of microthrombi within the intraosseous blood supply.
- The rise in pressure may eventually lead to rupture of the bony cortex, producing a cortical defect which drains into a subperiosteal abscess, rupture of the periosteum and spread of infection to the soft tissues –termed a cloaca.
- Over time, the reduced blood supply leads to frank bony necrosis, an area called a sequestrum, which provides a nidus for more pathogens.

How does this correlate with the expected findings on the imaging that you will request?

- With regard to imaging, I will request a plain radiograph in the first instance as it is a quick and accessible test, followed by an MRI.
  - I will expect radiological findings after 2–3 weeks of infection, including:
    - A periosteal reaction,
    - cortical irregularity, and
    - demineralization.
  - More chronic changes include:
    - sclerosis,
    - new bone formation, and
    - sequestrae.
  - MRI findings in the acute stage may include:
    - bone marrow oedema,
    - periostitis,
    - intraosseous and subperiosteal abscesses, and
    - sinus tracts from the bone to the skin surface.
  - Findings in the chronic stage may include:
    - peripheral enhancement of the sequestrum,
    - the involucrum, which is seen as a thickened shell around the sequestrum, and
    - a cloaca, which may be seen in acute or chronic cases, as a cortical defect which drains pus from the medulla to the soft tissues.

Both the X-ray and MRI show signs of osteomyelitis of the metacarpal head. During your intraoperative exploration and debridement, you find a purulent joint with evidence of joint destruction. How would you manage this?

- My concern is that he has developed osteomyelitis following septic arthritis. If his history is longer than 6 months, then I would suspect chronic osteomyelitis.
- I will obtain pus samples for Gram stain and culture, as well as bony and soft tissue samples for microbiology and histology – with the understanding that the microbiological picture may have been complicated by the numerous courses of antibiotics that he has already had.
- If osteomyelitis is confirmed on biopsy, then the plan is for:
  1. surgical eradication of the infection by excision of the bony sequestrum and surrounding infected soft tissue,
  2. management of a potential bone gap with an antibiotic spacer and external fixation, and
  3. soft tissue reconstruction – if required.
  4. This is followed by a 6-week course of IV antibiotics, with empirical therapy until culture directed therapy can be started if any microbial growth is obtained.

5. In addition, I will ensure that any predisposing patient factors are optimized, such as Diabetes or any other cause of immunosuppression.
6. Once the infection has been completely eradicated and stable soft tissue coverage has been achieved, then I will discuss options with the patient such as joint fusion or joint replacement whilst considering factors such as their:
    –   comorbidities,
    –   patient compliance – which I suspect will be poor given his history,
    –   occupation (and whether they are self-employed),
    –   dependence on the MCPJ range of motion, and
    –   their need to return to work and the speed of this.
    Whilst a joint replacement will restore MCPJ movement, it risks implant failure and the development of periprosthetic infection.

On the subject of hand infections, a poorly controlled diabetic patient presents with a 10-day history of a swollen hand with pus discharging from a point along the thenar crease. The patient does not recollect any trauma. What do you suspect and how would you manage them?

*   I suspect infection of the deep potential spaces of the hand such as the thenar space or midpalmar space. Given their history of poorly controlled diabetes, I am also concerned that they may possibly have:
    1. a sensory neuropathy with a potential foreign body or trauma that they didn't pick up on,
    2. a vascular or microvascular pathology which may be exacerbating the picture, or
    3. osteomyelitis in addition to the soft tissue infection
*   A focused history will establish their fitness for GA, their handedness, and their occupation and hobbies may also give me an idea regarding sources of potential trauma.
*   A focused exam will establish any neurovascular deficit and may help determine which space is affected. For example:
    –   A thenar space infection classically presents with a thumb held in abduction with pain exacerbated by flexion or opposition of the thumb, or
    –   A midpalmar abscess will present as pain on movement of the middle and ring fingers, and loss of palmar concavity.
    However, the clinical picture may be clouded by the fact that a number of spaces may be involved, and the patient's sense of pain may have been masked by a neuropathy.
*   I will supplement my examination with:
    –   a preoperative radiograph to evaluate for a potential foreign body and any signs of chronic osteomyelitis, and
    –   an MRI to confirm the spaces that may be involved, avoid missing a space that was not clinically obvious at the time, and avoid the morbidity of drainage of a space that is not necessary. In addition, any signs of osteomyelitis or a foreign body will be seen as well.

The MRI comes back confirming a thenar space infection. How will you drain this?

*   This is drained via a thenar palmar incision and a dorsal incision.
*   The palmar incision is transverse and proximal to the first MCPJ crease.
*   I will ensure I avoid the digital nerves and use a mosquito clamp to spread between the first and second metacarpals.
*   The dorsal incision is longitudinal on the dorsal aspect of the web between the thumb and index finger. I will spread to decompress the space behind the adductor pollicis and along the proximal radial aspect of first interosseous.

Let's consider another scenario: The trainee you are on call with lets you know that a patient is on their way to the emergency room, with an injured upper limb after being caught in a printing press for some time.

What would you be concerned about, giving the mechanism of injury?

I would be concerned about a limb-threatening severe crush injury, with the risk of compartment syndrome, rhabdomyolysis, with or without neurovascular or bony injuries.

How would you decompress this patient's forearm and hand?

- I will perform this urgently under general anaesthesia if the patient is fit for this. The alternative is an axillary block, but this may be slower to achieve.
  - I will decompress the forearm via two incisions:
    - a volar incision to decompress the volar compartment, that I will extend distally to also decompress the carpal tunnel, and
    - a dorsal incision to decompress the dorsal compartment and mobile wad.

      The volar incision starts just radial to FCU at the wrist, and extends proximally to the medial epicondyle. By incising lacertus fibrosus and the fascia overlying FCU, this allows me to retract FCU ulnarly and FDS radially, in order to open the fascia over the deep muscles of the forearm.

      The dorsal incision consists of a straight longitudinal incision extending from a point 2 cm distal to the lateral epicondyle towards the midline of the wrist. Here, I will dissect the interval between EDC and ECRB.
  - I will decompress the ten compartments of the hand via four incisions:
    - two longitudinal incisions over the second and fourth metacarpals that decompress the adductor pollicis, and the three palmar and four dorsal interossei,
    - a longitudinal incision on the radial side of the first metacarpal to decompress the thenar compartment, and
    - a longitudinal incision over the ulnar side of the fifth metacarpal to decompress the hypothenar compartment.
    - I will also perform a carpal decompression at this point, if I have not already completed that earlier as part of the forearm decompression.
- I will inspect all the muscles and debride any devitalized areas, then dress the wounds with a plan to return in 24–48 hours for a further look.

Please talk me through the long-term sequelae of an untreated compartment syndrome of the upper limb.

- This may result in a Volkmann's ischemic contracture with muscle contractures in the forearm, wrist, and hand that result from muscle necrosis.
- The classic presentation consists of a patient with elbow and wrist flexion, and a claw-like deformity of the hand with extended MCPJs and flexed IPJs, as well as thumb adduction.
- However, the picture varies between patients, and management will need to be planned on a patient-specific basis from:
  - dynamic splinting and tendon lengthening if finger flexors are only involved, to
  - tendon transfers if the wrist flexors are also involved, such as brachioradialis to FPL or an ECRL to FDP transfer, and finally
  - possible free muscle transfers in severe cases.

Case 1.3

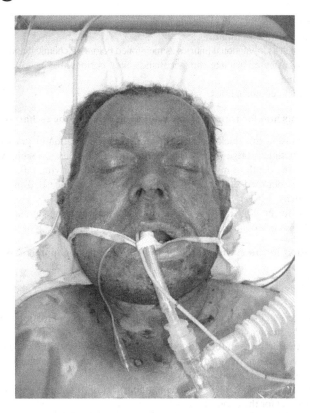

This man was trapped in a house fire and presents with full-thickness burns to the neck and venous congestion of the face in an emergency room. Based on that information, and the appearance of the photograph, what are your preliminary thoughts?

- I strongly suspect an inhalational injury based on the information you have given me, as well as evidenced in the photograph of singeing of his eyebrows, forehead hairline, possibly nasal hair, and swollen lips.
- I will manage him according to ATLS and EMSB principles, with urgent assessment and management of his airway by my anaesthetic colleague – which I can see has already been secured in this instance.
- In addition, I will consider an urgent escharotomy to address the venous congestion if the full-thickness burn to the neck is circumferential or near circumferential.

What would you do if your hospital does not have a burns centre?

- As he has an apparent inhalational injury, he may fit the criteria for transfer to a burns centre – if his cutaneous burns are 25% TBSA or more. If so, I will arrange this once:
  1. the airway has been assessed and secured as it has been here with an uncut ET tube – to accommodate swelling,
  2. any other injuries have been assessed and stabilized if required,
  3. resuscitation has been commenced, and
  4. an escharotomy is performed – if needed.
- If not, then I will discuss this with the burns centre, regardless of the cutaneous burn TBSA.

DOI: 10.1201/9780429399268-4

What are the other indications for transfer to a burns centre?

This is based on:

1. the affected TBSA – with more than 40% in adults (or more than 25% with an inhalational injury), 30% in children, and 15% in infants,
2. the type of burn (such as inhalational injuries as mentioned before, or chemical and electrical injuries),
3. any 'special areas' affected (such as the face, hands, feet, perineum),
4. extremes of age, and
5. concomitant medical comorbidities.

The burns centre accepts him for transfer. How would you perform the escharotomy of his neck?

- I will start and finish a full-thickness incision overlying the location of sternocleidomastoid to avoid inadvertently hitting large vessels and be mindful of the external jugular vein.
- I will ensure that the depth of my incision extends into the underlying fat, and the length of it extends 1 cm into unburned skin on either side-to ensure a full release, using local anaesthesia for the unburnt areas.
- I will then run my finger along the length of the incision to check for any remaining constrictions.
- Finally, I will dress the wound.

What is your indication for an escharotomy of the chest wall or abdomen? And how would you perform that?

- My indications include patients with full-thickness burns of the thorax or abdomen, which are:
  1. circumferential, or
  2. with consequent signs of compromised ventilation – even if not circumferential.
- With regards to the surgical technique:
  - I will place my incisions in the mid-axillary lines with a shield-like or square shape – with a horizontal component in the infraclavicular line, and across the abdomen below the costal margin if the abdominal wall is involved.
  - As with any escharotomy, I will pass from unburnt skin to unburnt skin down to fat, using local anaesthesia for the unburnt areas.
  - I will then check for any residual restrictions by running my finger along the length of the wound.
  - Finally, I will confirm with my anaesthetic colleague that ventilation has improved.
  - In children under the age of 2, I will ensure I release the abdominal burn in addition to the chest burn, as they rely on diaphragmatic breathing.

Please talk me through inhalational injuries.

- These are potentially life-threatening injuries, which may be:
  - supraglottic,
  - subglottic, or
  - systemic.
- They result in:
  - greater fluid loss (with up to 20% additional resuscitation fluid required), and possible:
  - bronchoconstriction and increased airway resistance, and
  - pulmonary interstitial oedema.
- It is crucial to have a high degree of suspicion based on the history, to achieve early diagnosis and management – as this is associated with an increase in mortality of 20% above that predicted on the basis of the patient age and burn size. This increases to 60% above the baseline if pneumonia develops.
- Suggestive factors include:
  - a history of a fire in an enclosed space or an unconscious patient in a fire,
  - symptoms-such as stridor, a hoarse voice, a brassy cough with carbonaceous sputum, or respiratory distress, and
  - signs – such as hypoxia, soot around the mouth and nose, singed facial and nasal hair – as per the photograph, and a swollen upper airway.

- I will arrange a fibreoptic bronchoscopy if I suspect it, in conjunction with my anaesthetic colleagues, to confirm the diagnosis.
- Supraglottic injuries are mainly thermal, and my management will be to assess and secure the airway along with my anaesthetic colleague, with early intubation before further swelling develops.
- Subglottic injuries are chemical injuries caused by the dissolved acidic products of combustion in the alveoli. These patients may require respiratory support with humidified oxygen, intubation to allow bronchial toilet, and possibly intermittent positive pressure ventilation (IPPV).
- Systemic injuries are caused by the toxicity of carbon monoxide (CO) or cyanide. Treatment consists of 100% oxygen in both cases, with the addition of vitamin B12 in patients with cyanide toxicity.

You mentioned carbon monoxide and cyanide poisoning. Please tell me more about these.

- Carbon monoxide is a poisonous gas caused by incomplete combustion of hydrocarbons, with three possible effects:
  1. it shifts the oxygen dissociation curve to the left with 250 times the affinity for haemoglobin as oxygen,
  2. it binds to the intracellular cytochrome system, producing sick-cell syndrome, and
  3. it causes a demyelinating brain injury – called Grinker myelinopathy, at very high levels of CO.

Neurological toxic symptoms appear at CO levels of 15–20% with headaches and confusion, progressing to hallucinations and ataxia at levels of 20–40%, with death at levels of 60%.

Treatment consists of 100% oxygen – delivered at 8 L/min through a non-rebreathing mask with a reservoir, to decrease the half-life of CO from 250 minutes in patients breathing room air to 40 minutes. This is maintained for 24 hours to cover for a secondary rise of serum CoHb, as cytochrome-bound CO is washed out 24 hours later. Ventilation is indicated for patients with decreasing GCS.

- Cyanide poisoning occurs when certain plastic materials burn, producing cyanide compounds which bind to, and inhibit cytochrome oxidase.

  Diagnosis can be difficult, but I will have a low threshold to consider this in patients with an unexplained metabolic acidosis that is inconsistent with the injury size and resuscitation status.

If so, I would confirm it with the following:

  1. A bedside diagnosis, by measuring the arterio-venous difference in oxygen saturation – with less than 10% being indicative of cyanide poisoning due to the inability of cells to extract oxygen from the RBCs.
  2. In addition, cyanide levels can be measured but this takes some time to process.

Again, treatment consists of 100% oxygen, but with the addition of vitamin B12 to chelate free cyanide molecules and aid their excretion.

Apart from patients with high levels of carboxyhaemoglobin and decreasing GCS that you mentioned, what are your indications for ventilating burns patients?

These are:

  1. respiratory distress,
  2. extensive burns to the head and neck,
  3. supraglottic oedema on fibreoptic examination, and
  4. for consideration prior to any transfer of a patient with a possible inhalational injury or potential airway loss.

Let us consider this patient's cutaneous burns: what is a thermal burn exactly? And what is its pathophysiology?

- This is a dynamic area of tissue damage that has been classified by Jackson into three zones of injury with:
  1. an inner zone of coagulative necrosis,
  2. an intermediate zone of stasis, and
  3. an outer zone of hyperaemia (that involves the whole body if more than 20% TBSA is affected).

- Its pathophysiology consists of local effects, and systemic effects if the burn covers more than 20% of the TBSA.
- Local inflammatory effects include:
  1. vasodilation, and
  2. increased capillary permeability, leading to:
     - decreased capillary oncotic pressure and increased tissue oncotic pressure – as albumin leaks out of the circulation, and
     - generalized impairment in cell membrane function leading to cell swelling.
- Systemic effects in those with a burn requiring resuscitation affect most organs, such as:
  1. Reduced cardiac output due to:
     - hypovolaemia causing decreased venous return,
     - direct myocardial depression caused by inflammatory mediators, and
     - increased afterload due to increased systemic vascular resistance.
  2. Pulmonary oedema due to:
     - increased capillary pressure and permeability,
     - left heart failure,
     - hypoproteinemia, and
     - direct injury following inhalational injury.
  3. Renal injury, with consequent:
     - decreased renal perfusion, and
     - increased ADH and aldosterone, with subsequent sodium and water retention.
  4. Hepatic and pancreatic injury, with consequent:
     - glucose intolerance,
     - increased metabolic rate and catabolism, and
     - growth inhibition in children.
  5. Gastrointestinal consequences, such as:
     - stress ulceration,
     - gut stasis and bacterial translocation, and
     - cholecystitis.
  6. Immunosuppression, and
  7. A systemic inflammatory response syndrome

What are your indications for fluid resuscitation? And what regimes are you aware of?

- This is indicated in burns that cover more than 20% TBSA in adults, or more than 10% in children – excluding erythema.

  These percentages of skin loss will lead to burn shock-induced renal failure caused by electrolyte shifts, an inflammatory response and evaporate losses – that is maximal at 12 hours post-injury, so fluid supplementation is required to prevent this.
- The Parkland formula is the most commonly used formula in the United Kingdom and is recommended by the ATLS and EMSB guidelines, but many others exist.

  It was originally described by Baxter and Shines in the 1960s following empiric experiments on burned dogs, and subsequent testing among burn patients. The original description was 3.7–4.3 ml of lactated Ringer solution/kg/% burn in the first 24 hours post burn.

  This was rounded to 4 ml in the ATLS protocol, with half of the fluid given in the first 8 hours after the injury, and the second half in the next 16 hours.

  However with time, many patients were found to be over-resuscitated with fluid creep occurring, resulting in complications that culminated in an increased risk of death.
- So, the concept of permissive hypovolaemia was developed where resuscitation is started at a lower end with 2 ml/kg/% burn, with titration based on clinical response. The aim is to give the least amount of fluid to ensure adequate tissue and organ perfusion, whilst avoiding the sequelae of over-resuscitation.

You mentioned fluid creep. What is that?

- This is a significant problem, with potentially life-threatening sequelae, where patients receive more fluid than is required, causing oedema.

- It is thought to be due to:
  1. the inaccuracy of all prescribed resuscitation formulae in large burns,
  2. the reluctance of many clinicians to reduce fluid infusions when urine output is high (possibly because they may be influenced by historical burn-related deaths due to under-resuscitation), and
  3. the influence of strict goal-directed resuscitation with inappropriate goals such as a particular urine output.
- This can lead to:
  1. airway swelling,
  2. pulmonary oedema,
  3. soft tissue oedema – causing limb and abdominal compartment syndrome, as well as an increased risk of pressure sores,
  4. elevated intracerebral and intraocular pressures, and
  5. an overall increased risk of death.

On the topic of fluids – What controversies of fluid resuscitation are you aware of?

- There is equivocal evidence for improved outcomes regarding:
  1. the type of fluid resuscitation (i.e. crystalloid vs colloid), and
  2. the timing of colloid administration.
- The proponents for the use of albumin cite the theory that large volumes of crystalloid decrease plasma protein concentration and further promote extravascular egress of fluid with consequent oedema, so replenishment of plasma protein using colloids would theoretically mitigate this effect. This was initially complicated by historical studies showing that albumin worsened mortality rates, but these have since been disputed by the Cochrane Injuries Group.
- With regard to the timing of albumin administration, there is a theoretical risk of protein and albumin leak – caused by the increased capillary permeability in the first 24 hours, which would further worsen the oncotic pressure, but again the evidence for this is equivocal.
- Some burn centres have now moved to using formulas where crystalloid is given for the first 8–12 hours – when capillary leak may be most pronounced, followed by colloid administration thereafter. There is some evidence that this protocol may decrease the overall volume of fluid required and reduce the risk of the complications of fluid creep.

You are the consultant burn surgeon: how would you personally avoid fluid creep in a patient who is admitted to your burn centre?

I will ensure that:

1. the true burn size is confirmed to avoid relying on a possible overestimation by the prehospital or ER team,
2. the patient's fluid response is constantly monitored and re-evaluated – as this is a dynamic process,
3. colloids are considered after the first 24 hours as a 'rescue' technique when crystalloid requirements become excessive,
4. early renal replacement therapy and hemofiltration are considered to offload any fluid, and
5. there is continual monitoring for oedema of the soft tissues, limbs, and the abdominal compartment – using regular bladder pressures when oliguria persists or when volume requirements become excessive (such as more than 500 ml per hour).

You titrate the fluid administration to attempt to prevent fluid creep but find a fall in the patient's urine output. How would you manage this patient?

- I will liaise with my critical care colleagues in the burns MDT to determine the cause of his low UOP, which may be:
  - hypovolaemia,
  - abdominal compartment syndrome, or
  - multi-organ failure.

- If the cause was found to be purely hypovolaemic, then I would administer a fluid challenge of 5 ml/kg and increase the fluid rate for the next hour by 150%.
- With regard to abdominal compartment syndrome, this is an intra-abdominal pressure of greater than 20 mmHg – measured by transduction of bladder pressure, with evidence of new organ dysfunction – such as oliguria, impaired mechanical ventilation, worsening metabolic acidosis or haemodynamic instability.

  I would manage this patient within the burns MDT in conjunction with my critical care and general surgery colleagues – with a decompressive laparotomy being the definitive treatment.

  However, I am aware of other treatments by the plastic surgery and critical care team that can be successful in lowering the pressure and avoiding laparotomy, such as:
  1. ensuring that escharotomies are performed on any full-thickness anterior trunk burns that haven't been excised yet,
  2. the use of increased sedation in mechanically ventilated patients, and
  3. the use of diuretics, if adequate intravascular volume is confirmed with pulmonary capillary pressure monitoring.

Are you aware of the hypermetabolic response? What is this and how can you modulate it?

- This is a response that occurs in patients with a thermal burn affecting more than 20% TBSA – mediated by the hypothalamic response, and consists of:
  1. increased metabolic rates,
  2. multi-organ dysfunction,
  3. muscle protein degradation,
  4. insulin resistance, and
  5. increased risk of infection.
- The classical description of the stress response after any severe injury consists of:
  - an initial ebb phase with a decrease in tissue perfusion and metabolic rate, followed by
  - the flow phase with increased metabolism and hyperdynamic circulation 2–3 days later.
- Modulation can be achieved by:
  1. achieving early wound closure – even with allografts, to decrease the metabolic rate, net protein loss and the incidence of sepsis,
  2. raising the ambient temperature to 28°C – to decrease resting energy expenditure, as the energy required for vaporization is derived from the environment rather than from the patient,
  3. early aggressive enteral feeding – to reduce translocation bacteraemia and sepsis, maintain gut motility and preserve the first-pass nutrient delivery to the liver,
  4. preventing infection, and
  5. the use of pharmacologic agents such as:
     - propranolol – to decrease the effects of catecholamine, such as catabolism, cardiac complications, and overall mortality, and
     - recombinant human growth hormone and IGF-1 – to decrease wound healing time, albeit with a risk of hyperglycaemia.

In addition to his inhalational injury, he has a 50% cutaneous burn. Why is nutrition important in the management of this patient?

- The aims of early feeding are to:
  1. minimize net protein loss,
  2. protect the gut from bacterial translocation,
  3. prevent gastric ileus, and
  4. avoid Gram-negative septicemia.
- An increased daily calorific requirement is needed as the basal metabolic rate increases dramatically during the acute injury phase and remains higher than normal for up to 1 year post injury. Oxygen consumption and CO_2 production steadily increase over the first 5 days post injury – with:
  1. an associated increase in protein, fat, and glycogen catabolism – with consequent weight loss, impaired wound healing, and immunity,

2. insulin resistance, and
3. altered carbohydrate metabolism with increased glucose uptake and gluconeogenesis.

- However, overfeeding should be avoided as it may lead to impairment of splanchnic oxygen balance and futile substrate cycling with peripheral lipolysis and central fatty deposition, and consequent liver fat deposition and hyperglycaemia.
- There are many formulae used to estimate requirements – based on the patient's body weight and size of the burn, such as the Sutherland and Curreri formulae, but indirect calorimetry provides the most accurate figure – aiming for feeding 1.2–1.4 times the measured resting energy expenditure.

You mentioned indirect calorimetry – What is this?

This is a method by which measurements of respiratory gas exchange are used to estimate the type and amount of substrate oxidized, and hence the energy produced by biological oxidation.

How will you choose to deliver his feed?

- I will arrange the insertion of a nasoduodenal feeding tube, which will achieve two goals:
  1. It provides the gold standard enteral nutrition, as it:
      – preserves mucosal integrity,
      – protects against bacterial translocation in the gut, and
      – is associated with improved regulation of the inflammatory cytokine response.
  2. In addition, it reduces the risk of aspiration pneumonia that may occur from gastric stasis-related regurgitation of food.
- I will only opt for TPN if he develops a prolonged ileus or becomes intolerant of enteral feeding, as it is associated with impaired mucosal immunity, enhanced endotoxin translocation, and up-regulation of TNF-alpha expression – which adversely affects survival.

Tell me – What are the principles of early surgery in burns management?

There is no true definition of early surgery, but most accept this to be within 7 days.

- The intra-operative goals are to minimize bleeding and heat loss:
  – Bleeding can be decreased by using multiple teams, preoperative infiltration, a limb tourniquet, adrenaline soaks, and fascial excision.
  – Heat loss is minimized by keeping the ambient temperature high. This avoids hypothermia-related coagulopathy.
- If performed within 24 hours, this reduces the patient's sympathetic drive – with the associated blood loss, and oedema.
- Priority grafting is indicated for the:
  – neck – if a tracheostomy is required, and
  – supraclavicular and groin areas – for central line access, followed by
  – grafting of the limbs, chest, and back – with an aim to achieve as much coverage as possible to minimize fluid loss and the patient's inflammatory response.

What are the possible methods of excision of his burns.

There are two methods: tangential and fascial excision.

- Tangential excision was originally described in partial-thickness burns, although full thickness burns can also be excised in this way. Excision occurs in layers until healthy bleeding tissue is encountered, but this is slower and can lead to more blood loss than fascial excision.
- Fascial excision occurs down to level of the fascia and is useful in massive burns or infected burns to decrease operative time and bleeding. It is also useful to limit bleeding in areas where a tourniquet cannot be used, but the disadvantage is a poor cosmetic appearance.

How will you manage his neck following the escharotomy?

- I may need to prioritize excision and grafting of his neck if he requires a tracheostomy to manage his inhalational injury.

- I will excise the full-thickness burn either in a tangential fashion or with diathermy down to platysma and narrowly mesh an autograft in the first setting to allow for early healing.
- Post-operatively, I will use a customized splint until scar maturity is achieved.
- This may need subsequent excision if a contracture develops.

You mentioned contractures – please describe your understanding of them, and the principles that you use to minimize their formation.

- These can be intrinsic and extrinsic in origin and may form a linear band, a broad band or joint contracture.
    - Intrinsic contractures occur where scarring directly involves the site affected by the contracture, whereas
    - extrinsic contracture is a contracture of normal structures that are pulled out of position by scarring distant to the site, such as cheek scarring causing an ectropion despite normal lower eyelid tissue.
- I will attempt to prevent them by using the same principles used to prevent hypertrophic scars, as minimizing scars will minimize contractures, such as:
    1. early excision and skin coverage, as this will decrease fibroblast activity,
    2. early splintage,
    3. external pressure garments or devices – with 20–25 mmHg required, preferably for nearly 24 hours per day until scar maturity is reached,
    4. early aggressive mobilization therapy – both active and passive,
    5. silicone gels and sheets, and
    6. consideration of steroid therapy, both as tapes and injections.

Please describe your management approach of contractures in general.

- My general surgical principles for release include:
    1. assessing for intrinsic versus extrinsic contracture – including joint contracture, and
    2. releasing limb contractures from proximal to distal.
- My indications for the timing of release include:
    - an urgent release for a severe contracture, such as a:
        - peri-oral contracture,
        - neck contracture, or
        - an upper eyelid retraction causing exposure of the cornea.
    - an early release within 6 months for:
        - a lower eyelid contracture causing ectropion,
        - an oral contracture,
        - a neck contracture, or
        - a limb contracture.
    - Contractures with no significant functional deficit can be released after that, ensuring I wait for 2 years for those with purely aesthetic issues to allow time for the scars to resolve as far as possible.

The patient survives and moves away. He returns to your clinic three years later with a broadband contracture of his neck. How will you manage him?

1. I will first establish how this contracture affects him and what his goals are from the release.
2. Next, I will consider the vertical and horizontal subunits, as well as the cervico-mental angle.
3. I will then proceed with a fish mouth incision release, resection of the platysma – which itself may be involved in the scarring and contracture, followed by
4. reconstruction of the vertical then horizontal subunits with either:
    - skin grafts with or without skin substitutes or
    - flaps, such as a local supraclavicular artery flap or a free scapular flap, depending on the extent of the affected area.

I will counsel him that the skin graft and skin substitute option carries a higher risk of recurrence; however, total flap reconstruction can cause loss of the cervico-mental angle and often needs thinning or liposuction.

What would you do if he doesn't have a large enough donor site to resurface the whole neck with regard to the flap resurfacing option?

- I will consider a chimeric free flap such as a scapular/parascapular flap if the back tissue is thin and pliable, or
- I will consider pretransfer expansion of the donor site.

Despite the inconvenience of expansion with regard to the time taken and the aesthetic deformity, this does offer multiple advantages in addition to the provision of tissue, as:

1. it produces a thinned and more pliable tissue, as a result of the fat atrophy,
2. it provides an improved vascularity of the flap due to the angiogenesis seen in expanded flaps – similar to that in delayed flaps, and
3. it allows direct closure of the donor site.

You mentioned delayed flaps. What do you mean by that? Please talk me through your understanding of the theory behind the phenomenon.

Answered in Case 3.8

Let us consider an additional scenario: the patient in the photograph has sustained an electrical contact injury on an industrial site which resulted in his clothes catching fire.

How are electrical burns any different from thermal burns, and how does that alter your management?

The pathophysiology and consequently the assessment and management of electrical burns are different.

- There are two theories regarding the progressive tissue necrosis found in electrical burns:
  1. The first states that the periosseous core of necrosis is due to the high resistance of bone and the consequent generation of heat. Muscle damage is due to the delayed thrombosis of vessels or the irreversible microscopic damage to muscle at the time of the burn.
  2. The second states that electroporation, with cell membrane breakdown caused by the excessive current, causes thrombosis and ischaemia in the absence of the heating effect.
- In the context of an ATLS/EMSB assessment,
  1. I will establish the voltage source from the history: as a high-voltage injury – as in this case, may result in systemic effects, in addition to the local destruction caused by low voltage injuries.
  2. I will assess:
     - the entry and exit wounds, and
     - the viability of his limbs, with the potential need for escharotomies or fasciotomies.
  3. For high-voltage injuries (>1000 V), such as here, I will also assess for:
     - cardiac arrhythmias,
     - myoglobinuria, and
     - peripheral neuropathy.
  4. In addition, I will ensure long-term patient follow-up as he is at risk of late-onset peripheral neuropathy, paralysis, and cataract formation.
  5. Lastly, I will assess and manage any thermal/inhalational burns as before.

FURTHER READING

1. Cartotto R. (2009). Clinics in Plastic Surgery (Burns), Vol. 36, Number 4. Saunders. Elsevier Health Sciences.

2. https://www.cobis.scot.nhs.uk/wp-content/uploads/2016/04/Paed-Guideline-CoBIS-Fluid-Guidelines-2016.pdf
3. Alderson P, Bunn F, Lefebvre C, Li WP, Li L, Roberts I, Schierhout G; Albumin Reviewers. Human albumin solution for resuscitation and volume expansion in critically ill patients. Cochrane Database Syst Rev. 2004 Oct 18;(4):CD001208.
4. http://www.bfirst.org.uk/wp-content/uploads/2020/08/Burn-Contracture-Surgery-handbook-Mr-S-Watson-Glasgow_UK.pdf
5. https://www.britishburnassociation.org/wp-content/uploads/2018/02/National-Burn-Care-Referral-Guidance-2012.pdf
6. https://ubccriticalcaremedicine.ca/academic/jc_article/Decreased%20Fluid%20Volume%20Burn%20Shock%20(Feb-05-09).pdf

Case 1.4

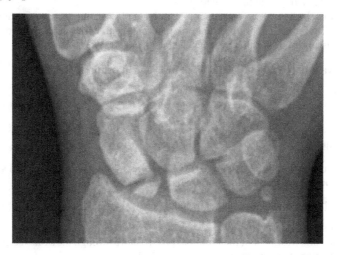

Please describe this radiograph.

This is the radiograph of a right carpus demonstrating a displaced fracture of the proximal pole of the scaphoid. In addition, if the radiograph is correctly orientated, then the patient is showing positive ulnar variance. This is associated with TFC tears and was historically thought to reduce the risk of developing Kienbock's disease – although this is now being challenged.

Please tell me about the anatomy of the scaphoid, and the relevance of this fracture.

- Over 80% of the scaphoid surface is covered with articular cartilage.
- The vascularity of the proximal pole depends entirely on intraosseous blood flow with a vascular watershed, which increases the risk of problematic union and avascular necrosis.
  - The proximal 80% of the scaphoid is supplied by the dorsal scaphoid branches of the radial artery that enter the only non-articular portion at the dorsal ridge of the waist.
  - The distal 20% is supplied by the volar scaphoid branches from either the radial artery or the superficial palmar branch that enter the bone at the distal tubercle.
- In addition, these fractures tend to occur in young adult men with a high impact on their return to work, sporting activities and quality of life.

This patient fell on to his outstretched hand 2 months ago. How will you manage him?

- In a patient who is fit for operative treatment, as most of these patients tend to be, treatment is based on:
  - the fracture personality (i.e. its' location and displacement),
  - the presence of non-union, and
  - any avascular necrosis.
- The proximal pole does appear to be somewhat sclerotic on the radiograph, which concerns me. I will investigate with a CT scan to provide the most precise definition of the osseous anatomy, and an MRI to determine the vascularity of the proximal pole.
- If there is any sign of AVN, then my preferred treatment option is open fixation via a dorsal approach with a vascularized bone graft from the 3,4 intercompartmental supraretinacular artery (3,4 ICSRA).
- If not, then fixation with a headless screw is indicated either percutaneously or open – both via a dorsal approach. However, I recognize that the small size of the proximal fragment may pose technical challenges to screw fixation and subsequent bone viability.

DOI: 10.1201/9780429399268-5

- I prefer to opt for the percutaneous approach in the first instance, as it avoids carpal ligament division, and interruption of the tenuous blood supply to the scaphoid, even if it may be more technically challenging than the open technique.
- If this fails, then I will revert to open internal fixation with a headless screw via a dorsal approach, as it provides improved exposure of the proximal pole with easier screw placement, but at the expense of disruption of the already tenuous blood supply.

You mentioned a vascularized bone graft. What are your indications for this?

These include:

- AVN,
- a non-union, and
- failed previous surgery.

You mentioned that you would use a bone graft from the 3,4 intercompartmental supraretinacular artery. Why did you choose that option? And what others are available?

The advantages of this dorsal pedicled option include:

- a reliable dorsal vascular anatomy,
- flap dissection and treatment of the proximal pole fracture through the same incision,
- avoidance of an unnecessary micro-anastomosis, and
- a technically simpler procedure to perform compared to volar grafts (that are more commonly reserved for correction of humpback deformity of the waist).

Other options include:

- the pronator quadratus pedicled bone graft,
- the 1,2 ICSRA and 2,3 ICSRA vascularized bone grafts, and
- free options – such as the medial femoral supracondylar bone graft and free DCIA option.

The patient moves abroad before his operation and returns 18 months later with a very painful wrist. You obtain a radiograph and CT, and this is reported as consistent with features of a SNAC wrist. What is this, and how would you manage that?

Scaphoid nonunion advanced collapse (SNAC) describes the specific pattern of progressive arthritis of the wrist following an established scaphoid nonunion.

- The natural history of degenerative changes first occurs at the radio-scaphoid area followed by mid-carpal and then pan-carpal arthritis.
- Management options include:
  - A radial styloidectomy and consideration for fracture reduction and stabilization for stage I disease (where arthritis is localized to the radial side of the scaphoid and radial styloid).
  - Options for stage II and III (where disease expands to the scaphocapitate joint and periscaphoid arthritis, respectively) include:
    - a proximal row carpectomy if there are no capitate head changes, or
    - a four-corner fusion – which retains some wrist motion and grip strength.
  - Salvage options include:
    - wrist arthrodesis (which reliably provides pain relief and good grip strength at the cost of wrist motion) or
    - wrist denervation, which is motion preserving.
    - Lastly, I am aware that total wrist replacement is being performed in certain specialized centres for pan-carpal arthritis, as an alternative to total wrist fusion, when the other options are no longer suitable.

Tell me how is that different from a SLAC wrist? And how would you manage that?

- Whilst the pathological sequential sequelae and management options are similar, the aetiology of the arthritis is different. In this case, SLAC refers to a Scaphoid Lunate Advanced Collapse and describes the pattern of arthritis seen following a chronic DISI deformity, itself due to SL

ligament injury. The DISI deformity refers to Dorsal Intercalated Segment Instability – with flexion of the scaphoid and extension of the lunate as the SL ligament no longer restrains the articulation.
- Management options include mostly salvage options based on the Watson classification stage.
  - For Stage I, with arthritis between the scaphoid and radial styloid, I would offer:
    - a radial styloidectomy and scaphoid stabilization to prevent impingement between the proximal scaphoid and radial styloid, or
    - denervation for pain relief.
  - For Stage II, with arthritis between the scaphoid and scaphoid facet of the radius, I would offer:
    - a proximal row carpectomy if there is a functioning radioscaphocapitate ligament (to prevent post-operative ulnar subluxation). This provides relative preservation of strength and motion.
    - If the radioscaphocapitate ligament function is lost, then I would offer a scaphoid excision and four-corner fusion.

This also provides relative preservation of strength and motion through the preserved articulation between the lunate and distal radius at the lunate fossa.

In addition, previous impingement-related problems with the Hubcap circular plate have been decreased with the more recent use of intraosseous screws.
  - For Stage III, with arthritis, I would offer:
    - wrist fusion for pain relief and stability, with the sacrifice of wrist motion, or
    - referral to a specialized centre that offers total wrist replacements.

You've mentioned some of the wrist ligaments. Please draw the extrinsic ligaments for me and describe your understanding of their anatomy.

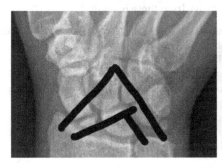 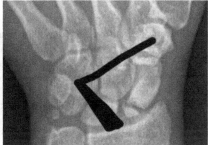

- The ligaments of the wrist are a complex system of extrinsic capsular and intrinsic intraosseous ligaments.
- The intrinsic ligaments lie between each of the carpal bones in the proximal and distal rows.
- The extrinsic ligaments are palmar and dorsal.
- The palmar ligaments are the more important stabilizers of the wrist and are arranged as proximal and distal double inverted Vs with the apexes centred on the lunate and capitate respectively – representing the 'greater' and 'lesser ligamentous arcs' – with the Space of Poirier between them as a potential anatomical weak spot that allows the escape of the distal carpal row from the lunate in perilunate dislocations.
- The dorsal ligaments are arranged as a horizontal V with the apex at the hamate starting at the radius and ending at the trapezium. The main two dorsal ligaments are the DRC (Dorsal RadioCarpal) and DIC (Dorsal IntraCarpal) Ligaments.

FURTHER READING

1. Kawamura K, Chung KC. Treatment of scaphoid fractures and non unions. J Hand Surg Am. 2008;33(6):988–997.
2. Karaismailoglu B, Fatih Guven M, Erenler M, Botanlioglu H. The use of pedicled vascularized bone grafts in the treatment of scaphoid nonunion: clinical results, graft options and indications. EFORT Open Rev. 2020;5(1):1–8.

Case 1.5

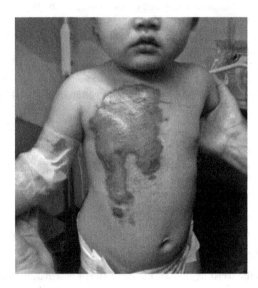

Tell me – How do paediatric thermal burn injuries differ from those in adults?

- Children have a proportionately greater surface area and reduced physiological reserves, including glycogen stores – resulting in increased insensible losses and hypoglycaemia.
  - Because of this, resuscitation fluid, if indicated, should be supplemented with additional maintenance fluid according to a weight-based maintenance table (consisting of 4 ml/kg/hour for the first 10 kg, followed by 2 ml/kg/hour for the next 10 kg, then 1 ml/kg/hour for the next 10 kg).
  - Also, additional carbohydrate is required to prevent potential hypoglycaemia.
- Lastly, the hypermetabolic response may result in blunted growth for 1–2 years post burn in children with burn sizes greater than 20% TBSA.

This infant has sustained a superficial partial-thickness scald as depicted in this photograph. How will you manage her?

- I will take a focused history assessing:
  - the timing and mechanism of the injury – ensuring that NAI is not a possibility,
  - any first aid given,
  - any comorbidities,
  - medications and allergies, and
  - up-to-date immunizations.
- My examination will include:
  - the surface area, which I estimate at about 4–5% according to the photograph, and
  - the depth, which is difficult to evaluate in a black and white photograph, but you have told me this is superficial partial thickness.
- As the TBSA affected is less than 10% in a child – which is the paediatric cut-off for resuscitation requirements – this injury does not require fluid resuscitation.
- A general anaesthetic is required for initial wound cleaning and deblistering, with early Biobrane application to optimize the future scar – as the burned area is confluent, as well as a formal wound assessment – including the use of a laser Doppler as per NICE guidelines.
- Once this has healed, then a pressure garment is required to minimize hypertrophic scar formation.

 DOI: 10.1201/9780429399268-6

How does a laser Doppler help with you with burn assessment?

- This provides non-invasive mapping of blood flow in an area of burned skin, which can improve the accuracy of burn wound depth assessment compared to clinical evaluation alone. In addition, it provides a calculated healing potential based on the blood flow image reported in three categories: <14 days, 14–21 days, and >21 days.
- It is particularly useful to differentiate between superficial dermal burns that can be managed with dressings, and deep dermal burn wounds that may require debridement to optimize the result and prevent hypertrophic scarring.
- It is also particularly useful in children – as in this case – because of the prevalence of mixed depth scald burns.
- It achieves this by rotating a mirror to direct a low-power laser beam at the burn wound area, which penetrates the full thickness of the dermis.

  Laser light scattered from moving blood cells in the tissue undergoes a Doppler frequency shift, the average of which is proportional to the average speed of the blood cells.

  Some of the scattered laser light is then collected by the mirror and then focussed by light collecting lenses on photodiode detectors.

  The resultant photocurrent is processed to calculate the blood flow in the tissue and this information is displayed as a colour-coded map of the burn area.
- Interpretation can be affected by infection, patient movement, old scars, and tattoos – none of which appear to be relevant to this little girl.
- Due to the changes in the inflammatory response and blood flow consequent to a burn, it is best to use it in the first 48–72 hours, but it can be used up to 5 days post injury.

How do you clinically differentiate a superficial from a deep dermal burn? And how do they heal?

- Superficial dermal injuries are pink, moist, and very painful – due to the sparing of nerve endings in the mid-dermis (although that is impossible to establish in children, as many will be distressed irrespective of the burn depth). In addition, skin blisters are often present in the injured area.
- Healing occurs within 2 weeks with rapid re-epithelialization by migration of epithelial cells from the deeper portion of the hair follicles, as well as from the sweat and sebaceous glands. However, the injured skin may result in a colour change due to hyperpigmentation – especially in non-Caucasian patients.

Why does hyperpigmentation occur?

This question is answered in Case 3.11.

Please continue.

- In contrast, deep dermal injuries involve an injury to the full thickness of the epidermis and the reticular dermis. These burns are typically dry, mottled pink, or even pale in deeper injuries. They are relatively insensate as the nerve endings are destroyed – but again this is difficult to establish in children. Skin blisters may still be present making it difficult to establish the depth.

  Healing is slowed due to the relative paucity of available cells for migration from the skin appendages with more than 3 weeks taken to heal, and a consequent increase in hypertrophic scarring.

What is a hypertrophic scar? And what is its pathophysiology?

Answered in Case 3.11.

What are the risk factors for the development of post-burn hypertrophic scarring?

These are patient and injury-related:

- Patient factors include:
  - female gender,
  - non-Caucasian skin types, and
  - children.

- Injury-related factors include:
  - burn sites of the neck or upper limbs,
  - the use of meshed skin grafts,
  - infection, and
  - prolonged healing time, especially more than 3 weeks.

You mentioned your estimation of the approximate surface area being 4–5%. How would you assess the surface area of burns in general?

- In patients with small burns, I use the template of the patient's palm and fingers for small, patchy burns, where the surface of the patients' hands with fingers adducted has been taken to represent approximately 1% of their TBSA, or
- In those with larger and patchy burns, I use tools that provide a graphical record of the extent of the burn, such as:
  - the Lund and Browder charts in children, or
  - the Wallace rule of nines in adults.
- In addition, I am aware of the development of specific apps to assist with this assessment.

You've mentioned the use of Biobrane earlier – What is this?

This is a bilaminar material with an outer silicone layer, and an inner nylon layer with porcine dermal collagen. The collagen peptides bind to the wound surface fibrin and so act as a dermal analogue – with spontaneous detachment once re-epithelialization is complete. Benefits of its use include:

1. faster re-epithelialization resulting in improved scar quality,
2. lower pain scores,
3. drainage of exudate via the pores,
4. in addition, the translucent quality allows the identification of any underlying infection.

However, one downside is that it requires a GA, as deroofing of blisters and debridement of wound debris are needed prior to its application.

How does re-epithelialization occur?

Answered in Case 3.11.

Tell me about burns dressings in general

- The ideal burn wound dressing, were it to exist, would fulfil the requirements of:
  - protection against trauma and infection,
  - reduction in heat and water loss,
  - the absorption of wound exudate, and
  - provision of pain relief.
  There is no level I evidence to show that a any particular dressing is associated with improved wound healing or a lower rate of infection.
- For small superficial burns, a dressing to encourage re-epithelialization is all that is required, such as the use of Mepitel with an overlying occlusive dressing to maintain a moist environment and prevent adherence to the wound. Confluent burns may be aided by Biobrane.
- For deeper burns or even very large superficial burns, then antimicrobial dressings are useful to attempt to prevent colonization. These are most commonly silver-based, or mafenide acetate is an alternative.
- Silver-based dressings such as Acticoat and silver sulphadiazine are popular as they have a relatively broad spectrum of cover, including Gram-positive and Gram-negative bacteria, as well as *Candida*.
  - Acticoat is easy to apply and remove, with different types that can be left in situ for up to 7 days, but requires activation with sterile water before application.
  - I am mindful of the fact that Flamazine and Flamacerium can make the assessment of burns more difficult, due to a pseudo-eschar (caused by the reaction of the polypropylene glycol carrier with the wound exudate). But this, in the right patient, can be useful as it is soothing, and can make dressings easier.

However, they are contraindicated in pregnant and breastfeeding women as well as infants less than 2 months old, due to the risk of kernicterus.

- Mafenide is a potent carbonic anhydrase inhibitor that also has a broad cover – especially Pseudomonas and Clostridium. In addition, it can penetrate a burn eschar.

However, it prevents the conversion of hydrogen ions to carbonic acid, leading to a metabolic acidosis if used continuously on extensive burns.

On presentation, your trainee notices odd-looking bruises on her back and buttocks of varying ages. Mum can't quite explain them and simply says: 'she just bruises a lot'. How would you proceed?

This may represent:

- a medical condition – such as a coagulopathy, or
- a non-accidental injury.

Both of these need admission and investigation by the paediatric team.
If medical reasons are excluded, then I will involve the paediatric safeguarding team as well.

What other features would make you suspect a non-accidental injury?

- Suspicious factors are those associated with:
  1. the type of burn, or
  2. those associated with the history and parental interaction.
- Those associated with the burn include:
  - immersion scalds affecting the extremities, or the buttocks and perineum – especially if uniform in thickness with a clear demarcation line,
  - those characteristically caused by abuse such as cigarette burns, imprints from hot objects such as irons, or
  - those with multiple injuries of varying ages – as in this case, which may be burns, bruises, or fractures.
- Factors associated with the history and parental interaction include:
  - an explanation that is incompatible with the injury sustained,
  - an unexplained delay in presentation, or
  - apparent lack of parental concern or parent/child bonding.

This little girl develops a pyrexia, a rash, diarrhoea, and vomiting. What do you suspect? And how will you manage her?

- I suspect she is developing toxic shock syndrome, which is a condition related to the production of TSST-1 toxin by many strains of staphylococcus aureus.
- I will manage her along with my paediatric colleagues with:
  - early targeted antibiotic treatment,
  - anti-TSST-1 toxin immunoglobulin or pooled gamma globulin, and
  - fresh frozen plasma.

Is this the same as toxic epidermal necrolysis?

- No, toxic epidermal necrolysis, along with erythema multiforme and Stevens-Johnson syndrome, are forms of an allergic skin reaction with diffuse blistering that can lead to loss of the body's entire epidermis in:
  - up to 10% loss in erythema multiforme,
  - 10–30% loss in Stevens-Johnson syndrome, and
  - more than 30% loss in toxic epidermal necrolysis, with a consequent increased mortality rate.
- Patients require treatment as per a major burn, with:
  - airway support and ventilation,
  - fluid and nutritional support,
  - ophthalmologic consultation for corneal loss, and
  - Biobrane and consideration of skin substitutes, including allografts and xenografts.

Let's move into the future – a 12-year-old girl attends your clinic having sustained a scald to the right side of the chest area in her infancy with consequent hypertrophic scarring. This is now restricting her breast growth with breast asymmetry, which is concerning her and her mother. How would you manage her?

- I will first establish if the contracture is extrinsic or intrinsic.
- Intrinsic contractures may mimic hypoplasia or aplasia of the breast.
- I will reassure the patient and her mum that contractures from a superficial or intermediate thickness burn – as I expect the scald to have produced, won't stop the breast growth but just conceals it. (As opposed to a severe deep injury that may have destroyed the breast tissue itself.)
- Unless there is severe asymmetry or psychological distress – I will monitor her regularly and allow the scar to mature, with the use of non-operative scar measures as required, prior to reconstructing the breast in early adulthood.
- However, in severe cases of asymmetry, or if there is significant psychological distress, then I will proceed with staged releases with dermal replacement and skin grafts throughout puberty. I would warn them that this may result in a 'patchwork quilt' appearance that will need a further reconstruction in early adulthood.
- Once breast development is complete, then any asymmetry can be approached along the lines of a breast reconstruction, with the possible need for breast envelope and or volume replacement depending on its severity.

FURTHER READING

1. Dziewulski P, Villapalos JL. (2012). Reconstruction of the burned breast. In Total Burn Care: Fourth Edition (pp. 623–630.e1). Elsevier Inc. https://doi.org/10.1016/B978-1-4377-2786-9.00055-2
2. Chipp E, Charles L, Thomas C, Whiting K, Moiemen N, Wilson Y. A prospective study of time to healing and hypertrophic scarring in paediatric burns: every day counts. Burns Trauma. 2017 Jan;5:3.
3. Cubison TC, Pape SA, Parkhouse N. Evidence for the link between healing time and the development of hypertrophic scars (HTS) in paediatric burns due to scald injury. Burns. 2006;32(8):992–999.
4. Engrav LH, Heimbach DM, Walkinshaw MD, Marvin JA. Excision of burns of the face. Plast Reconstr Surg. 1986;77:744–751.
5. https://www.nice.org.uk/guidance/mtg2/documents/moorldi2-burns-imager-a-laser-doppler-blood-flow-imager-for-the-assessment-of-burn-wounds-assessment-report-summary2
6. Pan SC. Burn blister fluids in the neovascularization stage of burn wound healing: a comparison between superficial and deep partial-thickness burn wounds. Burn Trauma. 2013;1,27–31.
7. Chipp E, Charles L, Thomas C, Whiting K, Moiemen N., Wilson Y. A prospective study of time to healing and hypertrophic scarring in paediatric burns: every day counts. Burn Trauma. 2017;5,3.
8. Nunez Lopez O, Cambiaso-Daniel J, Branski LK, Norbury WB, Herndon DN. Predicting and managing sepsis in burn patients: current perspectives. Ther Clin Risk Manag. 2017;13:1107–1117. doi: 10.2147/TCRM.S119938

Case 1.6

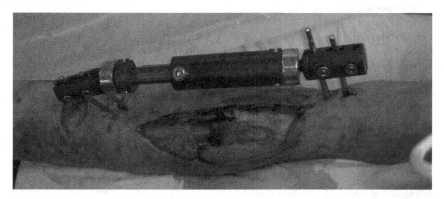

This patient is transferred from a holiday destination having suffered an open lower limb injury in an RTA two days prior to arrival. He was extricated from the wreckage a few hours after the accident. The transferring team informs you that he has a Gustilo and Anderson III B injury. They have managed him with prompt excision of the wound and external fixation and have temporized the wound with a negative pressure dressing.

What is the Gustilo and Anderson classification system?

- The clinically relevant differential of any lower limb trauma classification is whether the injury is low or high energy, but more recent evidence suggests that arterial injury also affects outcomes, even in the context of continued limb perfusion.
- The G&A classification includes three subtypes based on the energy transfer with types I and II as lower energy injuries, and type III as high-energy injuries – that is subdivided into three types: with A and B based on the adequacy of soft tissue coverage and bony exposure, and C based on the presence of 'an arterial injury requiring repair'.
- It is the most widely used as:
  - it is relatively simple, and
  - it provides prognostic information regarding future infection and non-union risk, with increasing risk in patients with higher scores.

However,
  - it has poor interobserver reliability,
  - the grade can only be confirmed following the primary wound excision, and
  - the III type injury is heterogenous and does not incorporate the presence of arterial injury in the context of continued limb perfusion. This is relevant as there is increasing evidence that this affects outcomes – as single-vessel limbs are associated with higher total flap failure rates, higher infection risk, as well as delayed healing times (as muscle recovery is affected by relative ischaemia).
    Based on that, there has been a suggestion for a further modification such that:
    - A G&A III B injury is defined as an injury that requires vascularized soft tissue reconstruction, with all three vessels intact.
    - A grade 'III B+' injury has a vascular injury but with at least one axial vessel patent that keeps the limb vascularized.
    - A grade III C injury is a devascularized limb, with all three vessels injured, that requires arterial repair for an acutely ischaemic limb.
- In view of the limitations I have discussed, I would also include information regarding:
  1. the mechanism of injury,
  2. the appearance of the soft tissue envelope,
  3. any likely bacterial contamination, and
  4. specific characteristics of the fracture.

DOI: 10.1201/9780429399268-7

What are the signs of a high-energy injury?

- Soft tissue signs include:
  - large multiple wounds,
  - crush injuries,
  - degloving, and
  - nerve or vascular injury.
- Bony signs include:
  - comminution,
  - injury to both the tibia and fibula at the same level, and
  - segmental injuries.

How would you manage this patient?

As with any transferred patient, I will start my assessment 'from scratch' with review of:

- any transferred notes and operative records,
- the patient's history,
- ATLS primary and secondary surveys, and
- a whole-body trauma CT and CTA of the affected limb.

If all seems to be in order, I will take him to theatre in the next scheduled joint orthoplastic list for exploration, and possible further excision of the wound if required, before planning the reconstruction.

Please talk me through your decision-making principles when planning the reconstruction.

There has been a historical debate regarding the superiority of fasciocutaneous or muscle flaps in lower limb reconstruction.

Some experimental data has shown that despite a higher blood flow in fasciocutaneous flaps, there is superior diaphyseal fracture repair with muscle flaps.

However, this has not translated into clinical evidence, so most surgeons, including myself, will make decisions based on practicalities such as:

1. the need for the reconstruction to withstand friction – such as on the sole of the foot or an amputation stump, which would be better served by a fasciocutaneous flap,
2. the presence of significant dead space that would be best served by a muscle flap,
3. any planned orthopaedic management – such as planned distraction that is best served by a muscle flap, or if future access is required – in which case a fasciocutaneous flap is preferable,
4. the need for a flap with a long pedicle to perform the anastomosis outwith the zone of trauma,
5. patient positioning and the preference to avoid intraoperative turning (for example, I will favour a flap from the subscapular axis if a lateral decubitus position is needed for a Godina approach), and
6. donor site morbidity.
7. Next, I will consider the choice of recipient vessels, the site of the anastomosis and the anastomotic pattern, be it end-to-end or end-to-side based on:
   - the zone of trauma, and
   - any vascular injury that is diagnosed on preoperative CTA as part of the trauma series.

   I prefer to use the posterior tibial vessels, accessed via the medial fasciotomy incision, as they are relatively protected compared to the anterior tibial vessels.

   I aim to perform two venous anastomoses – if possible, with at least one using the deep system, as this has been shown to decrease flap failure rates. If they are injured distally, then I would access them more proximally using a Godina approach.

What is the Godina approach? Please tell me how you would use it.

This is an alternative approach to access the posterior tibial vessels at the popliteal vessel division, with the possibility of following it distally according to need.

However, it does involve placing the patient in the lateral position – with the injured side down, so I would generally choose a flap from the subscapular axis when using this approach – if possible, to avoid turning the patient intraoperatively.

1. I will place a thigh tourniquet but not inflate it – unless required, followed by
2. a vertical longitudinal incision 1 cm medial to the midcalf line, from the level of the femoral condyles to the junction of the proximal 2/3 and distal 1/3 of the leg, whilst ensuring I preserve the short saphenous vein as a potential vein graft.
3. I will then divide the fascia exposing the two heads of gastrocnemius and the sural nerve in the midline groove, with sharp division at the avascular junction between the heads of gastrocnemius until the Achilles tendon is reached.
4. This exposes the popliteal vessels, which are seen passing under Soleus.
5. I will then divide Soleus, ensuring the venous branches are ligated.
6. Lastly, I will follow the popliteal vessel until the posterior tibial vessels are reached and these are followed as required – based on the zone of trauma and length of the chosen flap pedicle.

You mentioned a preoperative CTA – What is your rationale for that decision?

I am aware that its use is debated in young healthy patients with palpable pulses.

However, my rationale is that it provides useful information without the risks that were associated with an arteriogram (such as pseudoaneurysm, dissection, and haematoma), with benefits including the that include:

1. undiagnosed vascular injuries based on clinical examination alone, to confidently categorize a III B+ injury,
2. the detection of congenital variance of vascular anatomy – such as a Peronea Magna, and
3. In those at risk of potential atherosclerotic disease, it will also help with detection of this- which may alter my choice of recipient vessels if significant (with the understanding that the clinical presence of pedal pulses does not rule this out due to potential collateral circulation).
4. it may also give me an idea regarding the zone of trauma to allow quicker exploration and intraoperative decision-making.

It is also recommended in the updated UK lower limb standards – as long as it doesn't cause a delay to treatment – so I would routinely obtain it as part of the CT trauma series.

What are your thoughts regarding the timing of the reconstruction?

- I am guided by the UK standards for lower limb management, which suggests that we must aim to perform this at the earliest safe opportunity – within 72 hours of injury, unless patient factors dictate otherwise – as life must come before limb.
- This is balanced by the increasing risk of deep infection and technical difficulties encountered as the perivascular soft tissues become more oedematous, friable, and eventually fibrotic.
- This timing may also affect the chosen method of bony fixation as internal fixation should only be performed if definitive soft tissue reconstruction is achieved at the same time.

The patient's contralateral leg was bruised on arrival, but the trauma CT excluded any injury. His lower leg becomes tense and excruciatingly painful soon afterwards. His urine output drops, and he becomes mildly acidotic. You examine him and find that even attempted passive movement of his toes causes severe pain.

How would you manage him?

- I am concerned regarding compartment syndrome and the possibility of rhabdomyolysis – given his history. I will manage the suspected compartment syndrome with urgent fasciotomies using a two incision-approach.
- With regard to the rhabdomyolysis, I will share my concerns with the anaesthetic team and request an urgent intraoperative plasma CK level to avoid diagnostic delay.

What is the pathophysiology of compartment syndrome?

This is the elevation of pressure in a relatively fixed osseo-fascial compartment that eventually leads to vascular compromise – with reversible muscle damage occurring within 4 hours, and irreversible myonecrosis and nerve damage by 8 hours.

The exact mechanisms are not entirely understood – but the most popular model is the 'critical closure theory'. This is based on capillary collapse if the compartmental pressure exceeds the capillary perfusion pressure, resulting in muscle and nerve ischaemia.

The pathophysiological sequence of events is thought to include:

1. An initiating cause of elevated compartment pressure, such as bleeding or muscle swelling within a relatively fixed osseo-fascial compartment.
2. As the pressure increases, the veins become compressed causing fluid to move down its hydrostatic pressure gradient and out of the veins into the compartment, which increases the intra-compartmental pressure further.
3. Next, the traversing nerves are compressed, with paraesthesia as a first sign.
4. Lastly, as the intra-compartmental pressure reaches the diastolic blood pressure, the arterial inflow is compromised, which is a late sign of missed compartment syndrome.

Please draw a cross-section of the leg and use it to show me where you will place your fasciotomy incisions and tell me how you would perform the procedure.

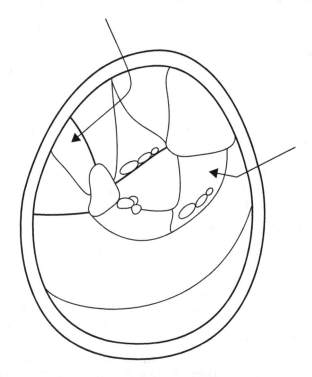

- I will decompress the superficial and deep posterior compartments with a full-length skin incision placed 1.5 cm posterior to the posteromedial border of the tibia, which I've drawn as the medial arrow.
  Once I have divided the skin and subcutaneous fat, I will release the fascia overlying the superficial compartment and then release the origin of soleus from the tibia to enter the deep compartment. As you can see from my diagram, the posterior tibial neurovascular bundle is at risk of injury at this point, as it is just deep to the investing fascia, so I will perform a full-length release of the fascia with care.
- The anterior and lateral compartments are decompressed by a full-length incision 2 cm lateral to the crest of the tibia, represented by the lateral arrow I've drawn.
  Once I have divided the skin and subcutaneous fat, I will fully release the anterior compartment then retract the compartment's muscles medially to access and fully release the anterior intermuscular septum, which separates the anterior and lateral muscle groups.

Why have you qualified the description of each fascial release as a 'full-length incision'?

The two common reasons for inadequate release of the compartments are:

1. short incisions that leave a residual constricting fascial band and
2. a failure to release the origin of soleus to decompress the posterior compartment.

Why do you use a two-incision as opposed to a single-incision approach?

Whilst I appreciate that a two-incision technique results in an additional wound, it has two advantages:

- Firstly, it avoids the morbidity of the required undermining of anterior and posterior skin with a single-incision approach.
- Secondly, it allows further decompression by allowing more muscle volume within the compartment to spill out.

How would your management have differed had the patient been intubated on intensive care, with a swollen leg?

I would be concerned regarding compartment syndrome, but I would have to rely on serial transducer catheter measurements of compartmental pressure to help me make the diagnosis.

I would decompress the leg if the measured compartmental pressure is either 30 mmHg, or within 30 mmHg of the diastolic pressure – for two consecutive hours.

What is the significance of 30 mmHg, and why 30 mmHg within diastolic pressure?

The capillary perfusion pressure is in the region of 25 mmHg (between 20 and 30 mmHg), so a compartmental pressure of 30 mmHg will theoretically cause capillary collapse.

The perfusion pressure of a compartment, also known as the compartment delta pressure, is defined as the difference between the diastolic blood pressure and the intra-compartmental pressure. If this is 30 mmHg, then capillary collapse will occur, even if the measured compartmental pressure may be less than 30 mmHg (such as in a hypotensive patient).

What are the contraindications to the surgical release of a limb with compartment syndrome?

These include

1. established myonecrosis, and
2. compartment syndrome of the foot.

The purpose of decompression is to rescue threatened muscle and nerve, so if these are already necrotic then there is no need to decompress. If anything, this would risk further morbidity – with infection and even death:

- If the diagnosis or presentation is delayed by more than 10 hours, I would obtain an MRI to evaluate the state of the muscles, as irreversible muscle damage is thought to start to occur at 8 hours. This will provide radiological confirmation regarding the progression of rhabdomyolysis to myonecrosis – with early ischaemic changes seen as a hyperintense signal on MRI, versus irreversible myonecrosis with complete lack of signal enhancement – in which case I would not operate.
- In addition, I would not operate if the diagnosis were delayed by 3 days, as widespread irreversible myonecrosis would have already occurred – with no need for imaging to confirm this.
- Lastly, I would not decompress a foot – even if acute – as morbidity of the procedure outweighs that of the sequelae, which is simply clawed toes.

His plasma CK results come back as 6000 IU/l, so your suspicion of rhabdomyolysis was correct. What is rhabdomyolysis and how do you manage it?

- As the name suggests, this is a condition where myocyte breakdown results in the leakage of intracellular contents – namely myoglobin, sarcoplasmic proteins, and electrolytes, into the extracellular fluid and circulation.

   This leads to renal injury, electrolyte imbalance – with potential cardiac arrythmias, acidosis, DIC, and compartment syndrome. Interestingly, it may also be caused by a missed compartment syndrome with ischaemic-induced muscle damage.

- Other causes of rhabdomyolysis include:
  - direct injury – such as crush injuries or
  - indirect injury – such as infections, metabolic and electrolyte disorders.
- Diagnostic indicators include:
  - CK levels greater than 1000 IU/l, and
  - serum and urine myoglobin – but these may not always be present.
- CK-MM increases within hours after the initial muscle injury with a peak at 24–72 hours then gradually declines over 7–10 days in a resolving injury, as it has a half-life of 36 hours. Persistently high levels would be suspect for continued muscle injury, such as a missed compartment syndrome.
- I will manage him along with my colleagues in critical care with:
  - early controlled large volume resuscitation to improve end-organ perfusion,
  - consideration of urine alkalinization – if alkalosis is excluded, to prevent precipitation of myoglobin in the distal convoluted tubule,
  - treatment of the identified cause and any sequelae, as well as
  - the possible consideration of the use of Mannitol – although this is debated and should be avoided with concomitant urine alkalinization, acute renal injury and oliguria.

This very unfortunate patient temporarily moves elsewhere to care for a sick parent then returns 18 months later with a draining sinus tract in the reconstructed leg.

What do you suspect is going on, and how would you manage him?

- I suspect chronic osteomyelitis. My management plan includes preoperative, intraoperative, and postoperative considerations:
  1. My preoperative aims include:
     - establishing a provisional diagnosis – with a focused history, examination, and imaging with a radiograph and CT,
     - staging – according to the Cierny-Mader classification, and
     - patient optimization – with a nutritional review, diabetic control-if required, and optimization of limb vascularity.
  2. The orthoplastic surgical aims include:
     - radical wound excision to remove all necrotic soft tissue and bony sequestrum, with
     - bone biopsies using a 'no-touch' technique to confirm the responsible organism – having stopped antibiotic therapy 2 weeks pre-operatively,
     - followed by an orthoplastic decision regarding reconstruction or eventual amputation.
     - Salvage reconstruction is considered in patients who are fit for and motivated for this. It entails:
       - skeletal stabilization,
       - dead-space management, and
       - the provision of vascularized soft tissue cover.
     - Amputation is indicated for failed salvage surgery, failed eradication of infection, and patients who are poor candidates for reconstruction.
  3. My post-operative management includes:
     - post-operative culture-driven IV antibiotics and
     - rehabilitation.
- The orthoplastic decision regarding reconstruction or eventual amputation is guided by patient factors and disease-related factors.
  1. Patient factors include:
     - comorbidities – such as diabetes and immunosuppression, which affect the bone healing potential,
     - their nutritional and smoking status,
     - their occupation, and self-employment status, and
     - patient psychology and social support structure – as they need to cope with a frame for 18 months.
  2. Disease-related factors include:
     - the virulency of the organism involved (with poor indicator organisms such a MRSA, candida, pseudomonas, and VRE),

- the vascularity of the limb, and
- quality of the bone determined by evidence of bone healing:
  - If more than 50% union is achieved, despite the infection, then this is a good indicator.
  - If there is no evidence of fracture healing, then this is considered 'poor biology', and is an indication for segmental resection and bone transport, or an amputation if the patient is not fit for or does not want salvage surgery.

You mentioned the Cierny-Mader classification. What is this?

This is the most commonly used classification system for osteomyelitis, which stratifies the disease and host condition:
- The anatomy of the osteomyelitic stages include:
  - medullary – with infection confined to the medullary cavity,
  - superficial – with involvement of the cortical bone only,
  - localized – with involvement of the cortical and medullary bone, but with only part of the bony diameter affected, and
  - diffuse – involving the entire thickness of the bone, with loss of bony stability.
- The host types include:
  - a 'normal' patient,
  - a locally compromised patient,
  - a systemically compromised patient, and
  - a patient with severe comorbidity – where the risk of treatment outweighs those of infection.

FURTHER READING

1. Eccles S, Handley B, Khan U, McFadyen I, Nanchahal J, Nayagam S. (2020) Standards for the Management of Open Fractures. https://oxfordmedicine.com/fileasset/9780198849360_Print%20PDF.pdf
2. Godina M, Arnez ZM, Lister GD. Preferential use of the posterior approach to blood vessels of the lower leg in microvascular surgery. Plast Reconstr Surg. 1991 Aug;88(2):287–291. doi: 10.1097/00006534-199108000-00019. PMID: 1852822.
3. Merle G, Harvey EJ. (2019) Chapter 3: Pathophysiology of Compartment Syndrome. In: Mauffrey C, Hak DJ, Martin III MP. (eds) Compartment Syndrome: A Guide to Diagnosis and Management [Internet]. Springer, Cham.
4. Stanley M, Chippa V, Aeddula NR, Bryan S, Rodriguez Q; Adigun R. (2022) Rhabdomyolysis. In: StatPearls [Internet]. StatPearls Publishing, Treasure Island, FL.
5. Stranix JT, Lee ZH, Jacoby A, Anzai L, Avraham T, Thanik VD, Saadeh PB, Levine JP. Not all gustilo type IIIB fractures are created equal: arterial injury impacts limb salvage outcomes. Plast Reconstr Surg. 2017;140(5):1033–1041.
6. Chummun S, Wigglesworth TA, Young K, Healey B, Wright TC, Chapman TWL, Khan U. Does vascular injury affect the outcome of open tibial fractures? Plast Reconstr Surg. 2013;131(2):303–309.

Case 1.7

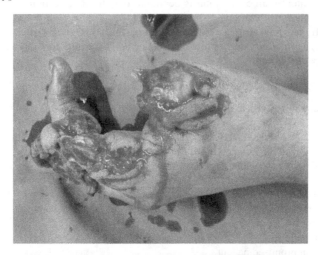

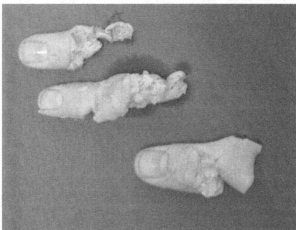

Please describe these photographs.

This is the photograph of a mangled left hand with amputation of the thumb, index, and middle fingers. The second photograph shows the amputate parts – with untidy wound edges, so this is not a sharp amputation. I am uncertain regarding the exact level of the amputation and would want to see radiographs to confirm this as well as exclude any other fractures.

What is your goal for patients with digital amputations?

The goal of replantation surgery, in the right patient, is successful restoration of function. Revascularization of an amputated part does not necessarily mean success – if the hand is stiff and painful.

What factors affect the outcome in extremity replants?

This is affected by:

1. general patient factors, such as:
   * physiological age,
   * any comorbidity, and
   * previous hand function.

DOI: 10.1201/9780429399268-8

2. factors related to the injury itself, such as:
   - the level of injury – with zone 1 having the best outcome, except if distal to the lunula as that is technically difficult and deficient of veins,
   - the ischaemia time – both cold and warm ischaemia times,
   - the mechanism of injury – with sharp versus crush and avulsion injuries, and
   - segmental injuries.

How will you manage this patient?

- I will ensure the amputates are transferred in a manner to decrease warm ischaemia time and avoid frost-induced tissue injury from direct ice, by transferring them in wet gauze placed in a sterile bag, which is itself placed in a bag that is half filled with saline and ice.
  On patient arrival:
- I will exclude and manage more pressing injuries as per ATLS in the first instance. With regard to their hand, I will obtain AP and lateral radiographic hand views and that of the amputates, to determine the bony levels of the amputations as well as any possible additional hand fractures.
- I will determine the factors that will establish the suitability of the patient for replantation.
- If they are suitable to go ahead, then I will counsel the patient regarding expected functional outcomes as well as risks and benefits.

    If the patient accepts this, then I will proceed with examination of the part for suitability for replant and tagging of the structures in theatre whilst the patient is anaesthetized (as a GA or axillary block). I will then proceed with addressing the structural injuries of each digit systematically.

- To save time, I prefer to repair each structural injury in all digits, before addressing the next structure to be repaired. So, I will proceed with:
  1. marking the position of possible vein grafts on the dorsum of the hand and the volar aspect of the wrist, prior to inflating the tourniquet, followed by
  2. midaxial incisions to explore the hand and tag the injured structures,
  3. examination of the arteries for signs of microscopical injury that indicate the need for excision and interpositional vein grafting – which I anticipate will be required given the nature of the injury in the photograph,
  4. reduction and fixation of all the fractures starting with the thumb, with consideration for bony shortening to avoid interpositional grafts, followed by
  5. flexor tendon repair of all digits, and
  6. letting the tourniquet down and completion all the arterial repairs – preferably of both vessels per digit, if possible, to reduce cold intolerance.
  7. This is followed by digital nerve coaptation of all digits.
  8. The hand is then turned over and the extensor tendons are repaired first, followed by
  9. the dorsal vein anastomoses – as the amputation levels appear proximal to the lunula (again with vein grafting if required), and lastly,
  10. removal of the nail plate as it decompresses the finger and provides access for leeching – if required.

Tell me – how does leeching work?

This is answered in Case 3.10.

Ok, please continue.

My post-operative regime consists of:

1. Keeping the patient warm, well hydrated, and pain free with:
   - an axillary infusion of Marcaine for pain relief and chemical sympathectomy, and
   - patient avoidance of caffeine or any form of Nicotine for the first week.
2. Broad spectrum antibiotics such as Co-amoxiclav that can be modified later if required

3. Hand elevation to 45% – or vertically if I am confident regarding the inflow and I have reconstructed both digital arteries, and splinting in the 'Intrinsic Plus position'
4. Perfusion monitoring with capillary refill, or a saturation probe if that is difficult
5. DVT prophylaxis starting 6 hours post operatively
6. Consider ation of leeching with antibiotic cover if the venous repair is tenuous, and finally
7. Post-operative low-dose Aspirin – of 75 mg for 10 days

How is this sequence changed in more proximal replantation? For example, at the wrist or forearm level?

Proximal level amputations involving significant muscle content will reduce the accepted ischaemia time, so I would place a temporary vascular shunt prior to bony stabilization.

I would also perform prophylactic fasciotomies at the end of the replantation if the warm ischaemia time exceeded 4 hours.

You mentioned signs of microscopic injury earlier. What are these and how would you manage this if encountered?

- The Cobweb sign describes the appearance of multiple laceration-like patterns on the vessel wall.
- The red line or red ribbon line sign is caused by a shearing force along vessels, which leads to separation of the intima from the media.
- Vessel anastomoses within these damaged sections lead to higher complication rates secondary to vessel thrombosis, so these are managed with resection and interpositional vein grafting.
- Vein graft donor sites include the dorsum of the hand or the volar aspect of the wrist. If a Palmaris tendon graft is also required, then I would prefer the volar wrist to minimize the number of extra scars.
  - I mark the position of the vein graft prior to inflating the tourniquet, followed by a gently curved incision overlying the vein.
  - The dorsal surface of the vein is then marked with blue dye to prevent subsequent twisting.
  - One end is marked with a Ligating clip to reverse it prior to the anastomoses, and
  - I will ensure both anastomoses are complete before releasing the clamps to reduce the chance of thrombosis.

You mentioned patient suitability for replantation. How do you assess for this?

By considering patient and injury-related factors:

- Patient factors include:
  - physiological age, occupation, hand dominance, and hobbies
  - general health – including vasoconstrictive medication and past medical history
  - pre-existing hand problems, and
  - suitability for long-term rehabilitation with:
    - their willingness to comply to rehabilitation,
    - the possible need for multiple revisional procedures, and
    - a possible lengthy time off work (with an average return to work time of 2–7 months).
- Injury-related factors include:
  - the mechanism of injury: such as sharp or crush injuries, and
  - the ischaemia time and storage.

You mentioned factors that are strong indications for replantation. Are there any others apart from those you have already mentioned?

Yes, these include:

- sharp proximal amputations (such as through the palm or wrist/forearm level),
- amputation of multiple digits,
- thumb amputations, and
- amputations in a child.

What is special about children in this case?

Replantation in children has improved outcomes as they are physiologically and psychologically resilient. This may be due to:

- low rates of acquired comorbidity,
- superior nerve regenerative capacity, as well as shorter regenerative distances,
- lower forces of motion,
- superior circulatory physiology – with lower rates of anastomotic thrombosis,
- axial growth overcoming scarring, and
- intuitive rehabilitation.

However, future growth distal to the original amputation level may be impaired.

And what is special about the thumb?

This digit represents 40–50% of the overall hand function.

It is important in precision grip function – such as key pinch, pulp-to-pulp, and tripod pinch, as well as assisting in power grasp.

You also mentioned contra-indications to digital replantation. What are these?

- Absolute contraindications include:
  - life-threatening concomitant injuries and
  - severe premorbid chronic illness, such as severe vascular disease with pre-existing limb ischaemia.
- Weaker indications for replantation include patient or injury-related factors. However, these are somewhat subjective with some debate between surgeons.
- My personal contraindications are:
  - patient factors, such as:
    - elderly patients with micro-arterial disease,
    - heavy smokers who are unwilling to stop,
    - severe untreated mental health disease which may complicate the rehabilitative process, in addition to the initial consenting process, and
    - uncooperative patients, or those unwilling to sign up to the post-operative rehabilitation.
  - injury-related factors, such as:
    - single finger amputation – particularly, at or proximal to the level of zone II in an adult,
    - multilevel segmental injury,
    - concomitant degloving,
    - widespread crush,
    - extreme contamination, or
    - ischaemia time of more than 24 hours.

Why do you give them Aspirin post-operatively?

I appreciate that the use of routine anticoagulation following any microsurgical procedure – including replantation – is controversial. There is no strong evidence that it improves patency rates. In addition, there is some evidence that post-replantation heparin has been linked to increased haematoma rates.

However, there is some evidence from animal studies that aspirin may improve patency rates and is less likely to cause harm – so a compromise is a low dose for a short period of time. However, I accept that some of my colleagues may differ on this – both with regard to its administration and duration.

How would you counsel patients regarding expected functional outcomes?

This will vary based on individual cases, but in general I will explain that:

- The replanted digit is expected to have decreased sensitivity, decreased grip strength and increased stiffness compared to the pre-injury digit.

- They may suffer from prolonged or permanent cold intolerance.
- They may be off work for at least 3 months, with the need for multiple revisional procedures such as neurolysis, tenolysis or to address non-unions.
- A 'late failure' of the procedure following successful revascularization is a painful stiff digit that interferes with their daily activities and requires a secondary amputation.

What is your general approach in a situation of multiple digital amputation, where not all amputates are available?

- Amputates should be replanted to the most useful stumps or in orientations most likely to succeed, to ensure maximal function.
- Heterotopic replantation, which is a concept of spare-part surgery, may be required to achieve that.
- Following the hand and amputate wound excisions, I will take the opportunity to evaluate what is available for replantation and how these can be best utilized.
- I will prioritize reconstruction of the thumb, followed by a discussion with the patient regarding their preference for:
  - a digit on the ulnar side of the hand – as a minimum, to enable power grip, or
  - the middle finger for fine pinching,
  - with index function as the most expendable of all the digits.

This patient's thumb replantation fails. He is left with a stump with a bony level through the proximal phalanx. How do you proceed, and what is your management algorithm?

This is disappointing both for the patient and myself, but I would have prepared the patient preoperatively for this possibility – especially given the injury mechanism and presentation as per the photographs.

1. First, I will determine if there are any additional reasons for failure – other than the zone of trauma and the mechanism of injury. These may be:
   - patient factors – such as an unknown coagulopathy,
   - intraoperative factors – such as a technical error or hypoperfusion, or
   - post-operative factors – such as vasoconstriction due to hypotension, hypothermia, pain, or Nicotine.
2. Next, I will determine the management plan with the patient – including:
   - the timing of the reconstruction – be it immediate or delayed, and
   - the technique, based on my reconstructive algorithm.
- If the reason for failure cannot be optimized or reversed, such as a previously undiagnosed coagulopathy, then I will proceed with a non-microsurgical reconstruction.
- If the reason for failure is reversible, or due to the zone of trauma, then I will suggest we aim for:
  - stump temporization with a pedicled groin flap, and
  - a delayed formal reconstruction once the inflammatory period has subsided and the patient is optimized.

    Advantages of this approach include a less thrombogenic patient, and the opportunity for the patient to be truly involved in the consent process. However, I accept that the anatomy will no longer be exposed and there will be more scarring to deal with at that point.

    If the patient cannot accept that and insists on an immediate reconstruction, then I would offer non-microsurgical options as the risk of another failure in the acute setting would be too high otherwise, due to the acute inflammatory process.

My selection algorithm is otherwise primarily based on the length of the remaining thumb to be reconstructed in the first instance. This is modified if the patient has specific considerations such as if there is a particular concern regarding:

1. cosmesis of the new thumb,
2. foot donor site morbidity, or
3. the need for improved interphalangeal joint mobility – such as in a pianist.

For injuries through the proximal phalanx with an intact MCPJ, as in this case, the options include:

1. distraction lengthening of the first metacarpal,
2. osteoplastic techniques such as:
   - a reversed pedicled radial forearm flap with a vascularized radius component or
   - a bone graft and pedicled groin, posterior interosseus artery or radial forearm flap.
3. Pollicization of an injured digit – unless the injured digit has been replanted, and
4. Toe transfer options, such as:
   - a wrap-around partial toe transfer – which gives the best cosmesis and sensibility, at the expense of IPJ motion,
   - a hallux transfer – which provides the best strength and range of motion, but with inferior cosmesis, and
   - a trimmed toe – which restores movement at the IPJ with good cosmesis.

The patient agrees to undergo a delayed reconstruction with a pedicled groin flap to manage the stump acutely, as you have suggested. Why did you opt for that?

This is because:

- I want to preserve as much length as possible – particularly for the thumb, so a flap is required as opposed to a terminalization.
- I also want to avoid complicating the secondary surgery, so I will:
  - preserve any local vascularity by avoiding free flaps, and
  - avoid local flaps to avoid further scarring.

You have described your reconstructive algorithm for injuries through the proximal phalanx.

Please talk me through the rest of your algorithm for thumb reconstruction in general.

As before, the algorithm is based on the length of the residual stump and any specific patient considerations.

- For injuries distal to the IPJ – there is little functional loss so I would consider:
  - restoration of the first webspace,
  - first metacarpal distraction lengthening, or
  - a toe transfer with a wrap-around or trimmed toe, which would restore length, sensibility, and a near normal appearance.
- For injuries proximal to the MCPJ, options include:
  - pollicization of the injured digit, with or without a toe transfer or
  - a second toe transfer.
- For injuries proximal to the first CMCJ, options include:
  - pollicization of the injured digit, with or without a toe transfer,
  - pollicization of a normal digit, or
  - a second toe transfer – as the MTPJ along with some MT can be harvested.

With regard to patients with additional specific considerations:

1. For those who are particularly interested in cosmesis: the two best options include a wrap-around transfer or a trimmed toe transfer.
   - A wrap-around partial toe only transfers soft tissue and nail from the hallux, so it would require bone from the amputate if this is still available, or an additional iliac bone graft to restore length.
   It offers the best cosmesis, and a sensate tip.
   However, disadvantages are potential graft resorption, and little or no movement at the level of the IPJ, which is a relatively minor functional compromise in most people.
   - If I can't use the bone from the amputate, and the patient doesn't want an iliac graft donor site, then I will offer a trimmed toe.
   Here, the hallux is trimmed with a longitudinal osteotomy, to the size of the contralateral thumb. This also has the advantage of restoring cosmesis without as much IPJ movement sacrifice.

2. For those who need to particularly maximize IPJ movement, the best option is a hallux transfer, but the patient should accept a lower cosmetic result of the new thumb and a relatively poor donor site cosmesis.

   In addition, this is not an option for those who need a CMCJ reconstruction as first MTPJ sacrifice would result in an unacceptable functional donor site morbidity. In this group, I will offer a trimmed toe transfer as the next best alternative.
3. For those who need to minimize foot donor site morbidity as much as possible – the metatarsal head should be preserved along with at least 1 cm of the proximal phalanx for 'push off'. In this case, a second toe transfer is best, but it is not as strong and stable as a hallux transfer.

The patient goes away to think about the options that you have offered but doesn't like the sound of any of them. He is a self-employed electrician and wants to go back to work soon. Whilst he did agree to a long rehabilitation at the time of the replantation – at the behest of his family, he now realizes that he just wants to get back to work as quickly as possible but needs to gain as much length as possible, to improve his precision grips. He asks if there is there anything else you can offer?

Another alternative is phalangization. The principle of this is to deepen the web with local tissue transfer, such as a Z-plasty or a dorsal rotational flap, to gain 1.5 cm of relative length. It is an option in those with at least half of the proximal phalanx remaining, with pliable web skin and a mobile first CMCJ.

It involves the release of the first dorsal interosseus and transfer of adductor pollicis insertion, which impacts on their mechanical advantage/power.

Despite it being a simple option, function is reduced compared to a reconstructed thumb and the web looks unnatural.

However, as he is looking for length and improvement of his pinch grip, as opposed to his power grip and cosmesis – this may be an option for him to consider if he accepts the downsides of the procedure.

How will you measure the outcome of any of these options, including replantation?

Apart from the viability of the replant, I will assess for subjective and objective measures, as well as patient reported outcome measures.

- Subjective measures include:
  - the patient's ability to resume work and
  - pain
- Objective measures include:
  - the resultant range of motion relative to normal,
  - sensibility using two-point discrimination testing, and
  - the measure of grip strengths.
- Patient reported outcome measures, which are hand specific, include:
  - the functional impact on the patient's hand function using the DASH and MHQ scoring system and
  - patient reported psychological sequelae and quality of life, e.g., using the HADS scoring system.

What are the DASH, MHQ, and HADS scoring systems that you've referred to? And why did you choose these tests in particular?

The DASH and MHQ systems – short for Disabilities of the Arm, Shoulder and Hand, and Michigan Hand Questionnaire – are the most frequently used patient reported outcome measures in hand surgery.

- The DASH questionnaire includes a 30-item scale relating to upper extremity function. These scales have been validated in the evaluation of impairments, activity limitations, and participation restriction to normal activities of daily living.
- The MHQ consists of 37 hand specific questions, divided into the following domains:
  1. overall hand function,
  2. activities of daily living,
  3. pain,

4.   work performance, and
5.   aesthetics and patient satisfaction with hand function.
- HADS – short for Hospital Anxiety and Depression Scale – is a good screening tool for identifying comorbid anxiety and depressive disorders in patients with musculoskeletal disorders.

What are the different grips that you have mentioned?

These are the movements used in normal hand function for activities of daily living.

- Power grips consist of:
  1.   cylindrical grip,
  2.   spherical grip,
  3.   hook grip, and
  4.   lateral prehension.

and
- Precision grips consist of:
  1.   tip pinch,
  2.   tripod (or chuck) pinch, and
  3.   key (or lateral) pinch.

FURTHER READING

1. Bakhach JY, Ghanem OA. (2017) Phalangization of the First Metacarpal With Dorsal Rotational Flap Coverage. In: Anh Tran T, Panthaki Z, Hoballah J, Thaller S. (eds) Operative Dictations in Plastic and Reconstructive Surgery. Springer, Cham. https://doi.org/10.1007/978-3-319-40631-2_103

Case 1.8

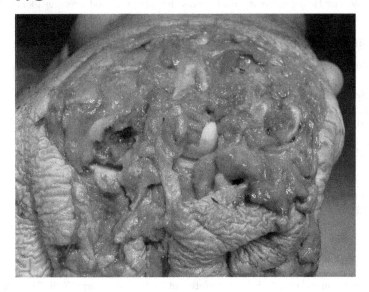

Please describe this photograph.

This is a photograph of the dorsum of a mangled hand with visible open fractured metacarpal heads and shredded overlying dorsal soft tissue. I am unsure as to the vascularity of the digits. I would need further views and radiographs for more information.

What are your general principles for managing a patient with a mangled hand? How would you apply them here?

- As with all trauma patients, I will manage this patient as per ATLS principles.
- With regard to the mangled hand injury, this is a high energy complex condition that is usually devastating for the patient and challenging to treat. It requires careful planning with a goal of achieving maximum possible function whilst aiming for an 'acceptable hand'.
- The first procedure is crucial and consists of:
  - wound excision to:
    - establish the exact nature and extent of the injury,
    - create a definitive plan, and
    - minimize the risk of wound sepsis.
  - I will not primarily repair soft tissue injuries unless there is a vascular injury, or undertake any internal fixation of fractures at this point until I have good skin cover.
  - I will then dress the wound, splint the hand in the position of function, and elevate with post-operative IV antibiotics.
- I will discuss my proposed plan with the patient including:
  - the planned procedures,
  - the rehabilitation required,
  - the possible complications, as well as
  - the possible requirement for secondary procedures.

This will provide a realistic picture to be agreed with the patient – as well as a 'road map' for both myself and the rest of the team.

- I will return to theatre in 24–48 hours, once the patient has agreed with the plan to:
  - fix any fractures
  - repair any nerve injury, and

DOI: 10.1201/9780429399268-9

    – re-establish soft tissue cover such as with an ALT free flap, if possible, as I can use the deep fascia to reconstruct the MCPJ capsules – which are at high risk of developing contractures according to the photograph
- Once the patient has healed, with mature scars and recovery of passive range of motion, I will address the extensor tendon repair with either:
  - tendon rods or
  - consider tendon transfers.

In addition, I expect the sagittal bands to be destroyed. These are important to maintain the central position of the extensor tendon so would need reconstruction also, and I would do this by creating a makeshift 'pulley' to centralize the tendon, similar to flexor tendon pulleys, using palmaris tendon if available or toe extensors.

- This is followed by post-operative therapy, which is an essential component to achieve the best function possible.

What do you mean by an 'acceptable hand'?

- This concept was proposed to introduce the minimal goal to aim for – from a functional and aesthetic point of view. I find it extremely useful to help me make difficult decisions and avoid burning bridges that may be subsequently required.
      It consists of a hand with a functioning thumb, three fingers with near normal length, near normal sensation, and a near normal ROM of the PIPJs.
- For the thumb to be functioning, it must be stable, opposable and of adequate length – at least up to the IPJ.
- At least two other digits are required for tripod pinch. They need adequate length and mobility to reach the thumb.
- To achieve this objective, I would consider three issues:
  1. the number of digits that may require reconstruction,
  2. the position of these digits, and
  3. aesthetic issues.

Please explain why you would aim for this. Why not aim for a hand with a thumb and four fingers? Or at the other extreme, why not accept a thumb and an opposing digit?

- The historical surgical goal of a thumb and an opposing digit provides a weak pinch and minimal grasping ability.
- A tripod pinch is presently considered by many to be the minimum requirement to provide a satisfactory result, as:
  - this provides a stronger pinch and dramatically improves the ability to grasp large objects, and
  - in addition, by aiming to reconstruct three fingers and the thumb, this also provides a more aesthetically pleasing hand.
- The decision to proceed to a four-digit reconstruction depends on the presence of at least one digital remnant in the hand, as I have to consider the donor site morbidity – which is significant, if two toes are sacrificed from the same foot.

What do you mean by the position of the digits?

- There is some debate regarding where toes and fingers should be ideally placed in a mutilated hand. Some recommend placing the toes in the:
  - middle position for fine pinching in the dominant hand and
  - in the fourth or fifth rays in the non-dominant hand to produce a larger span.
- However, what is accepted, is that the most important issue regarding toe placement is the presence and location of functioning joints of the hand, as transplanted toes rarely move.
      For example, in a hand where the index, middle, and ring fingers have been mutilated, I would place the toes at the position of the middle and ring fingers and remove the second ray to increase the webspace.
      This is because index function is most expendable, and a true tip pinch would be produced – as opposed to the more unstable mixed lateral pulp pinch, which would be potentially produced if the toe is placed at the position of the index finger.

Why are aesthetics important here? Surely only functional restoration should be aimed for in this complex situation?

The hand, like the face, is a cosmetically sensitive area for many. My goal is to produce a hand that is going to be used, and for this 'functional cosmesis' is essential – as there is evidence that the more natural looking the hand, the more likely the patient will use it.

I will discuss options with the patient to achieve the normal fingers' cascade – if possible, such as amputation of potentially functionless fingers and transposition of metacarpals to close gaps.

You seem to be planning delayed reconstructions. Why not proceed with immediate reconstructions with toe transfers?

There are two schools of thought regarding immediate or secondary reconstruction.

- Immediate reconstruction:
    - avoids scarring, with easier tissue plane dissection as well that of recipient vessels such as palmar arteries,
    - avoids intermediate interventions to achieve closure, and
    - allows the preservation of structures that would otherwise be sacrificed if the reconstruction is delayed.
- On the other hand, secondary reconstruction does allow an intervening mourning period, setting more realistic expectations and more opportunity to be involved in the consent process, with possible improved patient satisfaction (as is seen with patients following delayed breast reconstruction).
- I would use either approach depending on the physical and mental state of the patient: if they are physically optimized for a major procedure with good expectations, then I would proceed with immediate reconstruction. If either are in doubt, then I would delay until they have been addressed.

You mentioned counselling the patient for potential secondary procedures. What would you anticipate and warn your patient of in this situation?

Common sequelae of mutilated hands include:

- infection,
- prolonged swelling,
- intrinsic muscle scarring and contraction,
- sensory anomalies – from cold intolerance to numbness,
- CRPS, and
- the need for revisional procedures such as:
    - neurolysis,
    - tenolysis,
    - tendon transfers,
    - bone grafting for non-union, as well as
    - correctional osteotomies for malunion.

You've mentioned tendon transfers. What are the principles of this?

- The principles for successful tendon transfer consist of:
    1. good patient selection,
    2. optimal recipient site factors,
    3. optimal donor muscle factors, and
    4. good surgical technique.
- Patients must be well motivated to comply with post-operative therapy and informed regarding the nature and limitations of surgery.
- Recipient site factors include:
    1. good soft tissue coverage with mature scarring,
    2. a stable underlying skeleton,
    3. full range of passive ROM, and
    4. ideally, normal sensation.

- Donor muscle factors relate to:
  1. amplitude of motion,
  2. power,
  3. the plan for each transferred tendon to produce one intended action,
  4. the line of pull and expendability, and
  5. synergistic action.
  - Regarding the amplitude of motion, the donor muscle should have a similar excursion to that which it replaces.
    - Excursion of the wrist flexors and extensors is approximately 3 cm.
    - Excursion of the finger extensors is approximately 5 cm.
    - That of finger flexors is approximately 7 cm.
    This can be augmented by using tenodesis if the wrist is mobile.
  - With regard to power, donor muscles should have at least MRC grade 4 function as they lose at least one motor grade following transfer.
  - Consideration of the line of pull is important both for:
    - the donor muscles, as they should have a similar pull to those that they replace, and
    - the tendon transfer itself – such as avoiding an intervening pulley as it reduces power.
  - Synergistic transfers function better than asynchronous transfers, such as finger flexion and wrist extension, and vice versa.
  - Finally, only expendable muscles should be transferred.
  - With regard to surgical technique, I will:
    - use remote incisions,
    - ensure the recipient site and tunnel are ready before raising the muscle,
    - avoid compression of surrounding important structures such as nerves,
    - ensure I apply the correct tension, and
    - ensure a straight line of traction with adequate tension and a strong insertion.

How would you rehabilitate this patient?

I will start an early active movement regime with the physiotherapy team before discharge home.

Ok, so you have performed the ALT flap for coverage and performed tendon grafts to reconstruct the extensor tendons.

The patient develops an extensor contracture of the MCPJs with flexion of the IPJs. What do you suspect and how do you treat this?

I suspect scarring of MCPJs despite the ALT fascia reconstruction of the MCPJ capsules. I will manage this with dorsal capsulotomy of the MCPJs and hand therapy.

Let us consider another scenario – the patient returns with flexed MCPJs and extended IPJs – with difficulty flexing the PIPJs whilst the MCPJs are extended.

What do you suspect and how would you manage this?

The intrinsic plus position that you describe, leads me to suspect intrinsic tightness. This is a consequence of oedema, ischaemia to the intrinsics, and possibly poor mobilization.

I will confirm this with the Bunnell test – whereby passive flexion of the PIPJ is reduced with the MCPJ extended, compared to when the MCPJ is flexed.

I will first manage this along with the therapy team to stretch the intrinsics.

If this fails and is functionally problematic, then I will offer an intrinsic muscle release, with release of the lateral bands.

FURTHER READING

1. Del Pinal F. Severe multilating injuries to the hand: guidelines for organizing the chaos. JPRAS. 2007:60;816–827
2. https://emedicine.medscape.com/article/1243815-clinical

Case 1.9

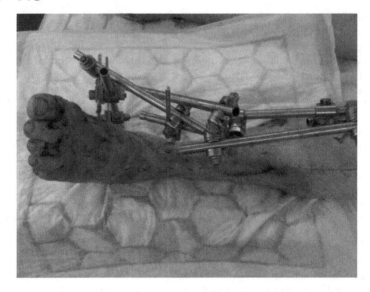

A patient with an open tibial fracture and degloving injury is transferred to your trauma centre as the patient sustained this injury on holiday. The transferring team informs you that the skin initially appeared viable during the primary excision so it was 'sutured back'.

On inspection after transfer, you find that much of this tissue has now demarcated. How will you manage this?

I will organize a return to theatre for a formal exploration under GA for excision of all devitalized tissue – both the demarcated skin and any potential underlying devitalized soft tissue. Once I am satisfied with this, then I will reconstruct this with either:

- a meshed split skin graft, dermal substitute – such as Matriderm – and overlying negative pressure dressing if the bed is graftable, or with
- a flap if the bed is non-graftable.

Please tell me about degloving injuries, and how would you manage them acutely.

- These are high-energy tangential shearing injuries in a plane superficial to the deep fascia that may be:
  - uni- or multiplanar, and
  - localized or circumferential.
- Uniplanar injuries sheer between the subcutaneous fat and the deep fascial plane.
- Multiplanar injuries cause disruption between and within the muscle groups, as well as between muscle and bone – with avulsion of trans-muscular and intermuscular perforating vessels that normally perfuse the skin.
- This leads to transection of perforating arteries and lymphatics that are traversing the fascial layers, resulting in:
  - a collection of blood, lymphatic fluid, and necrotic fat in the newly created potential space, and
  - decreased perfusion of the overlying skin.
- I would manage this acutely as with any lower limb open fracture – with systematic assessment of the skin and soft tissues from superficial to deep, and excision beyond the margin of viability. Vein thrombosis is a classic sign of skin devascularization and a helpful guide.

DOI: 10.1201/9780429399268-10

- However, I am mindful that necrosis of degloved tissues may evolve over time, as has occurred in this case. This is thought to be due to venous congestion and inflammatory cell infiltrate with proinflammatory cytokines and free radicals causing further damage over time.
- On occasion, when the soft tissue damage is difficult to assess, such as in multiplanar injuries, then I would bring the patient back for a second look within 24–48 hours, whilst still aiming for any open fracture coverage within 72 hours where possible.
- These patients are not candidates for a 'fix and flap' scenario.

You mentioned the primary wound excision of open lower limb fractures. How would you perform that?

- The term excision was popularized by military surgeons to describe debridement of open lower limb injuries.
- My objective is to produce a wound and fracture environment as close as possible to the local conditions found in a closed fracture environment, and hopefully match the infection rates of closed injuries.
- I will apply the following sequence along with my consultant orthopaedic colleague:
  1. A social wash, where the limb is washed with a soapy solution and a tourniquet is applied
  2. Limb prepping with alcoholic chlorhexidine, ensuring I avoid contact with the open wound, as well as pooling under the tourniquet
  3. Inflation of the tourniquet for the soft tissue debridement, to allow identification of key structures such as neurovascular bundles – especially in cases of extensive degloving
  4. Wound extension along fasciotomy lines to visualize deeper structures, deliver bone ends, and expose the full zone of injury
     The blood supply to the subcutaneous fat is relatively vulnerable and the zone of fat necrosis is often more extensive than that of the overlying skin.
  5. Next, I will assess the tissues systematically in turn, layer by layer from superficial to deep, and from the periphery to the centre of the wound. I will apply this compartment by compartment – excising any non-viable tissue that I encounter.

Tell me – how would you assess muscle viability here?

I use the four 'Cs' to assess muscle, although it can be difficult to assess this acutely. These consist of:

- Colour – which should be pink
- Contraction –when stimulated with forceps
- Consistency – with devitalized muscle tearing in the forceps during retraction, and
- Capacity to bleed

Ok. Please continue

  6. The tourniquet is then deflated and the bone ends delivered via the wound extensions to:
     - assess the capacity of the bone ends to bleed, with the 'paprika sign' representing punctate ooze in viable fracture fragments, whilst ensuring I have not mistaken bleeding from the medullary canal for this, and
     - remove any loose fragments of bone which fail the 'tug test'.
     - If this is uncertain, I will insert a hypodermic needle into the soft tissue attachment to test for bleeding, as an indication for the supply to the bone.
  7. This is followed by low-pressure lavage of the wound with Normal Saline.

Why not use high-pressure pulse lavage?

High-pressure lavage was the historical method of choice, but more recent guidelines have cited evidence that this is detrimental as it has been shown to cause:

- inoculation of dirt and bacteria into soft tissue and bone, and
- damage to the bony micro-architecture

If fragments of dirt are embedded in the bone, I will cleanse the bone with a scrubbing brush as this has been shown to be as effective as high-pressure pulse lavage, but without the risk of iatrogenic seeding.

Please continue

8. At this stage, the injury can be classified, and definitive joint reconstruction planned with my senior orthopaedic colleague – unless it is a severe multiplanar degloving injury, in which case I will bring the patient back in 24–48 hours if I am in any doubt as to the completeness of the excision.

9. If definitive skeletal and soft tissue reconstruction is not to be undertaken in a single stage, I will temporize the wound with then negative pressure wound therapy is used to temporize the wound – along with an antibiotic bead pouch applied if there is segmental bone loss, until definitive surgery is performed.

What is your understanding of the zone of injury?

- This concept was originally proposed for skin burns, with the term coined to define the area affected by an injuring force where tissue damage may not be immediately apparent from external view, and may even evolve over time, such as in severe degloving injuries.
- It may be defined by the soft tissue or bony injury patterns such as the:
  - fracture type,
  - the amount of comminution,
  - the area of crush, laceration, or shearing of the soft tissues, or
  - devascularization of the entire limb.
- It is clinically relevant, as it emphasizes:
  - emphasizes the need for appropriate wound extension to enable adequate inspection of the deeper tissues, and
  - the importance of planning the location of micro-anastomoses and local flaps outside of this zone – where possible.

  Interestingly, the historical debate regarding the superiority and safety of anastomoses distal versus proximal to the zone has now been debunked.

FURTHER READING

1. https://journals.lww.com/plasreconsurg/fulltext/2013/02000/does_vascular_injury_affect_the_outcome_of_open.24.aspx
2. https://books.google.com/books/about/Pathways_in_Prosthetic_Joint_Infection.html?id=vdt1DwAAQBAJ
3. https://oxfordmedicine.com/view/10.1093/med/9780198849360.001.0001/med-9780198849360-chapter-4
4. McGowan SP, Fallahi AKM. (2022) Degloving Injuries. In: StatPearls [Internet]. StatPearls Publishing, Treasure Island, FL. Available from: https://www.ncbi.nlm.nih.gov/books/NBK557707/
5. Prasarn ML, Helfet DL, Kloen P. Management of the mangled extremity. Strategies Trauma Limb Reconstr. 2012;7(2):57–66.

Case 1.10

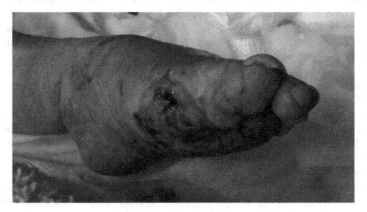

How would you describe this photograph?

This is the photograph of a sizeable ulcer on the plantar aspect of the midfoot. It is difficult to comment with certainty in a black and white photograph, but there appears to be necrotic areas. I note that the ankle is plantarflexed, which may be a result of glycosylation and shortening of the Achilles tendon in diabetic patients, or as is common in those who have been bedridden for long periods of time, or those with neuromuscular diseases.

This diabetic elderly patient has been brought in by her nursing home with a longstanding ulcer on the sole of her foot. She has just been transferred to them recently, and they are not sure how long she has had it for. She is not sure either. It has been discharging 'pus' since she arrived there.

How would you proceed?

- Given the history, my priority apart from addressing the diabetic foot ulcer itself, is to exclude malignancy, osteomyelitis, treatable peripheral vascular disease, and a Charcot arthropathy.
- I will manage this patient within an MDT consisting of a diabetologist, an orthopaedic foot surgeon, a vascular surgeon, and an occupational therapist.
- As her carers do not seem to have much information about her medical history, I will contact her GP, next of kin, and explore any hospital records for salient points in her history to establish:
  - how the ulcer started,
  - the timeline,
  - any previous treatments for it,
  - how the diabetes is managed, and if it is well controlled,
  - any sequelae of her diabetes, such as:
    - neuropathy,
    - peripheral vascular disease, and
    - renal disease, and
  - any other medical comorbidities to determine her fitness for a GA (or multiple GAs), and whether she is on any anticoagulation that needs to be stopped, or immunosuppressants that may affect subsequent wound healing.
- My examination will include assessing for:
  - the depth and size of the ulcer – with a 'probe-to-bone' test to evaluate the depth with relation to bone – as diabetic ulcers down to bone have a much higher chance of osteomyelitis,
  - sensation – including examining for a stocking distribution of sensory loss, and
  - infection – both of the ulcer itself, and signs of systemic sepsis.

DOI: 10.1201/9780429399268-11

- Given the history of possible mental impairment – as she was not sure of her history, I will assess her ability to consent by assessing her ability to understand, retain, and weigh the information and communicate her thoughts. If I am concerned, then I will take all practicable steps to help support this process by involving the trust's independent mental health advocate as per the Mental Capacity Act of 2005, as well as involving any persons she would like involved such as close family members or friends, her GP, and establish if she has appointed a Power of Attorney or an advanced directive concerning any future treatment.
- I will then exclude malignancy with numerous deep tissue biopsies.
- With regard to investigating for osteomyelitis, I will request a plain radiograph in the first instance, as I expect signs to be present with a long-standing picture.
- I will also request standing X-rays of both feet to help diagnose a Charcot arthropathy.
- With regard to investigating for vascular insufficiency, I will first palpate for dorsalis pedis and posterior tibial vessels – with the understanding that pulses may be palpable in the presence of chronic vascular insufficiency due to the development of collateral circulation. So, I will supplement my clinical findings with a duplex study to investigate this and look for loss of the normal triphasic waveform indicating early vascular disease. ABPIs are not indicated in this context as they are often falsely elevated in diabetics due to calcification in diabetic neuropathy.

What is the pathophysiology of diabetic foot ulcers?

This is classically due to:

1. peripheral neuropathy,
2. peripheral vascular disease, which may be macro- or microvascular, and/or
3. pressure points from a change in foot shape, e.g., a Charcot foot collapse.

   They have a higher rate of developing osteomyelitis when infected, most probably due to the ischaemic environment and the depressed immune response due to the glycosylation of white blood cells.
- With regard to peripheral neuropathy:
  - autonomic nerve dysfunction affects the microcirculation of the skin – opening arteriovenous shunts, and allowing blood to bypass the high-resistance vessels of the skin capillary bed. This further decreases nutrient blood flow to the skin and compounds the ischaemic effect of peripheral vascular disease.
  - Motor neuropathy leads to:
    - gradual denervation of intrinsic muscles of the foot, and
    - resulting claw foot from MTPJ hyperextension, loss of transverse and longitudinal arches, and metatarsal head prominence.
    - This causes a pressure effect, which is amplified by the loss of sensation.

Are you aware of the pathophysiology that causes the neuropathy in the first place?

Yes, there are several pathophysiological theories for axonal degeneration, but the most important is the metabolic theory – where saturation of the glycolytic pathway shunts excess glucose into the alternative polyol pathway, the end-products of which decrease membrane Na/K ATPase activity, impair axonal transport, and cause structural breakdown of the nerve.

Please continue.

- With regard to peripheral vascular disease, this is four times more prevalent than peripheral neuropathy and progresses more rapidly. The pathophysiology is thought to also be due to advanced glycation end products causing:
  1. up-regulation of pro-inflammatory cytokines that play a role in the progression of atherosclerosis, by creating a prothrombotic environment, platelet dysfunction, and plaque rupture, and
  2. the promotion of oxidative stress by increasing the production of reactive oxygen species. This leads to:
     - endothelial dysfunction, and
     - lipid peroxidation, which further up-regulates the expression of pro-inflammatory cytokines.

The distribution of vascular disease is also unique, classically affecting vessels distal to the popliteal artery and sparing the pedal arteries. Therefore, it is amenable to distal bypass to the dorsalis pedis or the peroneal or posterior tibial artery.

You've mentioned the microcirculation of the skin and AV shunts. Please tell me more about its anatomy and normal regulation of this – in the absence of a neuropathy.

- The blood supply to the skin is almost 60 times its nutritive requirements and has a primarily thermoregulatory function.
- The cutaneous microcirculatory anatomy is organized in two parallel plexuses with:
  1. a superficial subepidermal plexus consisting of arterioles, venules, and capillary loops – located in the superficial papillary dermis that is involved in oxygenation and nutritional exchange, and
  2. a deeper plexus consisting of arterioles, venules with connecting AVAs – located at the junction between the reticular dermis and hypodermis that is involved in thermoregulation – as blood flowing through AVAs bypass the capillary bed and allow heat to be dissipated.

  AVAs are either densely innervated glomerular structures called indirect AVAs or much less convoluted structures that are sparsely innervated structures called direct AVAs.
- Microcirculation is controlled by myogenic, humeral, neural, and temperature factors to maintain a constant flow.
  - The Bayliss myogenic theory states that increased intraluminal pressure results in constriction and decreased intraluminal pressure results in dilation.
  - Neural control acts by increasing arteriolar tone to decrease cutaneous blood flow, and increasing precapillary sphincter tone to reduce blood to the capillary network. Decreased AVA tone results in more non-nutritive blood flow bypassing the capillary bed.
    - Vasoconstriction is mediated by a sympathetic mechanism that includes co-transmitters such as neuropeptide Y and ATP
    - Vasodilation is mediated by:
      - a cholinergic mechanism that includes co-transmitters such as Vasoactive Intestinal Peptide and
      - axonal reflexes that mediate vasodilation through Calcitonin gene-related peptide and Substance P.
  - Humoral factors such as adrenaline/noradrenaline cause vasoconstriction. Vasodilation is caused by cellular hypoxia with low oxygen saturation, high carbon dioxide, and acidosis.
  - Lastly, high temperature produces cutaneous vasodilation and increased flow which bypasses the capillary beds for thermoregulation.

Thank you – let's go back to our patient with possible Charcot foot collapse. Please tell me about that.

- This is a progressive condition characterized by:
  - joint dislocation,
  - pathological fractures, and
  - destruction of pedal architecture.
- It is thought to be due to:
  - the loss of protective sensibility to the joint,
  - increased osteoclast activity due to the changes in bone blood flow brought on by the autonomic neuropathy, and
  - glycosylation and consequent ligamentous laxity and collapse of the arches.
- Patients present with a warm swollen foot, which may be painless.
- Periosteal erosions may be seen before the development of fractures several weeks after foot swelling.
- After some months, during which bony resorption continues, the swelling and warmth begin to resolve.
- The midfoot is a common site of Charcot neuro-arthropathy, which can result in midfoot collapse with a plantar bony prominence and 'rocker' foot.
- The aims of MDT management include:
  - strict glycaemic control to be achieved by the diabetologist,
  - any correctable vascular disease to be treated by the vascular surgeon,

- – medical treatment with bisphosphonates to decrease osteoclastic activity,
- – excisional surgery to remove bony prominences,
- – rest and immobilization in a total-contact cast until the disease activity subsides (unless ischaemia, or infection, is present – as I suspect may be the case in this patient), then specialized footwear to pad prominences and spread pressure.

What is total contact casting?

- This is the recognized gold standard treatment for diabetic foot ulceration and a Charcot foot. It is made of non-fibreglass tape that is designed to:
  - – offload pressure on the plantar aspect,
  - – increase total surface area of the midfoot and forefoot during weightbearing, thereby reducing peak pressures,
  - – shorten the wound healing time, and
  - – increase patient compliance as it cannot be removed by the patient.
- However, contraindications to its use include infection and ischemia.

Let's go back to our patient. What signs would you expect to see on the radiograph, in the case of osteomyelitis?

- Osteopenia,
- erosion of cortical bone – often in the heads of metatarsal and midfoot bones,
- cortical lysis,
- periosteal thickening, and
- bony sequestration.
  However, these can be very subtle and non-specific, and with similar signs in early Charcot joint arthropathy.

You find that the radiograph does show these signs. How will you proceed?

- An MRI may be helpful but the result of this will not be conclusively diagnostic, as any signal changes are not specific.
- So the gold standard investigation is a bone biopsy, as it provides microbiology – including the biopsy of the intrinsic muscles and surrounding soft tissues as confirmation of spread of osteomyelitis.
- I will ensure I use a 'no-touch technique' to avoid contamination.

Tell me – How does an MRI work?

- Magnetic resonance imaging employs powerful magnets to produce a strong magnetic field and force protons in the body to align with that field.
- Sensors detect the energy released by the protons after they are temporarily stimulated by a radiofrequency current that is pulsed through the patient.
- Intravenous contrast agents, such as gadolinium increase the speed at which protons realign with the magnetic field, with a brighter image produced by faster proton realignment.

What would you do if she has had an open reduction and internal fixation in the past following an ankle fracture?

This would be a contraindication to an MRI, so I would request a three-phase bone scan using Technetium-99 with or without a SPECT to improve the anatomical functional correlation with 3D images. But an intraoperative biopsy is required to confirm the diagnosis – as before.

You find that osteomyelitis of the midfoot is confirmed on bone biopsy – how will you proceed now?

This may be a limb-threatening condition and treatment is challenging.

In an elderly patient who is bedridden with other comorbidities, such as in this case, I would suggest a more conservative approach, with surgical excision of the affected soft tissue, and management of the bony infection with long-term culture-driven antibiotics until the MRI changes subside. This may be performed under regional block if a GA is a concern.

What would you do if this were a young fit patient?

I would suggest a staged approach with:
- excision of the affected soft tissue and bone, followed by insertion of an antibiotic spacer, and
- culture-driven antibiotics for 6–12 weeks, and then
- reconstruction with a vascularized bone graft, such as a free fibula, to arthrodese the midfoot.

When planning the reconstructive options, I would obtain a preoperative CTA of the limb to determine the best recipient vessel.

If there were no adequate recipient vessels, then I would refer the patient to my vascular surgery colleagues for consideration of a femoral-distal revascularization in the first instance, which would allow an end-to-side anastomosis onto the recipient vessel.

FURTHER READING

1. Yang SL, Zhu LY, Han R, Sun LL, Li JX, Dou JT. Pathophysiology of peripheral arterial disease in diabetes mellitus. J Diabetes. 2017 Feb;9(2):133–140.
2. Gouveri E, Papanas N. Charcot osteoarthropathy in diabetes: a brief review with an emphasis on clinical practice. World J Diabetes. 2011;2(5):59–65.
3. Cancelliere P. A review of the pathophysiology and clinical sequelae of diabetic polyneuropathy in the feet. J Diabetes Metab Disord Control. 2016;3(2):21–24.

Case 1.11

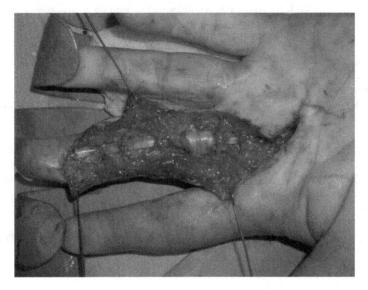

How would you describe this photograph?

This is an intraoperative photograph of the volar aspect of a patient's left hand which has been placed in a lead hand, with a tendon rod in situ in the middle finger, as well as reconstructed pulleys which appear to have been accessed via Bruner incisions.

What is the blood supply of tendons, and how do they heal?

- There are two sources of blood supply:
    - the first is via diffusion through synovial sheaths, which is the more important source distal to the MCP joint, and
    - the second is via direct vascular perfusion by the vincular system.
- Tendon healing occurs via two pathways:
    - an intrinsic pathway – involving epitenon and endotenon tenocytes, and
    - an extrinsic pathway – by invasion of inflammatory and synovial cells from the surrounding sheath and synovium, which contributes to adhesions and scarring.
- As with all tissue healing, it occurs via an inflammatory, proliferative, and remodelling phase.

Please talk me through two-stage tendon repairs.

- This two-stage technique allows reconstruction of the FDP tendon in patients who are unsuitable for a primary tendon repair, or in whom this is contraindicated, and who satisfy the following:
    - a full range of passive range of movement with stable joints,
    - adequate soft tissue cover with stable scars, and
    - the motivation to comply with hand rehabilitation protocols.
- The principle involves:
    1. initially placing a silicone rod, and reconstruction of the pulley system – if required, to allow for the formation of a pseudo tendon sheath in the first stage, followed by
    2. replacement of the rod with a tendon graft in the second stage.

DOI: 10.1201/9780429399268-12

How would you achieve this? Please describe your surgical technique.

- For the first stage:
  1. As in the photograph, I will first expose the flexor sheath via Bruner incisions extending into the palm, then excise the old tendon remnant, insert the silicone rod, and fix it to the distal FDP stump.
  2. This is followed by reconstruction of the A2 and A4 pulleys – if required, ensuring that the implant glides smoothly and does not buckle with passive flexion. This can be achieved by a variety of techniques, but I prefer a triple wrap of the phalanx deep to the extensor mechanism, using the excised tendon remnant as a graft. This will save palmaris or other tendon grafts for the second stage.
     - I recognize that the ideal graft for reconstruction of the pulley system would have an intrasynovial lining on the tendon gliding surface. So, my usual preference for pulley reconstruction in circumstances – other than two-stage tendon repairs, is to use a graft from the extensor retinaculum of the wrist as it is thinner than tendon grafts and offers an excellent gliding surface. However in this case, I prefer to make use of tissue that will be discarded.
     - Other techniques include using a portion of FDS or the contralateral palmaris – for a reconstruction through (1) drilled phalangeal holes or (2) to the remnants of the destroyed pulley.
     - I will ensure the pulleys are not too loose or too tight with radiographs of the digit on extension and flexion at the end of the procedure: bowstringing of the rods would indicate that the pulleys are too loose, and buckling of the rods would indicate that the pulleys are too tight, and need revision.
  3. Rehabilitation following the first stage ensures stable wound healing and maintenance of full passive ROM of the joints.
- The second stage occurs 3–6 months later, and consists of:
  1. rod replacement with a tendon graft via proximal and distal incisions, whilst ideally keeping the pseudo sheath intact,
  2. distal fixation of the graft via a bone anchor,
  3. tensioning of the graft to obtain slight overcorrection of the normal cascade, and
  4. proximal repair with a Pulvertaft weave in zone III if possible, or otherwise in zone V.
     It is essential that the tension is correct to prevent a lumbrical plus finger if the tendon graft is too long, or a quadriga effect if too short.

Please explain what you mean by a Lumbrical plus finger, as well as the quadriga effect that you have mentioned.

- A lumbrical plus position is manifested by an intrinsic plus attitude where attempted flexion of the finger causes paradoxical extension of the IPJs.
  The pathophysiology is a contraction of a long FDP that is transmitted first through the lumbrical muscle, then to the expansion hood of the extensor tendon and lateral band, causing extension of the IPJs.
- The quadriga effect refers to a flexion lag in fingers adjacent to a finger with a shortened FDP tendon, owing to a common muscle belly for the small, ring, and middle FDP, so excursion of the combined tendons is equal to the shortest tendon.

What sized silicone rod would you use?

I will choose a size corresponding to the diameter of the FDP tendon, and that will pass freely through the flexor sheath. Ultimately this will be replaced with a palmaris tendon graft – if present, which is thinner than the original FDP.

What do you mean by patients 'who are unsuitable for a primary tendon repair'?

These are patients with:

1. tendon retraction and shortening – as would be expected if the injury is more than 2 weeks old – except in Leddy and Packer injuries type II and III,

2. segmental tendon loss,
3. local active infection, and
4. failed primary repairs if re-repair is not possible.

What are Leddy and Packer injuries, and why would they affect the acceptable timeline for primary repair?

This refers to a classification of closed FDP tendon avulsion injuries with five types described, based on the level of the tendon end, and the presence of a fracture. The tendon is retracted into the palm in all types except type II and III where they are caught in the pulley system at the level of the PIPJ and DIPJ respectively – preventing the extent of retraction and shortening that would occur otherwise:

- Type I indicates retraction of the FDP tendon to the palm.
- The tendon ends in Types II and III are at the level of the PIPJ and DIPJ respectively, which would allow delayed repair as myostatic shortening does not occur to the same extent.
- Type IV is a double avulsion consisting of a bony fragment and retraction of the tendon into the palm, and
- Type V represents a ruptured tendon with bony comminution.

You mentioned contra-indications for a one-stage tendon reconstruction, what are these?

- an inadequate tendon sheath and pulley system
- an unstable bony skeleton, and
- inadequate skin coverage

What do you mean by an 'inadequate pulley system'?

Any injury to the pulley system that requires reconstruction to prevent tendon bowstringing, such as:

- 25% of A2,
- 75% of A4, and
- 25% of both A2 and A4

What complications will you warn your patient about?

- I will counsel the patient that it will take at least 1 year to complete the reconstruction and rehabilitation, and that this may take even longer if complications occur.
  It is essential for them to sign up from the outset to investment of their time and effort for the duration of the process.
- Complications include:
  - neurovascular injury,
  - infection,
  - implant extrusion or migration,
  - pulley breakdown,
  - rupture of repair,
  - consequences of incorrect tensioning as discussed before (such as lumbrical plus, quadriga effect),
  - skin flap necrosis,
  - adhesions causing flexion contracture, and
  - CRPS.

How would you manage a patient who is unwilling to accept a two-stage reconstruction? What are the alternatives for the patient, if they are unable or unwilling to accept this option?

Options include:

- doing nothing,
- an arthrodesis,

- tenodesis of the distal stump to prevent hyperextension, or
- finally, amputation may be considered in extreme situations in a patient where the digit is interfering with their work or is at high risk of injury.

Where would you obtain the tendon graft for in the second stage?

My options are the following: palmaris longus if present, or plantaris longus, or alternatively the extensor tendons of the toes.

If plantaris is not clear clinically, then I would obtain a preoperative USS.

How will you rehabilitate this patient?

This is variable across different units, but my unit's programme is to:

- start patients on a controlled mobilization programme one week after surgery – with passive flexion and active extension;
- active ROM exercise is started at three weeks, and
- unprotected digital motion is allowed at six weeks.

How would you measure the success or failure of the procedure?

- Apart from objective measures, I will assess for patient subjective measures such as their return to work and hobbies, as well as hand specific PROMs as – ultimately, it is a success if the patient can use it and is satisfied, and a failure if not.
- There is some debate regarding outcome scores following flexor tendon repair, but I will measure:
  - the active and passive range of motion of each joint,
  - the palm-to-pulp distance (which is the distance between the fingertip and the distal palmar crease in maximal flexion),
  - pinch grip (or pulp-to-pulp pinch), and
  - power grip strength of the hand measured using a pinch gauge and hydraulic dynamometer.
    I will ensure measurements of the injured side are compared with the uninjured hand and expressed as a percentage of it.
- The functional results are classified according to the Buck-Gramcko rating. This is a scoring system that scores pulp to pinch distances, the total active flexion, and the extension deficit.
- Hand specific PROMs include:
  - the functional impact on the patient's hand function using the DASH and MHQ scoring systems and
  - patient reported psychological sequelae and quality of life, e.g., using the HADS scoring system.

This is discussed further in Case 1.7

Case 1.12

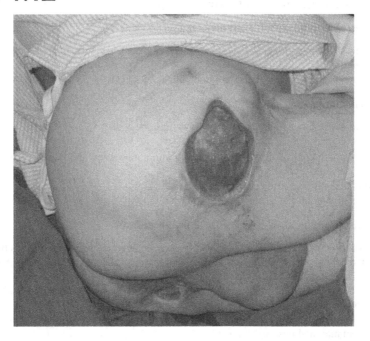

Please describe this photograph.

This shows a right trochanteric pressure sore and left ischial pressure sore.

It is difficult to comment with certainty on the base of the wounds in a black and white photograph, but both appear to be clean.

The base of the wound appears to be covered with granulation tissue, which would suggest chronicity.

I also note scars around the trochanteric sore which extend on to the anterior aspect of the left thigh, which may or may not represent a previous attempt to reconstruct the pressure sore.

In addition, the trochanteric sore is not centred on the trochanter – but lying on the posterior aspect of this, which suggests to me that there is poor-seated posture.

What is the pathophysiology of chronic wounds?

- These are wounds that fail to progress through the linear and overlapping phases of acute wound healing. Some areas of the wounds may be stuck in different phases and the cells are phenotypically altered.
- The pro-inflammatory environment promotes matrix metalloproteinases (MMPs), which suppress cell proliferation and angiogenesis, as well as increase the degradation of the extracellular matrix.
- The most common clinical examples are pressure ulcers – such as in this patient, venous ulcers, and diabetic ulcers.
- The pathophysiology includes a 'unifying hypothesis of chronic wound pathogenesis' based on causative factors which include:
  1. local tissue hypoxia,
  2. pressure-induced repetitive ischaemia-reperfusion injury (for e.g., in chronic ulcers with altering levels of local hypoxia as the pressure is varied on or off the area),
  3. bacterial colonization of the wound,
  4. an altered cellular and systemic stress response in the aged or immunosuppressed patient, and
  5. local wound radiation, chronic stress, and prolonged cytokine exposure leading fibroblasts to lose their proliferative potential, and for keratinocytes at the periphery to lose their ability to migrate as they become unresponsive to activation signals.

    DOI: 10.1201/9780429399268-13

You've mentioned MMPs. What are these?

MMPs are a family of zinc-dependent endopeptidases secreted as inactive zymogens capable of degrading virtually all extracellular components and basement membrane proteins at neutral pH.

So how does bacterial colonization contribute to chronic wounds?

The host immune response to bacteria is inflammation with the release of proteases and oxidants from leucocytes, which degrades cytokines and the ECM.

You mentioned the ischaemia-reperfusion injury. What is its pathophysiology?

- This is the same process that leads to the no-reflow phenomenon that is responsible for the failed salvage of flaps, despite restoration of adequate blood flow.
- In the setting of chronic wounds, these events occur in multiple cycles resulting in eventual tissue necrosis.
- The pathophysiology is thought to be due to:
  - ischaemia-induced endothelial cell swelling and membrane disruption, with
  - reperfusion-induced overproduction of reactive oxygen species, and
  - activation of the inflammatory cascade with platelet aggregation.

You mentioned the cellular stress response in the aged. Please tell me about that.

Fibroblasts in the aged have a higher expression of stress response genes than those of the young, and they fail to upregulate or proliferate under hypoxic conditions. In addition, TGF-Beta is less effective at inhibiting the production of MMPs in aged cells.

So, how will you manage this patient?

- I will take a focused history to identify:
  - any precipitating causes, with extrinsic or intrinsic etiological factors,
  - the nutritional status of the patient,
  - any comorbidities,
  - intercurrent infections,
  - social circumstances, and
  - any previous treatments including surgery undergone to manage these.
- My examination will focus on the:
  - pressure sores with evaluation of:
    - the depth – according to the National Pressure Ulcer Advisory Panel Stage, and
    - the presence of infective or necrotic tissue, which doesn't appear to be the case here
  - the health of other pressure points and any other areas at risk, and
  - possible donor sites if surgery is contemplated.
- My management is primarily non-surgical in the first instance with involvement of other members of the MDT – as required – to:
  - address any reversible causes,
  - optimize risk factors – including nutrition,
  - ensure pressure relief – with pressure mapping and pressure-relieving devices, and
  - ensure bedside excision of any necrotic tissue.
- Pressure sores have a high recurrence rate so I will reserve surgery for those who are fit for surgery and in whom non-operative management has failed despite patient compliance.
- If surgery is contemplated, I will ensure that any procedure does not burn any future reconstructive bridges.

Why not operate as a first option?

I expect the wounds to heal in an optimized patient – except in patients with stable neurological problems. If a patient is not optimized, then the surgical wound would breakdown anyway.

Can you expand on the staging classification you mentioned earlier?

The National Pressure Ulcer Advisory Panel Stages are classified into stage I–IV based on the depth of injury: from stage I representing non-blanching erythema of intact skin to stage IV representing full-thickness tissue loss down to muscle and deeper structures.

In addition, there are two additional stages: 'unstageable' – if the base is obscured by eschar or slough, and 'suspected deep tissue injury of unknown depth' if the skin is intact, with suspected deep tissue injury.

Can you tell me about the extrinsic and intrinsic causal factors you mentioned before?

- Extrinsic factors are external forces on the skin, such as:
  - shearing forces,
  - pressure, and
  - friction.
- These are exacerbated by intrinsic predisposing patient factors that are either:
  - systemic: such as sensory loss, Diabetes, extremes of age, peripheral vascular disease, and malnutrition, or
  - local: such as incontinence, skin maceration, local infection, and joint contraction.

How would you address these factors as part of your non-surgical management?

- Shearing forces are mechanical stresses parallel to a plane acting in opposite directions, e.g., the superficial and deep fascia being pulled in different directions, causing ischaemia by distorting the perforator vessels.

  This can be prevented by ensuring correct patient transfer methods.
- Pressure produces ischaemia by compressing vessels, with pressure twice that of capillary arterial pressure for 2 hours resulting in irreversible ischaemia in animal models.

  So I will ensure an immobile patient is turned every 2 hours, and pressure dispersion techniques are used, such as:
  - foam padding of bony prominences,
  - the use of alternating air cell mattresses, and
  - addressing any spastic joint contractures.
- Friction is caused by the rubbing of the skin against another surface such as bed sheets. It won't cause a pressure ulcer in itself, but will damage the skin and may act synergistically with pressure and shearing forces to create the sore. This can be prevented by correct patient transfer and skin care such as:
  - minimizing moisture and
  - managing any incontinence – with consideration of urinary or faecal diversion.

Other measures include:

- Other measures include the identification and management of malnutrition including micronutrients such as:
  - albumin,
  - Hb level,
  - Vitamins A, C, and
  - Zinc.

Tell me – what are your thoughts on negative pressure therapy in this scenario. Would you use it here to temporize the wounds?

No, I wouldn't unless a partner or carer is comfortable applying it and changing the dressings – particularly if frequent changes may be necessary to manage the volume of exudate.

Whilst it does encourage healing of a clean wound, its long-term use is generally impractical in the community – with recurrent loss of vacuum and a reliance on an overworked and increasingly scarce community nursing team – so it is a less effective option than more conventional dressings.

In addition, it may create a pressure point if the patient lies on the tube.

Let's return to the patient in the picture. He has had a spinal injury and you've addressed all these factors – how will you manage the wounds themselves?

- The wounds appear to be free of eschar and slough, but despite that, I expect the granulation tissue to be contaminated.

- Given the scar on the right thigh, I will request:
  - the details of previous operative procedures as that may affect my surgical options, as well as
  - plain radiographs to delineate the bony anatomy involved such as subluxed or dislocated hip joints, or a previous Girdlestone procedure that may explain the slightly odd location of the trochanteric pressure sore, and
  - an MRI and CT if there is concern of more extensive bone involvement: with an MRI to identify signs of osteomyelitis and CT for any signs of bone destruction
- My general surgical plan will consist of:
  - soft tissue and/or bony excision of the granulation tissue including surrounding scar and any necrotic bone, and
  - reconstruction that is aimed at:
    - managing the dead space, and
    - addressing the skin defect, without undue tension, whilst displacing the scar from bony prominences.

As is best practice, I will choose a flap with geometry that allows further advancement or rotation to manage any future recurrence.

- My intraoperative considerations include:
  - patient positioning on the operating table, and
  - their subsequent rehabilitation position whilst healing, so I will avoid turning the patient where possible, especially onto the operated wound.

I prefer to address one pressure sore at a time and will start with addressing the larger of the two, unless the patient prefers to start with the other one – if particularly problematic.

- Staging the surgery will facilitate rehabilitation and reduce the burden of recovery from the surgical insult. An incidental benefit may even be that the smaller of the two wounds may even heal spontaneously during the post-operative period as the inflammatory burden is decreased.
- So in this case, I will start with the trochanteric pressure sore if the patient agrees by planning a reconstruction with a rotation flap based on the hamstring perforators.

  A TFL rotation advancement flap is another option – but I am concerned that this flap may be compromised or may have been previously used given the location of the overlying scar.
- Once this is healed, then I will address the ischial sore.
  - I prefer to use a buttock rotation flap – planned as large as possible to allow re-rotation if required in the future.
  - The other option is a medially based posterior thigh V-Y advancement rotation flap; however, these can retract with resultant wound dehiscence, and the scar is close to the ischium with the potential for further breakdown.

How would you plan a buttock rotation flap if you needed to?

1. I will first plan the donor site in the area with the most skin laxity available.
2. Next, I will Doppler the IGAP or SGAP perforators that I will include in the flap.
3. I will triangulate the defect, with an ideal apex angle of 30 degrees – but ensure the triangulated area is exaggerated to intentionally displace the scar further from the ischium to try and reduce the risk of recurrence.
4. I will plan as big a flap as is possible with the radius of the semicircle at least equal to 3× the side of the triangle, and a circumference at least 5–8× the side of the triangle. My pivot point is the perforator cluster for either the IGAP or SGAP perforators.
5. Further advancement rotation can be gained with a back cut if needed, as this transfers the pivot point towards the defect, with the understanding that it does decrease the blood supply to the flap.

Let's change the scenario – how would you manage a medically fit patient with a temporary cause of immobility – such as a head injury and deep structure exposure?

The intensivists tell you that the patient is optimized, and they are keen for you to operate to expedite their rehabilitation.

This may be open to debate. There is no indication to rush to operate as I hope the wounds will heal as the patient recovers and they start to mobilize. I will only intervene if the wound healing plateaus.

FURTHER READING

1. Huang C, Leavitt T, Bayer LR, Orgill DP. Effect of negative pressure wound therapy on wound healing. Curr Prob Surg. 2014;51(7):301–331.
2. National Pressure Ulcers Advisory Panel. (2014). New 2014 Prevention and Treatment of Pressure Ulcers: Clinical Practice Guideline.
3. Ahuja RB. Mechanics of movement for rotation flaps and a local flap template. Plast Reconstr Surg. 1989 Apr;83(4):733–737.

Case 1.13

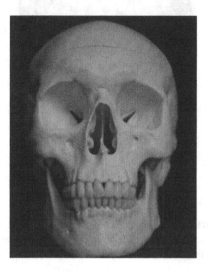

What are Lefort fractures? Please draw the fracture lines for me on this skull illustrations below and talk me through them.

Lefort described three classic patterns of maxillary fractures, which are a useful way to think of them, even if real-life injuries result in a mixture of these patterns, which are frequently asymmetrical.

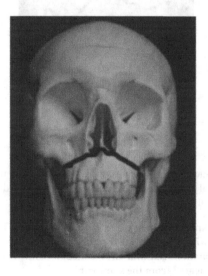

A Lefort I fracture separates the tooth-bearing maxilla from the midface and results in a clinically mobile upper alveolus.

It extends from the pyriform aperture through the nasal septum, lateral nasal walls, and anterior maxillary wall, then continues through the maxillary tuberosity and pterygoid plates.

DOI: 10.1201/9780429399268-14

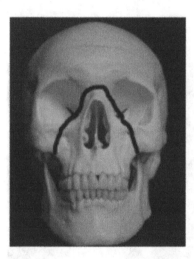

A Lefort II fracture is a pyramidal fracture that results in a mobile central midface. It extends through the frontonasal junction along the medial orbital wall, usually passing through the inferior orbital rim at the ZM suture and continues posteriorly through the tuberosity or pterygoid plates.

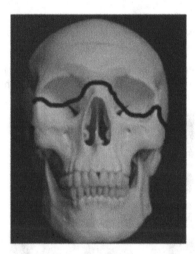

A Lefort III fracture is a craniofacial disjunction resulting in a completely mobile midface and lower orbit. It extends through the frontonasal junction along the medial orbital wall and inferior orbital fissure and then out through the lateral orbital wall.

The Emergency Room consultant calls you as there has been a major RTA involving multiple vehicles: they are expecting a patient with a pan-facial fracture, who has had to be extricated from a car. They inform you that your maxillofacial and ENT colleagues will manage the other more injured passengers that have been extricated from the same car.

Please tell me – What are your thoughts on the way there?

As with all trauma patients, I will assess and manage this patient according to ATLS principles, and I will organize my thoughts according to the most pressing possible emergencies – given the limited history:

- The mechanism of injury leads me to presume the patient has a cervical spine injury – until proven otherwise, particularly as there are more injured passengers in the same vehicle: so, I will immobilize the C-spine until any injury is clinically and radiologically excluded, whilst managing the airway.

- The airway may be compromised by:
  - retrodisplacement of the tongue with a mandibular fracture,
  - a retro-displaced midfacial fracture,
  - massive haemorrhage or oedema, or
  - foreign bodies such as dentition.

Suctioning will help visualization.

- As I am concerned regarding the C-spine, I will not manage this patient sat up until the C-spine injury is clear. Until such time, I will manage any airway obstruction with progressively more invasive manoeuvres such as:
  - a jaw thrust,
  - guedel airway,
  - an endotracheal intubation performed by my anaesthetic colleague, or
  - a surgical airway if this fails.

I will not attempt to disimpact a midface fracture, as this may precipitate bleeding – unless the bleeding appears to be coming from the maxilla – in which case manual reduction may stem an acute haemorrhage.

In addition, I will not use a nasopharyngeal airway as they may have a cribriform plate fracture.

- I may need to deal with facial haemorrhage, and it is important to cross-match early.
  This may be from:
  - superficial vessels – such as facial or temporal artery branches, or
  - deeper vessels such as branches of the maxillary artery.
    - Superficial vessels may be managed with direct pressure and ligation.
    - Deeper bleeding will need tamponade, which can be achieved with packing the nose and/or the mouth with due consideration not to further displace midfacial fractures.
    - If the patient has a C-spine collar on, the midface may be braced with bite blocks between the maxilla and mandible, the latter of which is supported on the collar.
    - If bleeding cannot be controlled through these measures, I will consider immediate transfer to theatre, and potential ligation of the external carotid artery.
- I will also be concerned regarding a neurologic injury as head injuries are frequently associated with significant facial trauma.
  - On that note, I will pay particular attention that hypoxia, hypercarbia, and hypotension are minimized to avoid a possible secondary neurologic injury by maintaining an appropriate cerebral perfusion pressure.

You've mentioned a surgical airway – Please tell me what you mean by that.

The quickest method of obtaining a surgical airway is a cricothyroidotomy. Definitive airway management may require a formal tracheostomy, but this should not be considered a first-line emergency procedure as it is time consuming and may delay securing a definitive airway.

What do you mean by a definitive airway?

This is a cuffed tube which may be inserted nasally, orally, or via the neck in a tracheostomy. The cuff stops anything else except gases, such as oxygen, from entering the lungs.

How would you perform a surgical cricothyroidotomy in this trauma patient?

1. In a supine patient with C-spine immobilization, I will ideally use a prepackaged cricothyroidotomy kit.
2. I will palpate for the inferior thyroid notch and cricoid cartilages to locate the cricothyroid membrane.
3. I will then insert the wide bore needle that is provided and aspirate air into a saline-filled syringe.
4. I will use a Seldinger technique with a dilator to widen the access and insert the airway,
5. before finally securing the cuffed tube.

Alternatively, if a pack is not available:

1. I will perform a transverse skin incision over the cricothyroid membrane and then through the membrane,

2. I will use a dilator to widen the stoma, and then
3. insert a cuffed tube.

You arrive in the ER, and they have already completed the primary survey. What next?

- I will complete the secondary survey to identify any craniofacial trauma that was not identified in the primary survey.
- I will take a focused history from the patient-if conscious or from witnesses, to elucidate:
  - their past medical history with medication and allergies,
  - confirm the mechanism of injury,
  - the timing of it,
  - any loss of consciousness, and
  - any symptoms – specifically from the top of the head and working my way down.
- I will inspect and palpate for soft tissue and bony injuries starting on the scalp, paying particular attention to injuries that may be obscured by hair.
- Moving down to the upper, middle, and lower face – I will look for:
  - lacerations,
  - a haematoma,
  - contour deformities, and
  - bony steps – specifically the contours of the orbit, nose, zygoma, and mandible, followed by
  - assessment of the stability of the midface and mandible to clinically demonstrate fractures, which may be indicated by new malocclusion or limited mouth opening.
    - midfacial instability is identified by holding the anterior maxilla between my thumb and forefinger and applying gentle pressure and palpating for movement at the nose, infraorbital rim, and ZF sutures
    - mandibular instability is identified by flexing the left and the right sides of the mandible.
  - Loose or absent teeth may indicate dentoalveolar injury
  - Rhinorrhoea may signal a possible base of skull fracture
- Next, I will perform a neurological assessment of the face – in a conscious patient to examine their trigeminal and facial nerve function – and
- an ear examination to assess for gross hearing loss – in a conscious patient – and observe for other indicators of a base of skull fracture such as:
  - mastoid bruising,
  - bleeding or otorrhea within the external auditory canal, or
  - rupture of the tympanic membrane.
- I will perform an eye examination, with assessment of:
  - subconjunctival haemorrhage, as an indication of midfacial fracture,
  - position of the eye – with proptosis, enophthalmos, hypoglobus, and telecanthus indicating possible periorbital fractures,
  - pain,
  - acuity,
  - ocular mobility – specifically unilateral restriction of movement or diplopia as possible indications for orbital floor fracture,
  - pupil responses, and
  - periocular structures (including the lids, ducts, and glands).
    I will involve my ophthalmology colleague for further assessment if any globe injuries are demonstrated.
- I will also ensure the patient has a trauma series with a CT head and facial bones specifically to evaluate for any facial fractures.

The patient is intubated and the CT scan demonstrates a mandibular condylar neck fracture, a Lefort II fracture, and a retrobulbar haemorrhage.

How would you manage the retrobulbar haemorrhage?

This is a sight-threatening emergency.

I will call my Ophthalmology colleague for support but in the meantime, I will perform an emergency lateral canthotomy and cantholysis, which is a bedside release of the inferior crus of the lateral canthal ligament to decompress the orbital nerve.

Mannitol and Acetazolamide may be used to support the surgical decompression.

How will you perform the lateral canthotomy and cantholysis?

1. I will first identify the lateral canthus. There is no need for LA in an intubated patient.
2. I will crush the lateral canthus with artery forceps for 1–2 minutes to reduce incisional bleeding, then, cut through the crushed tissue with tenotomy scissors to perform the canthotomy.
3. I will then pull the lower eyelid away from the globe with straight artery forceps.
4. Next, I will 'strum' the tissue under the canthotomy with the scissors to identify the inferior crus of the lateral canthal ligament and divide it with tenotomy scissors. This will feel like a 'band under tension' prior to division.

Are you aware of the principles of Lefort fracture management?

This is managed with an ORIF with miniplate fixation. Surgical approaches to the midfacial skeleton include:

- a transoral approach,
- a lower eyelid approach: which may be subciliary, midtarsal, as well as transconjunctival,
- an upper blepharoplasty approach to the lateral orbit and ZF suture, or
- a coronal flap approach.

You notice the patient has a persistent clear nasal discharge whilst you assess them. How do you proceed?

- I am concerned regarding CSF rhinorrhoea – especially if it doesn't appear to clot or dry. This may occur with a base of skull fracture with a dural tear.
- I will investigate this with:
  - a Ring test at the bedside,
  - a Beta transferrin test, and
  - an MRI with contrast.
- I will involve my neurosurgical colleagues early, and specifically check the CT for involvement of the anterior and posterior tables as well as a pneumocephalus, with the understanding that it cannot exclude a nasofrontal ductal injury.
- The treatment algorithm is based on:
  - involvement of the anterior and posterior table,
  - confirmed presence of a CSF leak, and
  - the likelihood of ductal obstruction.
- Minimally displaced fractures of the frontal sinus may be managed conservatively.
- Displaced anterior table fractures may be managed conservatively or have surgical intervention, as this will primarily result in an aesthetic deformity with limited functional implications.
- Displaced posterior table fractures should be managed surgically in conjunction with a neurosurgeon and may include cranialization of the sinus to prevent an intracranial mucocele.

You've mentioned the Ring test. What is this?

- This is a bedside test to quickly identify suspected CSF.
- One drop of blood and one drop of the fluid are placed simultaneously on filter paper. The blood coalesces in the centre, leaving an outer ring of CSF.
- This is reliable for detecting CSF but it is not exclusive, so needs to be confirmed with a β-2-transferrin test, which is a carbohydrate-free form of transferrin that is almost exclusively found in the CSF.

    It is important to analyze a simultaneous blood sample in parallel with the leakage fluid to avoid the risk of false positives due to genetic variants or excess alcohol use.

Case 1.14

Please draw the brachial plexus and talk me through your understanding of its anatomy

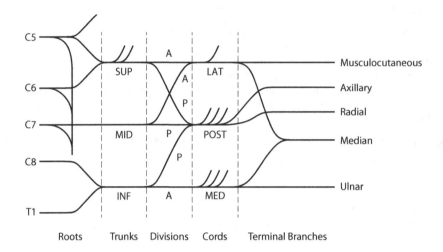

The brachial plexus is a nerve network with motor and sensory components that control the composite function of the upper limb. It consists of spinal roots, trunks, divisions, cords, and terminal branches – with named nerves arising from the roots, trunks, and cords but not the divisions.

As you can see in my diagram:

- The spinal roots most commonly arise from the C5-T1 dorsal and ventral rootlets between the anterior and middle scalene muscles.

  Occasionally, fibres are received from C4 and T2 – with a prefixed plexus including a contribution from C4, and a postfixed plexus including a contribution from T2. The long thoracic nerve arises very proximally from C5/6/7 nerve roots to supply serratus anterior, and the dorsal scapular nerve from C5 root to supply the rhomboids.
- The superior, middle, and inferior trunks are formed from the upper two, middle and lower two roots, respectively. These are located in the posterior triangle of the neck. The nerve to subclavius and the suprascapular nerve (C5/6), which supplies the supra and infraspinatus muscles, both arise from the superior trunk. The trunks then divide deep to the clavicle.
- The lateral cord is lateral to the axillary artery and consists of the anterior divisions of the superior and middle trunks. The lateral pectoral nerve arises here and supplies pectoralis major.
- The medial cord is medial to the axillary artery and consists of the anterior division of the lower trunk. The medial pectoral nerve, the medial brachial cutaneous nerve, and the medial antebrachial cutaneous nerve arise here.
- The posterior cord is posterior to the axillary artery and consists of the posterior divisions of all the trunks. The upper and lower subscapular nerves, and the thoracodorsal nerve-supplying latissimus, arise here.
- The terminal branches consist of the musculocutaneous nerve which arises from the lateral cord, the ulnar nerve arising from the medial cord, and the radial and axillary nerves from the posterior cord. The median nerve has lateral and medial roots arising from the lateral and medial cords, respectively.

DOI: 10.1201/9780429399268-15

Please describe your understanding of peripheral nerve anatomy.

- Neuronal cell bodies have dendrites to receive presynaptic neurotransmitters, and axonal projections that end in axonal terminals. They reside in:
  - the dorsal root ganglia – with regard to sensory spinal nerves, and
  - the ventral spinal cord – with regard to motor spinal nerves.
- Connective tissues surrounding neuronal axons provide a vascularized connective tissue scaffold consisting of:
  - the endoneurium, which encases each individual axon,
  - the perineurium, which encases fascicles, and
  - the epineurium, which encases the nerve proper.
- The vasa nervorum provide nutrient blood supply to the axons. It originates in the epineurium, then branches in the perineurium, and forms a capillary plexus in the endoneurium.
- Myelinated nerves are ensheathed in a layer of myelin – produced by Schwann cells. This limits ionic transfer along the axon to the nodes of Ranvier, enabling saltatory conduction.

You mentioned nerve conduction. How does this occur?

- Action potentials are initiated by the presynaptic release of a neurotransmitter, such as Acetylcholine that increases the permeability of ion channels.
- This changes the electrochemical gradient, which in turn produces a rise in the resting membrane potential of −70 mV, until the threshold potential of −55 mV is reached, and depolarization occurs.
- This activates voltage-gated ion channels allowing an inward flow of sodium or calcium ions – depending on the nerve type, producing a rapid rise in voltage, and causing further sodium or calcium channels to open.
- This reverses the polarity of the plasma membrane, and the ion channels then rapidly inactivate.
- As the sodium channels close, sodium ions can no longer enter the neuron, and they are then actively transported back out of the plasma membrane.
- Potassium channels are then activated, and there is an outward current of potassium ions, returning the electrochemical gradient to the resting state.
- After an action potential has occurred, there is a transient negative shift, called the afterhyperpolarization – during which the nerve cannot be stimulated.

Saltatory conduction allows the action potentials to transmit along the only uninsulated areas along the axon, termed the nodes of Ranvier, to speed transmission from 10 m/s in an unmyelinated nerve to 150 m/s in a myelinated nerve.

What is your general approach to a patient who presents with a brachial plexus injury?

- These patients require a multidisciplinary team long-term approach.
- Broad objectives include:
  1. establishing a diagnosis,
  2. creating a treatment plan,
  3. controlling pain – which is often significant in patients with preganglionic injuries,
  4. ensuring adequate therapy to maintain a passive ROM and prevent contracture, and
  5. ensuring psychological and social support.
- In a patient who is stable from an ATLS point of view, the two points that are crucial to the surgical strategy are:
  - whether an injury is pre or post ganglionic, or a mixture of both, and
  - the anatomical level of the injury.
- The three tools available to help me diagnose the injury are:
  - clinical assessment, supported by
  - radiology and
  - neurophysiology.

However, the definitive extent and severity of the diagnosis of injury can only be established at surgical exploration.

- Once the level and extent of the injury is established intraoperatively, a reconstructive plan is made based on:
  - the remaining intact nerves,
  - the patient's age, and
  - comorbidities.
- Physiotherapy input is vital to maintain and optimize the passive range of joint motion both before and after surgery.
- With regard to my clinical assessment, this consists of:
  1. a focused history,
  2. an examination structured along the 'Look Feel Move' system,
  3. myotome and dermatome testing, and finally,
  4. charting the sensory and motor exam – as graded per the MRC classification, using a number of standard charts available to facilitate this.
- With regard to the history, I will determine:
  - the time interval from injury,
  - the mechanism of injury energy transfer, and associated injuries,
  - the patient's age, handedness, previous injuries, and level of pain,
  - their occupation – if employed, and hobbies, and
  - any comorbidities – if applicable, although most of this population are young and healthy.
- I will structure my examination according to the 'Look Feel Move' approach, and
- I will start by noting:
  - how the limb is held or if it is entirely flail – which would denote a total palsy,
  - any muscle atrophy – which won't be present in the acute phase,
  - the presence of Horner's syndrome – which denotes a preganglionic injury,
  - any bruising or swelling within the posterior triangle, and
  - winging of the scapula – which indicates a proximal injury such as an avulsion injury.
- Next, I will:
  - perform a sensory dermatomal exam: including touch, pain and 2-point discrimination, to determine whether sensory loss is in a root, cord, or individual nerve distribution – followed by
  - a Tinel-Hoffman test within the posterior triangle – with a positive test denoting a post-ganglionic injury and a potentially better prognosis, since that lends itself to nerve grafting.
  - Finally, I will palpate for the peripheral pulses and perform an Allen's test.
- Key muscle tests whilst facing the patients' back include testing for:
  - Trapezius function (supplied by the spinal accessory nerve and C3,4) by asking the patient to shrug their shoulders. This may be a donor nerve or future muscle transfer.
  - Rhomboid function (supplied by the dorsal scapular nerve, C4,5) is tested by asking the patient to push their shoulder blades together. Paralysis indicates a proximal injury such as root avulsion.
  - Serratus anterior function (supplied by the long thoracic nerve, C5,6,7) is tested with the classic 'wall-press' test.
    However, if they are unable to lift their arm then I will ask the patient to push their shoulder forward against resistance as an alternative.
    Winging of the scapula points to a possible preganglionic lesion.
  - Latissimus dorsi function (supplied by the thoracodorsal nerve, C6,7,8) is tested – by supporting the patient's arm in the flexed position and asking them to push down onto my hand, whilst feeling for muscle contraction with the other hand.
    Another way to test this in a patient with a paralysed arm is to palpate the muscle whilst the patient coughs.
  - Deltoid function (supplied by the axillary nerve, C5,6) is tested – by asking the patient to flex, abduct and extend their shoulder to test the anterior, middle, and posterior parts.
- Standing from the front, I will test for:
  - The clavicular and sternocostal heads of pectoralis major (supplied by the lateral and medial pectoral nerves, respectively).
    - Clavicular head function (supplied by C5,6) is tested by asking the patient to touch their contralateral shoulder and palpating for evidence of contraction. Atrophy or paralysis may imply a lateral cord injury.

- Sternocostal head function (supplied by C7,8,T1) is tested by asking the patient to push against their hip and palpating the axillary fold. Atrophy or paralysis may imply a medial cord injury.
- Rotator cuff function with Supraspinatus and Infraspinatus (supplied by the suprascapular nerve – C5,6), Teres minor (supplied by the axillary nerve C5,6) and Subscapularis (supplied by the upper and lower subscapular nerves, C5,6,7):
  - Supraspinatus is tested by asking the patient to initiate abduction at the shoulder in the scapular plane with the thumb pointing downwards.
  - Infraspinatus is tested by asking them to flex their elbows and externally rotate their shoulder in adduction against resistance.
  - Teres minor is tested by again asking them to flex their elbows and externally rotate their shoulder, this time in abduction.
  - Finally, Subscapularis is tested by asking them to bring their elbows forward whilst pressing their abdomen. Wrist flexion on the affected side is a positive sign.

What are your indications for surgery?

These include:

1. all high-energy neurological injuries – as their level and extent of injury can only be confirmed intraoperatively,
2. those with a suspicion of avulsion injury,
3. iatrogenic injuries and sharp injuries, and
4. those with a low-velocity injury, such as a shoulder dislocation, in whom there is no clinical or neurophysiological evidence of improvement after serial examinations.

What are your reconstructive goals in a pan-plexus injury?

The two most important goals are:

1. reconstituting elbow flexion – to allow hand to mouth function, and
2. shoulder stabilization – to support power across the elbow.

It is rarely possible to restore complete function to the hand in a significant global plexus injury in adults.

What about your thoughts on the timing of exploration and repair?

- This is somewhat controversial, with differing protocols across the world.
- Most UK centres will advocate for early surgery in high-velocity injuries, as there are basic science and clinical studies to support better outcomes with early surgical intervention in brachial plexus injuries.
- The advantages of early exploration include:
  1. the absence of scar tissue and consequent ease of dissection,
  2. the ability to stimulate distal nerves for accuracy,
  3. earlier timing for nerve regeneration, and
  4. preservation of motor and sensory cells, as emergent repair minimizes sensory and motor neuronal cell death, as well as fibrosis in the distal nerve.
- However, I am aware that proponents of delayed surgery (up to 3–6 months post injury) cite:
  1. more accurate identification of the lesion due to Wallerian degeneration and neuroma formation (in post ganglionic lesions),
  2. a non-contaminated wound, and
  3. reported cases of unexpected recovery with conservative management.
- My own indications include:
  - Urgent surgical exploration – as soon as is safe to do so for those with:
    - open injuries,
    - sharp penetrating trauma,
    - iatrogenic injuries, and
    - those with an expanding hematoma or vascular injury.

  – Early surgery – preferably in the first 2 weeks in:
  ▪ High-velocity injuries,
  ▪ suspicion of avulsion injury, and
  ▪ progressive neurologic deficits.
  – Delayed surgical intervention for up to 6 months may be indicated in patients with:
  ▪ partial upper plexus involvement and low energy mechanism, such as a shoulder dislocation, and
  ▪ a plateau in neurological recovery.

You mentioned preganglionic injuries. What signs would point you to this?

These are clinical, radiological, and neurophysiologic signs– with

- Clinical signs including:
  1. Horner's syndrome,
  2. paralysis of rhomboids,
  3. winging of the scapula,
  4. a phrenic nerve palsy,
  5. severe deafferentation pain,
  6. the absence of a Tinel's sign in the supraclavicular area, and
  7. history of a high-velocity or high-energy injury.
- Radiological signs include:
  1. CXR signs include a raised hemidiaphragm, with possible fractures of first and second ribs.
  2. USS signs may show an immotile diaphragm.
  3. C-spine X-ray signs include fractures of the transverse processes.
  4. MRI signs include:
     – a pseudo meningocele with avulsion of the roots,
     – empty nerve root sleeves,
     – a cord shift away from the midline, and
     – transverse process fractures.

In a purely preganglionic injury, nerve conduction studies will demonstrate persistent sensory conduction within the peripheral nerve with absent motor conduction (unless there is also a co-existent post ganglionic injury, which is often the case).

Let's consider the following scenario: a young man is referred to you with a flail arm after coming off a motorbike at speed. He was a pillion passenger. His initial injuries included a head injury which has been managed conservatively, a fractured clavicle, ipsilateral fractured ribs and a haemopneumothorax, as well as a femoral fracture and a perineal burst injury.

He has been stabilized, has had a chest drain, and an intramedullary nail to his femur. His perineal wound has been temporized and a temporary colostomy performed.

His GCS is now 15. There is no Horner's syndrome.

In addition, you note the motor function of the rhomboids and serratus, but no other function present.

How would you manage his brachial plexus injury?

- This patient has a pan plexus injury which I suspect is highly likely to be preganglionic – bearing in mind the high-energy injury and the fractured clavicle – even in the absence of a Horner's sign.
- I will investigate this with an MRI and USS diaphragm and ensure a complete clinical examination as I described earlier.
- Neurophysiology will not be useful at this early stage.
- After ruling out concurrent life-threatening injury, I will plan for an exploration as soon as possible.
- Surgical options depend on whether there are root avulsions:
  – The mainstays of surgery for a postganglionic injury are nerve grafts.

- – Options for preganglionic injuries include nerve transfers. Typical transfers for upper plexus injuries (to reanimate shoulder and elbow flexors) are:
  - the accessory to suprascapular nerve,
  - a radial triceps branch to the axillary, and
  - a double fascicular transfer for elbow flexion (which consists of transfer of a fascicle of ulnar nerve to biceps and a median nerve fascicular transfer to brachialis).

Other sources of nerve transfer are intercostal nerves, usually used for transfer to the musculocutaneous nerve. However, I would be wary of using these nerves in the presence of a lung injury, phrenic nerve injury, and rib fractures.

If there is a single root intact (usually C5), then this can be used as a source for a graft. In the presence of lower root avulsions, the ulnar nerve can be raised as a source of vascularized graft, either free or pedicled.

Let's consider another scenario: a young man is referred to you with a flail arm after coming off his motorbike at speed a year ago. His initial injuries included a head injury which has been managed conservatively.

You note Horner's sign. In addition, you note the motor function of the rhomboids and serratus but no other function present.

How would you manage his brachial plexus injury?

- This patient has a pan plexus injury which is likely to be preganglionic due to the Horner's sign, the high-energy injury, and the fractured clavicle.
- Investigations will include an MRI, USS diaphragm, neurophysiology, and clinical examination.
- Had this patient presented acutely, I would have managed him with early exploration and reconstruction rather than nerve grafts, as there is evidence of a preganglionic injury. However, at 12 months post injury, salvage procedures are indicated as motor endplates begin to permanently degenerate within weeks of injury. At one year post-injury, nerve surgery would be futile.
- The only option available to reanimate the limb would be introduce new muscle, either free or pedicled.
- My primary goals are to establish:
  - Shoulder stability with a shoulder fusion, given that Serratus is functioning.
  - Elbow flexion may be achieved using a free *Gracilis* powered by the accessory nerve. If this is routed under the mobile wad, it can be attached to finger extensors to allow concurrent finger extension.
- Finger flexion may be achieved by a second *Gracilis* motored by the intercostals (but this may not be possible due to the rib fractures).
- Wrist position may be improved by fusion in due course.

FURTHER READING

1. Menorca RM, Fussell TS, Elfar JC. Nerve physiology: mechanisms of injury and recovery. Hand Clin. 2013;29(3):317–330.
2. Burnett MG, Zager EL. Pathophysiology of peripheral nerve injury: a brief review. Neurosurg Focus. 2004 May 15;16(5):E1. doi: 10.3171/foc.2004.16.5.2. PMID: 15174821.
3. Romero-Ortega M. (2014) Peripheral Nerves, Anatomy and Physiology of. In: Jaeger D, Jung R. (eds) Encyclopedia of Computational Neuroscience. Springer, New York, NY.

VIVA II

Case 2.1

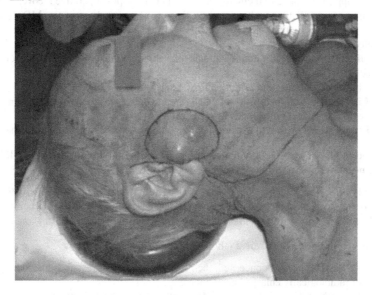

Please describe this photograph

This is an intra-operative photograph of an intubated patient with preauricular subcutaneous swellings and markings consistent with planned excision, as well as a likely parotidectomy and neck dissection.

How would you proceed if this patient presented to you in clinic?

The goals of my clinical assessment are to establish:

1. possible differential diagnoses,
2. the patient's general fitness for treatment, followed by,
3. histological confirmation of the diagnosis, and
4. the presence and extent of any further spread via imaging.
- My differential diagnoses for a preauricular mass include:
  - a primary parotid tumour – which may be benign or malignant,
  - parotid metastases – usually from a skin cancer primary, or
  - rarer causes such as lymphoma.
1. With regard to the differential diagnosis, I will elucidate factors that are suggestive of malignancy with a directed history and examination looking for:
  - rapid progression,
  - pain,
  - duct obstruction, infection, or bleeding, and
  - compression or invasion of surrounding structures with:
    - facial nerve involvement,
    - trismus,
    - ear problems, or
    - dysphagia due to deep lobe involvement.

  I will then clinically exclude skin metastases by enquiring about any past skin cancers within the head and neck, and examining for any new lesions, or scars from previous excisions.
2. Regarding their general fitness for treatment, I will establish:
  - their comorbidities,
  - alcohol and smoking dependency,

DOI: 10.1201/9780429399268-17

  – any anticoagulation or immunosuppressant therapy,
  – exercise tolerance, and
  – social support available to them, to help them plan their post-operative recovery.

     My assessment will be supplemented by that of other members of the MDT such as the
anaesthetist and clinical nurse specialist, and possibly the care of the elderly physician if required,
with frailty scoring – if relevant.

3. Next, I will obtain histological confirmation of the suspected diagnosis with ultrasound-guided
   Fine Needle Aspiration, and then
4. I will establish the presence and extent of any further spread – with:
   – MRI imaging, which is used to establish the local extent of the tumour and any spread to
     locoregional cervical lymph nodes, and
   – a CT chest, which is used to exclude any lung metastases or a synchronous primary tumour.

What would you do if you are strongly concerned regarding a malignant differential, but the FNA comes back as negative?

If I am concerned from a clinical or imaging point of view regarding malignancy, then I will discuss this in an
MDT setting and suggest a repeat biopsy or a core biopsy. There is no test that is 100% accurate, and FNA has
up to a 10% failure rate. This is why the multidisciplinary correlation of findings is of fundamental importance.

The core biopsy comes back as equivocal – how will you proceed?

• If both I or the MDT are still concerned, then I will request an ultrasound-guided biopsy of any
  clinically or radiologically enlarged neck nodes.
• If that is also equivocal, and both I or my MDT colleagues are sufficiently concerned, then I will
  suggest to the MDT that I proceed with a superficial parotidectomy with frozen section control in
  the first instance. I will only continue with any subsequent operative steps, such as a possible total
  parotidectomy and/or neck dissection, if the frozen section is positive for malignancy.

How would you manage the facial nerve – when would you resect it?

My indications for nerve resection are:

1. preoperative radiologically evident invasion of the nerve by tumour, or
2. intraoperative macroscopic nerve involvement.

     Otherwise, I will plan for a nerve-sparing parotidectomy – be it superficial or total – and rely on
radiotherapy to treat any potential microinvasion, as well as 'close tumour margins'.

How do you perform a nerve-sparing parotidectomy?

• This procedure involves a dissection of the parotid tissue and tumour off the facial nerve using a
  facelift incision approach.
• There are two key points that allow me to perform it safely:
  1. the first is to safely locate the facial nerve using antegrade and retrograde approaches, and
  2. the second is to maintain excellent haemostasis throughout the procedure, as a bloody field
     will increase the inadvertent injury to the nerve branches. This is achieved with dissection
     of the nerve branches with Mosquito forceps and low-setting bipolar cautery of the parotid
     tissue above it – preferably by my assistant for maximized time efficiency.
• With regard to safely identifying the facial nerve, I will first ask my anaesthetic colleague to
  ensure that muscle relaxation is avoided completely, or at least limited to one bolus on induction,
  as the use of a nerve stimulator may be required.
• To find the nerve, my preferred method is to use an antegrade approach, but if this proves to be
  difficult – for example, if there is a large, fixed tumour or if this is in a radio-recurrent field, then
  I will use a retrograde approach or a combination 'siege' approach.
• There are three anatomical landmarks that have been described in the antegrade approach:
  – the tragal pointer,
  – the tympanomastoid suture, and
  – the styloid process.

I prefer to use a combination of the cartilaginous tragal pointer, and the tympanomastoid suture. The tragal pointer is encountered first as it is more superficial. I expect to find the nerve about 1.5 cm deep to this point; however, this is not entirely accurate as the cartilage is mobile, so I supplement the approach with the tympanomastoid suture. This is a palpable ridge located 4–5 mm above the nerve – with the advantage of being fixed. Lastly, another option would be to follow the posterior belly of digastric back to the styloid process, with the nerve located antero-inferior to this.

- The retrograde approach consists of following any of the distal branches back to the main trunk. The more easily identified branches are the buccal branches and the marginal mandibular nerve, which may have more than one branch.
  - The buccal branches are located alongside the parotid duct, which itself is located along a line connecting the intertragal notch and a point midway between the upper lip and alar base. Locating the duct may be aided by cannulation from inside the mouth, with the orifice opposite the second upper molar, but this is rarely necessary except in trauma cases.
  - The marginal mandibular branch (or branches if more than one) is most easily found as it runs superficial to the facial vessels just below or along the lower border of the mandible.

You mentioned nerve stimulators. Do you use one to locate the nerve?

- This is a controversial topic.
- I routinely use the stimulator in the instance of recurrent disease as I expect tissue planes to be altered. With regard to primary cases, I would reserve the use of the stimulator if I were in any doubt.
  This is because:
  - there is a false positive and false negative risk with its use – although the figures for these have not been quantified exactly in the literature, and
  - there is no evidence to show that its use decreases facial nerve injuries.
    However, I recognize that proponents cite the possibility of increased medicolegal protection in the event of an injury, especially in other countries.

You see this man in clinic 6 months following a superficial parotidectomy and neck dissection, and he mentions that he has developed copious 'sweating' from his cheek when he eats. He remembers you mentioning this risk pre-operatively. How do you manage him?

- His symptoms are consistent with that of Frey's syndrome, which is due to the aberrant regeneration of severed parasympathetic fibres between the otic ganglion and the skin. I will treat this with chemodenervation, which is successful in controlling symptoms in the vast majority of cases.
- In the rare event that it is not, surgical options consist of lipofilling, the interposition of dermal grafts, or a superficial temporoparietal fascia transfer.

Let's consider another scenario: the patient's facial nerve is infiltrated on preoperative imaging and is planned for a radical parotidectomy. How would you manage this?

- This patient will likely require adjuvant radiotherapy, so I will plan to offer concomitant reanimation prior to this – to avoid the high risk of wound healing problems if I were to operate in an irradiated field. In addition, my choice of reanimation should withstand radiotherapy, so I personally prefer to avoid nerve-based options, although I appreciate that this is contested.
- My preference is to offer a Labbe temporalis myoplasty as it achieves immediate postoperative movement – albeit with an initial 'mandibular' smile (where the patient must clench their teeth to achieve this).
- However, I will warn the patient of the drawbacks, including:
  - a less predictable excursion of movement,
  - the need for rehabilitation to eventually transform an initial 'mandibular' smile to a 'voluntary' smile (without the need for teeth clenching), and
  - the likelihood of some radiotherapy-induced fibrosis of the temporalis tendon, but this can usually be managed with stretching as part of their facial therapy.

- The alternative is a nerve-based procedure such as:
  - a cable graft if the facial nerve stump is available, or
  - nerve transfers – such as a nerve to masseter transfer,
      with the potential for the addition of an overlying protective flap such as an ALT, to theoretically reduce the effect of radiation damage.
- The disadvantage of these options is a longer wait for neurotization and return of movement, which may be delayed even further with radiotherapy.
- Regarding the cable grafting option, potential donors include the sural nerve or the saphenous nerve, amongst others. These may or may not be vascularized, with the theory that vascularized grafts may better withstand the effects of radiotherapy, but there is no strong evidence for this.
- The resultant lagophthalmos is managed with an upper eyelid platinum chain weight.

Please talk me through a Labbe temporalis myoplasty

- This is a lengthening temporalis myoplasty based on a temporalis tendon transfer from the coronoid process to the nasolabial fold without an interpositional graft, by relying on anterior rotation of the muscle to achieve the required lengthening effect and resulting reproduction of upper lip and modiolus movement on contraction of the muscle.
  1. A zigzag approach to the temporal fossa is used to expose the temporalis muscle.
  2. The temporalis is then mobilized with a 1 cm strip of aponeurosis left on the temporal crest and then freed from the masseter.
  3. A coronoidectomy is performed to safely transfer the temporalis tendon insertion to the nasolabial fold without damaging it.
      Access for this was originally described via a zygomatic osteotomy, but this was since revised with an approach via the nasolabial fold, which avoids the morbidity of an osteotomy. An intraoral approach is a third option.
  4. The tendon is then delivered to the nasolabial fold, where it is unfurled and sutured to reproduce a smile type that is symmetrical to the contralateral side.
  5. The original strip on the temporal crest is now used to receive the sutures for reinsertion of the muscle origin, with appropriate tensioning.

How do you locate the nerve to masseter intraoperatively?

Answered in Case 3.16

FURTHER READING

1. Guerreschi P, Labbe D. Lengthening temporalis myoplasty: a surgical tool for dynamic labial commissure reanimation. Facial Plast Surg. 2015 Apr;31(2):123–127.
2. Kimata Y, Sakuraba M, Hishinuma S, Ebihara S, Hayashi R, Asakage T. Free vascularized nerve grafting for immediate facial nerve reconstruction. Laryngoscope. 2005 Feb;115(2):331–336.

Case 2.2

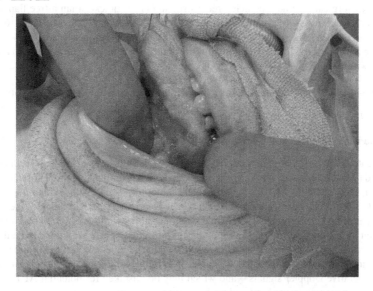

This patient presented to the Head and Neck service with an ulcerative lesion on the lateral and ventral aspect of his tongue that has been preoperatively staged as a T2 N1 M0 SCC. Your resective maxillofacial colleague discusses resection and a neck dissection with him. How will you reconstruct this?

- In a patient who is fit for a free flap reconstruction, then I will opt for thin flaps to maximize the functional result, such as:
  - a RFFF if his modified Allen's test is normal, as the tissue is very thin, or
  - a thin ALT if he has adequate perforators – as it provides thin pliable tissue with a good donor site.
- If he is not a candidate for a free flap, then I will discuss a pedicled pectoralis major transfer.

You mentioned a patient being a poor candidate for a free flap. What do you mean by that?

This refers to:

- severe patient comorbidity with unacceptably high risk of general anaesthestic and post-operative complications,
- a coagulopathy which cannot be optimized preoperatively,
- severe peripheral vascular disease,
- the unavailability of donor sites, or
- the unavailability of adequate recipient vessels.

What are the disadvantages of a pectoralis major flap? Why isn't this your first choice – and why would you subject the patient to a potentially longer procedure with a free flap anyway?

A pedicled pectoralis major flap is not my first choice due to:

- the mechanical effect of the weight of the flap,
- the chest donor site morbidity – with an increased risk of atelectasis and post-operative pneumonia – especially in the elderly and those with pre-existing chest comorbidities, and
- the unsightliness of the muscle bulk at the level of the clavicle and neck.

DOI: 10.1201/9780429399268-18

- In addition, it is important to save this flap as a 'life-boat' for possible future recurrences, as the patient's general medical health may deteriorate such that that they are no longer fit for a free flap.

With regard to surgical timing, a pedicled reconstruction is not quicker than a free flap as concurrent raising of the pedicled flap is not possible during the resection – so in fact – the time taken to raise the flap is at least equal to, or even longer, than the time taken for a routine micro-anastomosis.

However, the advantage is a lower risk of flap failure and consequent need for a return to theatre for flap re-exploration, with its additional GA risks.

What about the use of a local submental flap? You didn't mention that as a pedicled option.

No. This is not an option here, as it is not oncologically safe to do so.

How would you raise an ALT?

- I will locate the perforators preoperatively using a pencil Doppler, starting halfway between the ASIS and lateral patella, and moving proximally and distally until adequate perforator signals are identified. If there are no ALT perforators, then I prefer to proceed with another flap rather than use the TFL – which is the traditional ALT lifeboat, as it is bulkier than I would like, especially for the ventral part of the reconstruction and floor of mouth – with likely functional implications.
- I will then follow the perforator via a septal or intramuscular course until the descending branch of the lateral femoral circumflex vessels are followed back to the femoral artery and vein.
- I will am aware that small subcutaneous vessels in extremely thin patients may give misleadingly high preoperative Doppler signals – and which may be mistaken for potential ALT perforators. This is not uncommon in the head and neck cancer population.
- If unsure in such a patient, I will 'save a RFFF' by asking the anaesthetist to keep a forearm free of IV and arterial lines, for a potential RFFF if the ALT was not suitable.

And what about a radial forearm flap?

- I will first perform a preoperative modified Allen test to check the patency of the palmar arch, the radial and ulnar arteries, and will only proceed with a RFFF if this is normal.
- This can be raised supra – or subfascially – but I prefer to use a subfascial approach as it is quicker and easier to teach my junior colleagues. Also, I have found that the supplementation of Matriderm to the SSG reconstruction of the donor site has virtually eliminated the complication of tendon exposure – which used to be the main disadvantage of subfascial dissections.
- I start the dissection under tourniquet control, from ulnar to radial until palmaris or the median nerve is encountered – in the absence of a palmaris tendon.
- Then, the flap is raised from the radial side: the cephalic vein is dissected and included in the flap, the superficial radial nerve branches are protected, and the radial artery and commitantes are dissected from distal to proximal.
- The tourniquet is then deflated once the dissection of the radial artery at the level of the wrist is completed.
- The radial artery is followed until its origin, and the venous commitantes and cephalic vein are then followed to the confluence of the superficial and venous systems to avoid two venous anastomoses. In the small number of cases where they don't meet, then two venous anastomoses are unavoidable.
- Donor site closure options other than a SSG and Matriderm include:
  - a FTSG, or
  - a local flap closure such as a Y-V or Hatchet flap – if laxity of tissues allows.

What are your preferred recipient vessels in the neck?

- The facial artery is my preferred recipient artery, as it usually has the largest calibre of the external carotid branches that are easily accessible.
- If not, then other options include:
  - the superior thyroid,
  - the lingual artery – which I will refrain from using until other options are exhausted – unless it is divided anyway as part of the resection,
  - the occipital artery, and

- the transverse cervical artery, if the pedicle length allows this.
- The last option is the external carotid artery, as a last resort if its branches are not suitable or available.
- With regard to the vein, I prefer to use a venous coupler to the base of the common facial vein. By dividing it a couple of millimetres from the IJV, an end-to-side set up is created without the need for a venotomy. The advantage being that the IJV has a high suction pressure with minimization of venous stasis and thrombosis, as well as minimizing any possible kinking or twisting of the recipient vein. If this is not available, then I will explore other IJV tributaries or perform a 'true' end-to-side anastomosis on to the IJV with a venotomy.

You mentioned that you would aim to avoid using the lingual artery – where possible if it hasn't been divided as part of the resection. Why is that?

- The left and right lingual arteries are the main blood supply to the tongue.
- Using this as a first-line recipient vessel would put the tongue vascularity at risk if both sides were used (e.g., with eventual bilateral head and neck flaps), or if one is used for a flap and the other side is divided as part of a subsequent resection.
- Therefore, I would reserve its use unless all other options are exhausted.
- If the lingual artery is ligated as part of the resection, then the proximal stump becomes my second-line option if the facial artery is not available, as it is usually of good size.

How will you apply the coupler in an end-to-side anastomosis onto the IJV?

My first key steps are to ensure the venotomy edges are everted at 12 and 6 o'clock in the first instance, as these are the two key areas that will be most under tension if left until the end, and at risk of a 'leak' with an end-to-side anastomosis.

Once these are secure, the rest of the coupler insertion is routine.

Is there any situation where you wouldn't use a coupler?

Yes, in the case of extreme vessel size mismatch (more than 2 mm), then I would hand sew the venous anastomosis, but this is uncommon.

What would you do if the facial artery is the most suitable recipient artery in terms of vessel size match, but the stump – left at the end of the neck dissection was too short, and barely visible under digastric to comfortably perform your anastomosis?

Delivering the facial artery stump from under the digastric tendon and retracting the tendon itself upwards with self-retaining hooks such as 'Fishhooks', adds a couple of centimetres in length and usually solves this issue. This usually requires the micro-ligation and division of small branches.

If that is still too short, then I would first consider other recipient vessels, followed by the option of division of the digastric tendon itself, which would add almost a centimetre of exposed facial artery.

How do you safely transport the flap pedicle from the oral cavity into the neck?

1. I will create a tunnel to comfortably pass the largest Hegar dilator between the defect and the neck. I then double check that I can comfortably pass at least two of my digits, and
2. then pass a large Penrose drain in this tunnel and clamp the distal aspect in the neck.
3. Next, I will fill the drain with normal saline before feeding the pedicle vessels into it, whilst ensuring it is not twisting on insertion by observing for Bonney's blue marks that are applied prior to flap division.
4. Finally, I will ask my assistant to withdraw the drain gently in the neck until the vessels are seen and delivered safely, and I will check they are not twisted.

   I am also aware of an alternative method where a large saline-filled liposuction tube is used on gentle suction.

The ALT and radial forearm flaps are not available to you: what other options do you have?

The reconstruction requires a thin flap to contour adequately in the floor of mouth so other options include an MSAP flap – if it is thin –or a Serratus free flap.

What about the neck dissection – what are your indications for neck dissections in general?

The purpose of a neck dissection is to control regional spread, so each case is judged on an individual basis and an MDT plan is made, but my general indications include:

1. established nodal disease (be it clinical or radiological),
2. those at risk of occult nodal metastasis (>T2 tumours),
3. those requiring a free flap reconstruction (so an 'access neck dissection' is performed), and
4. patients where nodal surveillance is predicted to be difficult (such as those with a thick neck) or adequate follow up is impossible (e.g., due to their chosen lifestyle).

The patient's son comes with him to clinic. He has done some online research on the treatment of Head and Neck SCC and asks about how HPV status affects the prognosis in head and neck SCC patients.

I will explain that the main protective effect occurs in oropharyngeal SCC (such as tonsillar and tongue base tumours) with close to a 60% decrease in risk of death from oropharyngeal SCC in HPV positive patients compared to their HPV negative counterparts. There is also a protective effect in oral cancer – as in this patient – but to a lesser extent.

So how would this patient's HPV status affect their treatment plan?

It won't. The UK HN guidelines suggest that this should only be undertaken in clinical trials. There is current research on the safety of titrating the treatment modality to prognosis, e.g., reducing the intensity of radiotherapy regimes in HPV positive patients to decrease the morbidity of their treatment, in view of their relatively good prognosis.

What is the pathophysiology of HPV infection and how is it linked to cancer?

- High risk HPV strains associated with HN SCC include HPV 16 and 18. These express viral oncoproteins (such as E6 and E7), which target the degradation of p53 and the pRb retinoblastoma tumour suppressor protein.
- HPV-associated head and neck SCC accounts for about 70% of oropharyngeal SCCs and up to 10% of oral SCCs.

Tell me, what are other predisposing risk factors in oral SCC?

- Smoking and alcohol remain the most common risk factors.
- Less common factors include premalignant lesions such as erythroplakia and leukoplakia.
- Less common still, are inherited conditions such as Fanconi Anaemia and Li-Fraumeni syndromes.

Please tell me about the use of SLNB in oral SCC patients.

- This is part of NICE guidance in the treatment of T1-T2 N0 M0 patients who may otherwise have undergone a potentially unnecessary selective neck dissection – as 80% of patients will be node negative on pathology.
- By sampling the sentinel node, the morbidity of a neck dissection is avoided in node-negative patients. This technique is also particularly useful for staging the contralateral neck.
- However, it is important to note that the technique is limited in floor of mouth tumours due to the 'shine through phenomenon', whereby the primary is very close to the lymphatics.

The patient's son has also read about SLNB and oral cancer. He asks whether his father can be offered this treatment to avoid the morbidity of a neck dissection. How do you proceed?

- I will explain that this technique is not indicated in his father's case for two reasons:
- It is only useful in a patient with a small primary and an N0 neck, as the purpose is to avoid a neck dissection in the patient cohort who is unlikely to benefit from it (so for the 80% of patients in the T1/T2 N0 cohort).
- In this case, his father already has nodal disease so he will need this treated with surgery or radiotherapy.

- In addition, he needs a free flap reconstruction, so an 'access neck dissection' would be required anyway, even in the absence of clinical nodal disease.

You've mentioned the morbidity of a neck dissection. How will you counsel a patient due to undergo this?

- Specific risks depend on the type of the neck dissection, but assuming that I will counsel the patient for a selective level I–III neck dissection as would be expected here, then I will explain that the lymph glands need to be removed from the neck as there is evidence of cancer spread.
- I will warn them regarding the risks of bleeding and infection, nerve injury to the spinal accessory nerve, marginal mandibular and great auricular nerves most commonly affected, numbness of the skin flap of the neck, as well as the risks of a seroma collection. Chyle leaks are rare with this type of neck dissection but still possible.

You've mentioned the 'type of neck dissection'. Please talk me through your understanding of neck dissections in general.

- These are comprehensive or selective.
- Comprehensive neck dissections include:
  - radical dissections, where levels I–V are resected as well as the IJV, SCM, and the accessory nerve,
  - modified radical dissections, where levels I–V are resected, in addition to one or two of those three additional structures, and
  - an extended radical dissection, which includes resection of levels I–V, in addition to structures such as the paratracheal or mediastinal nodes.
- Selective neck dissections include the resection of specific nodal levels according to characteristic patterns of spread of various tumours, such as I–III for intraoral SCCs, or I–IV for laryngeal SCCs.

Let us consider another scenario: how would you deal with a patient referred by their GP with a palpable neck node but with an unknown primary?

- This patient is best seen in a dedicated 'neck lump clinic'.
- Clinical examination will include:
  - examination of the skin and scalp of the head and neck, and
  - examination of the nose to the hypopharynx, including rigid and flexible endoscopy, by my ENT colleague.
- Investigation includes:
  - ultrasound guided histopathological investigation – preferably with a core biopsy rather than an FNA,
  - PET CT full body scan, and
  - GA panendoscopy from the paranasal sinuses to the proximal oesophagus, as well as bilateral tonsillectomies.
- Treatment consists of:
  - locoregional control with a modified radical neck dissection,
  - adjuvant chemoradiotherapy for T0 N1 disease with extra capsular spread, or T0 N2/N3 disease, and
  - a 5-year follow-up.

Why would you prefer a core biopsy in this instance rather than a FNA as a first-line biopsy?

- The clearer histological picture that can be obtained with a core biopsy is even more important here than in other scenarios, as this may help determine the potential origin of the primary.
- In addition, immunohistochemical techniques may be able to exclude certain sites.

FURTHER READING

1. De Bree R, de Keizer B, Civantos FJ, Takes RP, Rodrigo JP, Hernandez-Prera JC, Halmos GB, Rinaldo A, Ferlito A. What is the role of sentinel lymph node biopsy in the management of oral cancer in 2020? Eur Arch Otorhinolaryngol. 2021 Sep;278(9):3181–3191. doi: 10.1007/s00405-020-06538-y. Epub 2020 Dec 28. PMID: 33369691; PMCID: PMC8328894.
2. Tanaka TI, Alawi F. Human papilloma virus and oropharyngeal cancer. Dent Clin North Am. 2018 Jan;62(1):111–120.
3. https://bahno.org.uk/_userfiles/pages/files/ukheadandcancerguidelines2016.pdf
4. Mackenzie K, Watson M, Jankowska P, Bhide S, Simo R. Investigation and management of the unknown primary with metastatic neck disease: United Kingdom national multidisciplinary guidelines. J Laryngol Otol. 2016 May;130(S2):S170–S175.

Case 2.3

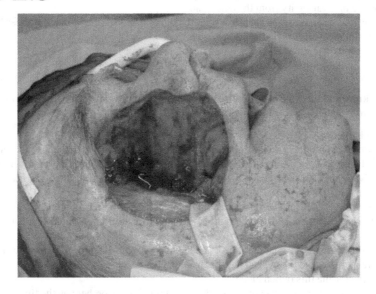

Please describe this photograph

This is an intraoperative photograph of an intubated patient with a north-facing nasal tube in the left nostril and a defect on the right side of his face which appears to include that of a right-sided hemi-maxillectomy, and right orbital exenteration.

How would you reconstruct this?

In a patient who is fit for a free flap, then my first choice is a chimeric fibula flap with a skin paddle and soleus, to reconstruct the palate as well as the external cheek and orbital component. This will allow the possibility for future dental restoration.

The alternative is a large soft tissue free flap such as a chimeric ALT flap with Vastus Lateralis, a rectus abdominis, or an LD.

Whilst soft tissue-only reconstructions are acceptable, I will need to counsel the patient that this will not allow future dental implant restoration and will result in some facial collapse with time.

How would you proceed if this patient has a severe mental health illness which has necessitated periods of inpatient admission at a mental health facility?

This raises two potential scenarios to address:

- The first is to establish if his illness affects his capacity to consent to the procedure.

    If I am concerned regarding his ability to understand, retain, weigh the information, or communicate his decision, then I will take all practical steps to help support the process by involving the trust's independent mental health advocate as per the Mental Capacity Act of 2005, as well as involving any persons he would like involved such as close family members or friends, or members of his mental health team/GP if they are well known to him, and establish if he has appointed a Power of Attorney or an advanced directive concerning any future treatment.
- The second is to ensure his mental health illness is controlled enough to allow him to undergo a long procedure with the associated physiological and emotional stress, or whether he needs further urgent input from his psychiatric team to optimize this as much as possible, as well as optimising his post-operative support structure – whilst ensuring that this does not delay his cancer treatment. The head and neck specialist nurse will play a crucial role to coordinate liaison between the MDT, the patient, the mental health team, and the GP to achieve this in a timely fashion.

DOI: 10.1201/9780429399268-19

What are your reconstructive goals here?

- My primary goals are to:
  1. separate the oral cavity from the defect, and
  2. fill the dead space, ensuring I obliterate the ethmoid or sphenoid sinus if they have been breached.
- My additional ideal aims include:
  1. bony reconstruction to allow for future dental restoration, and
  2. future orbital prosthetic reconstruction.

This patient is known to have a coagulopathy with two proximal DVTs in the last 2 years, and a more recent PE 6 months ago. How would you reconstruct this defect?

- This is a challenging scenario:
  - If his clotting profile cannot be optimized with the help of the haematologist, then a free flap would have a high failure rate. In addition, it carries the risk of needing a further procedure to salvage the flap, with additional GA time – further increasing his high risk of another DVT and PE.
  - So, I will consider an obturator plate and prosthesis – although I anticipate that it may be challenging to achieve a good result as there is no lateral anchoring point for it, but my colleagues in the prosthetic department may be able to achieve that.
  - The alternative is a combination of local flaps such as a temporalis muscle flap and a contralateral extended forehead flap, but I anticipate that it may be difficult to fully reconstruct the defect using this option alone:
    - A pectoralis major myocutaneous flap is not a great option here as the limit of its reach would be the very lower aspect of the defect – if that. It also has the tendency to be 'pulled back' in the first few weeks post-operatively due to the weight and effect of gravity – with the risk of future dehiscence if it is stretched to its maximum reach on the table – even if it doesn't appear to be under tension at that point. Again, it would be too high for a pedicled LD.
- I will warn the patient that they may be RIG-dependent post-operatively, if complete separation of the oral cavity from the defect is not achieved.

The prosthetic department inform you that they will be able to create a prosthesis for this patient. How will you counsel the patient regarding this?

- I will explain that a reconstruction carries a high risk of failure due to their comorbidities, but that a prosthesis – like any option – brings its own set of advantages and disadvantages.
- The advantages include:
  - a shorter intra-operative procedure and post-operative recovery period, which is particularly important given their history of a PE and DVTs,
  - the restoration of dentition, and
  - the possibility for a very high aesthetic result.
  - In addition, it may aid ongoing cancer surveillance as the tumour bed will remain in full view.
- However, disadvantages include:
  - speech issues – with an expected degree of hypernasality,
  - swallowing issues – with some nasal leakage,
  - they will have to take care of their prosthesis and ensure it is clean,
  - it may be uncomfortable, and
  - it is likely that they will need readjustments.

Please tell me – how would you perform a level I-III selective neck dissection?

- A neck dissection is a procedure where the lymphofatty tissue is resected from around the important structures to be preserved (very much like resecting Dupuytrens disease from around the neurovascular structures or resecting parotid tissue off the facial nerve).
- So, in level I, I am mindful that the structures to protect are the marginal mandibular nerve, the lingual nerve, and hypoglossal nerve along the mylohyoid floor.

- In level II, the same applies to the spinal accessory nerve, and hypoglossal nerve – where it crosses the external carotid artery.
- In level III, there are no specific nerves structures at risk apart from the vagus nerve when the carotid sheath is stripped.
- There is also a risk of vascular injury in all levels.
- During the preoperative team brief, I would have requested that neuromuscular relaxants are avoided after induction and discussed the tube positioning – such as a nasal tube in this patient. I prefer a south-facing nasal tube to avoid the risk of alar rim pressure necrosis that may occur with a north-facing tube.
- Once the patient is on the table, I will ensure supine patient positioning with a bolster under their shoulders to allow adequate neck extension, with the head resting in a head ring and turned to the contralateral side.
- I will then double check the nasal tube positioning, and that it is well padded – if north facing.
- There are numerous incisions described with the principles being:
  1. the incision should allow adequate access to the required levels that are to be excised, and
  2. to avoid long distally-based flaps, as this may affect their vascularity.

     I use a proximally-based half visor flap starting at the mastoid and extending down to the inferior aspect of level III – to expose level III adequately – and then extending back up to a point 3 cm below the submental triangle (as extending it further anteriorly to the mandibular border will result in a more noticeable scar in that area – that is unnecessary for access to level I).
- This is raised in the subplatysmal plane until the submandibular salivary gland is identified. I will also identify the external jugular vein and great auricular nerve superficial to the SCM.
- Next, I will address level I:
  1. Regarding protection of the marginal mandibular nerve, I will use two manoeuvres:
     - The Hayes – Martin manoeuvre, where the facial vein is divided at the level of the lower border of the submandibular gland and retracted superiorly. This protects the nerve as it runs superficial to the facial vessels and the capsule of the gland.
     - In addition, I will dissect the superficial leaf of the submandibular gland fascia and retract it superiorly to protect the nerve further along its course.
     - I do not make a point of purposefully visualising or dissecting the marginal mandibular nerve to avoid a risk of neuropraxia.
  2. Next, I will dissect the submandibular gland and lymphofatty tissue, and ask my assistant to retract the free margin of mylohyoid to deliver the deep lobe of the gland.

     Inferior traction of the gland will allow visualization of the submandibular duct and the ganglion which links it to the lingual nerve. Once I see the lingual nerve, then I can safely divide both the duct and the ganglion to deliver the whole specimen from this level. The hypoglossal nerve is seen at the floor of the mylohyoid. The facial artery is either divided just above the posterior belly of digastric or preserved – especially if a local flap is planned such as a buccinator or FAAM flap, which won't be the case here.
  3. Next, I will unsheathe the SCM by dividing the fascia along its length and asking my assistant to retract this medially with three artery clips. I will ask my assistant to also retract the SCM laterally to visualize the carotid sheath, which I incise. I will sharply strip the specimen from the IJV along its length – starting in level III – as injury to the IJV in this level is easier to deal with than at the skull base in level II. I will ligate and divide tributaries of the IJV as I go along. The posterior limit of the dissection is marked by the cutaneous branches of the cervical plexus – which are preserved, and the inferior limit is the omohyoid.

     I will then continue my dissection along the IJV up to level II until I encounter the accessory nerve. This is superficial to the vein in just under 70% of people, deep to the vein in about 30%, and runs through the vein in about 3% of people.
  4. I will ensure I preserve the accessory nerve, then proceed to complete the dissection of level II – off the deep muscles of the neck.
  5. I will deliver the neck dissection specimen – which is marked and orientated with sutures.
  6. I will complete the procedure by ensuring haemostasis – including a Valsalva manoeuvre, and ensuring the specimen is marked on a specimen board.
  7. At this point, I will dissect the chosen recipient vessels for the free flap transfer.

Let us consider another scenario – this patient is fit for a free flap. The senior fellow is performing the neck dissection, whilst you are raising the flap. They ask for your help as there is sudden copious bleeding from level II where they have started the neck dissection, and they are unsure where it is from. How would you manage this?

- I will let the anaesthetist know and obtain control by a mixture of pressure and suction in the first instance to locate the source.
- Once identified, then I will use Satinsky clamps on either side of the injury and proceed to repair it.
    If the injury is at the level of the skull base and I am unable to clamp the proximal side, then:
    - I will let the anaesthetist know of my finding, and
    - attempt to prevent an air embolism by asking for the patient's head to be dropped and clamping the distal end.
    - I will then place the trainee's finger on the 'hole' and ask them to apply pressure whilst I ensure that the rest of the neck dissection is completed.
    - Once I am satisfied with that, then I will plug the defect with the SCM.
- I will then check with the anaesthetist that it is safe to continue with the reconstruction.

FURTHER READING

1. https://www.legislation.gov.uk/ukpga/2005/9/contents
2. Fagan J. Selective neck dissection. Open Access Atlas of Otolaryngology, Head & Neck Operative Surgery. *(Excellent illustrated step-by-step guide through neck dissections for trainees)*. https://vula. uct.ac.za/access/content/group/ba5fb1bd-be95-48e5-81be-586fbaeba29d/Selective%20neck%20 dissection%20operative%20technique.pdf

Case 2.4

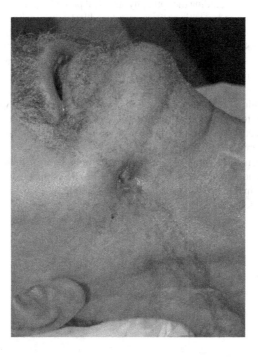

This patient presents to the head and neck clinic after relocating from another geographical area. He had resection of an intraoral tumour and adjuvant radiotherapy 6 years ago.

How will you manage him?

- The photograph shows what appears to be a draining fistula. My concern is to exclude:
  - tumour recurrence, and
  - osteoradionecrosis (ORN).
- I will take a focused history which includes:
  - The progression to fistulization, and any mucosal involvement,
  - history of recent dental extractions,
  - the TNM stage of the original tumour,
  - any sequelae to radiotherapy such as trismus and consequent malnutrition, as well as
  - any other PMH such as smoking, excessive alcohol intake or comorbidities.
- My examination will include:
  - examination of the external tract,
  - an intraoral exam looking for obvious recurrence, mucosal ulceration, and nodules,
  - any trismus, and
  - palpable lymphadenopathy.
- My investigation will include:
  - an OPG, CT, and MRI.
  - If unclear, a PET can differentiate between recurrence and ORN.
- I will investigate any palpable or radiologically enlarged lymph nodes with ultrasound-guided FNA.

What is ORN?

- Osteoradionecrosis is a slow-healing radiation-induced ischaemic necrosis of bone with associated soft tissue necrosis of variable extent, which occurs in the absence of local primary tumour necrosis or recurrence of metastatic disease.

DOI: 10.1201/9780429399268-20

- It occurs in up to 10% of irradiated head and neck cancer patients, and usually develops 6–12 months following radiation, but it may develop spontaneously at any point.
- There are several theories regarding the pathophysiological process, the summary of which includes:
  1. The development of endarteritis obliterans-induced ischaemia, with
     - endothelial, osteoclast, and osteoblast cellular damage that is either:
       ○ from direct damage by radiation, and/or
       ○ from indirect damage by reactive oxygen species and free radicals produced by injured endothelial cells.
     - These trigger an acute inflammatory response which generates a further release of free radicals resulting in further destruction of endothelial cells and vascular thrombosis.
  2. The damaged osteocytes and osteoblasts may survive until they attempt to divide when mitotic death occurs – which may be months or years post radiotherapy – or it may never divide unless stimulated by trauma.
  3. Therefore, there is a slow loss of bone cells after radiotherapy, with a consequent slowing down of the remodelling process, which leads to the risk of bone necrosis.
- Predisposing factors include:
  - tumour size and location,
  - radiation dose,
  - local trauma such as surgery or dental extractions,
  - infection,
  - immune defects,
  - malnutrition, and
  - decayed teeth.

What are your indications to treat ORN operatively?

These include:
- fistulation,
- mucosal damage,
- impending fracture, and
- recurrent infections and uncontrolled pain.

Otherwise, I will manage the patient conservatively with close observation and strict oral hygiene.

Why is the relevance of teeth extraction?

This is a common cause for the progression of ORN:
- Dental caries, periodontal disease or root lesions can lead to bone infection and progression to ORN because of low vascular patency and inability to repair irradiated tissues.
- The extraction process itself may then provide the traumatic stimulus to activate the mitotic death of cells that have been lying dormant.

The head and neck MDT preoperative pathway includes a preoperative dental assessment and teeth extraction during the cancer resection – if required, so that healing occurs by the time of radiotherapy – with the avoidance of post-radiotherapy inflammation and trauma.

The investigations exclude a recurrence and confirm ORN of the mandible. Now what?

- The patient will require segmental resection of the affected areas, with a free fibula and skin paddle reconstruction if the patient is fit for this.
- If the patient is not suitable for a bony reconstruction, then a large soft tissue reconstruction such as an ALT is an acceptable option, or a myocutaneous pectoralis major if they are unfit for a free flap.

You proceed with a fibula reconstruction. How would you plan the reconstruction of a significant mucosal ulceration as well as the skin fistula?

- Both the mucosal and skin defect can be managed with:
  - one skin paddle (with de-epithelialization of the intermittent skin bridge), or
  - two paddles if two adequate perforators are present.

- The alternative is the use of soleus for the intraoral segment, with a backup plan for an additional free flap, if adequate perforators are lacking, such as a RFFF or a thin ALT.

What about the theory of using ipsilateral free fibula flaps for intraoral soft tissue reconstruction and the contralateral side for extraoral soft tissue reconstruction? Would you use an ipsilateral or contralateral fibula in this case?

- That is a mostly historical concern:
    - If the septum is sufficiently mobile, it doesn't matter as the soft tissue paddle can be rotated intraorally or extra orally.
    - If it isn't, then a large enough skin paddle can be taken to allow proper positioning, and the flap can be inset with the proximal end inset medially or laterally to allow for intraoral or contralateral reconstruction.
- In practice I choose the side of the fibula donor site based on the results of the preoperative CTA. If both are equal, and the signal of both perforators are equally good, then I choose the contralateral side to allow for more physical space in the operating room for both my team and that of the resective surgeon.

You mentioned a preoperative CTA. Why do you use this? Why not simply rely on palpable pedal pulses?

There is some debate regarding preoperative imaging, especially in young healthy adults. However, I find a preoperative CTA useful as it allows me to:

1. exclude a peronea magna artery – thought to occur in 5% of people – where the peroneal artery is the dominant blood supply to the leg and foot,
2. exclude subclinical chronic peripheral vascular disease – which may be tipped into acute ischaemia by removing a feeding vessel. It is possible to have palpable pulses in the presence of chronic vascular impairment due to collateral circulation. I am aware that some have tried to elucidate this clinically with a pedal modified Allen test (where the anterior tibial artery is occluded when feeling for the posterior tibial vessel and vice versa), but this has not been shown to be accurate or reliable.
3. Lastly, it is also useful to see the level of vessel branching and consequent length of the pedicle – which is particularly important in larger reconstructions (and consequently shorter pedicles), as well as the quality and diameter of the peroneal vessels on both sides.

Are you familiar with the CAD/CAM planning system for bony reconstructions? What are your thoughts on this?

- This refers to the integration of computer-aided design (CAD) and computer-aided manufacturing (CAM) to create patient-specific cutting jigs using 3D reconstructions of fine cut CTs of the patients' mandible and fibula – with the following advantages:
    - more accurate mandibular and fibular osteotomies – both with regard to the exact position as well as the ideal angle, and
    - reduced operative time, especially for patients requiring multiple osteotomies to contour the flap.
- However, the technique does have disadvantages, such as:
    - the inability to allow for potential tumour growth between the time of planning and the day of surgery,
    - the inability to take the skin perforator anatomy into consideration, which may affect the osteotomy level, and
    - a 10–14 day turnover to create the jig, so it is not suitable for patients who need expedited surgery.

How do you raise an osteocutaneous free fibula flap 'free-hand', without a CAD/CAM system?

- I will position the patient supine with an uninflated high thigh tourniquet, a jelly pad under the buttock, and a padded bar as a foot support – allowing hip and knee flexion.

- I will then mark the flap by drawing a line from the head of the fibula to the lateral malleolus, with the proximal and distal osteotomy levels at 6 cm from either anatomical point, to protect the common peroneal nerve and the ankle syndesmosis respectively.
- Next, I will confirm the location of the Doppler perforator signals along the peroneal intermuscular septum, which is made more apparent by flexing the knee and hip to allow the muscle to fall away due to gravity.
- The incision is made along the anterior skin paddle mark and continued just beyond the bony resection levels. I will then visually confirm the position and quality of the chosen perforator(s). This allows me to move the position of the skin paddle proximally or distally if the true perforator location does not correspond to the Doppler signal.
- The aim of the procedure is to dissect the muscles off the fibula in a 360-degree fashion moving through the lateral compartment ensuring I preserve the superficial peroneal nerve, then the anterior, and posterior compartments – whilst leaving a 2 mm cuff of bone or less – to minimize donor site morbidity.
- Once I incise the anterior intermuscular septum, then I will place a rib elevator around the bone to allow a safe osteotomy without endangering the pedicle, starting with the distal osteotomy to allow the more critical proximal osteotomy to be performed under less tension. There is historical controversy regarding the resection of a bony segment or the creation of osteotomies at angles to allow easy removal of the bone, but there is no evidence for the need for either, so I prefer to simply create 90-degree osteotomies.
- The osteotomies allow the bone to be rotated to continue the dissection and expose the interosseous membrane which is then incised.
- I will slow down at this point until I identify the pedicle distally and ligate it, then follow it proximally whilst continuing the muscular dissection.
- I will only complete the posterior skin incision once the required size and shape of the soft tissue paddle are confirmed following the resection.

How will you manage his airway?

- I anticipate that the post-operative swelling in this patient will remain very anterior and spare the floor of mouth, so the likelihood for the need for a tracheostomy is not high.
- However, I will consent the patient for this possibility, and then jointly re-assess the need for this at the end of the procedure, along with my resective consultant colleague and the consultant head and neck anaesthetist.
- In this way, the shared airway is managed in a multidisciplinary manner.
- I am aware that there is debate regarding routine airway management following intraoral reconstruction – with a wide variation in practice across the United Kingdom. Some units routinely keep patients intubated and ventilated overnight to allow any overnight swelling to subside, others encourage routine tracheostomies for all patients.
- Considerations on making that decision include, not only patient and surgical factors, but also the healthcare environment such as ITU availability, anaesthetic support, and ward staff expertise, which may partly account for the variation in practice between units.
- The ideal practice is to correctly identify those who will require a tracheostomy and limit this to those who will need one – to avoid any unnecessary associated morbidity – whilst ensuring a safe post-operative airway.
- Measures taken to ensure safety include a standardized approach to preoperatively identify patients who are anticipated to require a tracheostomy and those who are less likely to need it. Those who will definitely require one undergo this at the start of the case. All other patients are reassessed at a 'pause' at the end of the procedure, with a default stance for a tracheostomy if any doubt is expressed by a member of the surgical or anaesthetic teams regarding the safety of going without.
- Where elective tracheostomy is not immediately indicated, then immediate extubation and the use of a high dependency post-operative environment, or less commonly, delayed extubation to the following day, are appropriate. Additional security in the immediately extubated patient may be achieved with staged extubation wires.

Why not simply accept routine tracheostomies for all patients or routine overnight ventilation until the swelling subsides?

- Tracheostomies – whilst essential to secure the airway in some – also carry risks such as:
  - blockage and displacement of the cannula,
  - failure to decannulate,
  - increased risk of pneumonia,
  - the risk of cross-contamination of the neck incision with dehiscence, infection, and fistulation – be it tracheoinnominate, tracheo-oesophageal, or tracheocutaneous, and
  - there is evidence that it is associated with increased patient hospital stays.
- Routine overnight ventilation of this patient group also carries the risks associated with prolonged intubation and sedation – especially in elderly patients – who frequently have cardio-respiratory morbidity, with complications including:
  - increased cardiovascular instability requiring inotropic support,
  - agitation, and
  - prolonged ICU stay.
- Therefore, there is a need to avoid unnecessary tracheostomies as well as protracted intubation.

So, how do you preoperatively identify those who will require an elective tracheostomy?

There are patient and surgical factors:

- Patient factors include:
  - significant obesity,
  - hypoventilation syndrome or severe sleep apnoea,
  - likely poor cough, or
  - increased aspiration risk

Previously, the use of CPAP masks risked compression of the pedicle or flap, but there are now alternative devices such as OPTIFLOW which can support such patients post-operatively.

- Surgical factors include:
  - large tumours – particularly close to the midline and posterior,
  - significant involvement of the tongue – especially posteriorly,
  - bulky reconstructions,
  - bilateral neck dissections,
  - previous radiotherapy, and
  - anticipated prolonged surgery with increased fluid requirements or blood loss.

You reassess him at the end of the procedure, and you decide to opt for a tracheostomy. Please describe how you will perform that.

- As part of the preoperative team brief, I would have requested for:
  - a tracheostomy set to be available, along with a cricoid hook, suction, and bone nibblers in case the cartilage is severely calcified, as well as
  - a cuffed non-fenestrated tube with an introducer and inner tube – size 7 in women and size 8 in men.
- I would have preplanned the skin marking by ensuring the neck incision does not communicate with this to avoid cross contamination of the neck wound – even if the chance of performing a tracheostomy was preoperatively deemed to be low – as in this case.
- The anaesthetist will be aware of the decision as they are part of the decision making 'pause'.
- I will re-confirm the appropriate size of the cuffed tube with the anaesthetist based on their ET tube size and will test the cuff for any leaks at this point.
- Important principles for a safe tracheostomy include:
  1. ensuring strict haemostasis at each tissue plane,
  2. ensuring my assistant understands that they have a crucial role by pulling equally on the lateral and medial retractors to prevent me being diverted off the trachea, and

3. ensuring I palpate the trachea between my thumb and index at each tissue plane to avoid veering off the trachea. This is especially important in a patient with a particularly fat neck or with a trachea that is not central.

- With regard to the procedure itself, this involves:
  - a horizontal skin incision overlying the third tracheal ring, and dissection of the subcutaneous fat,
  - vertical division of the plane between the strap muscles, and lateral retraction of these.
  - The thyroid isthmus is then retracted superiorly to expose the trachea. If this is not possible, I will use diathermy dissection through the isthmus.
  - I will then ligate the thyroid ima artery and inferior thyroid veins.
  - Once the cricoid is identified, I will expose the third ring, and then
  - warn the anaesthetist that I am about to create the tracheostomy.
  - I will create a defect in the third ring – just over 1 cm in diameter and ask the anaesthetist to retract the tube to allow me to introduce the tracheostomy tube – then swap the introducer for the inner tube.
  - I will then inflate the cuff with 10 cm of air and connect the tube to the anaesthetic tubing and ask the anaesthetist to confirm a CO_2 trace.
  - I will then secure the tube using a 4/0 silk and divide the gap in the phalange that is used for the tracheostomy tape, to discourage the nursing team from using it as that may compress the free flap pedicle in the neck. I will then place a U-shaped tracheostomy sponge to protect the underlying skin from compression from the plastic phalange as well as tracheostomy secretions.

How will you instruct your team to take care of the tracheostomy?

It is important to ensure:

1. protection of the skin from maceration and excoriation with daily inspection and dressing changes, and the use of Duoderm or Cavilon if there are severe secretions,
2. regular suction to manage increased secretions,
3. identification and prevention of tube blockage with 4 hourly inner tube inspections and saline nebulizer humidification, and
4. protection of the neck incision from tracheostomy secretions to prevent neck wound cross contamination, maceration, and breakdown.

The intraoral swelling subsides a few days following the tracheostomy.

How do you ensure safe decannulation?

- I will ensure that the patient is stable from a cardiovascular and respiratory point of view, then ask the Speech and Language Team (SALT) to check he has a safe swallow and strong enough cough to manage his oral secretions.
- An uncomplicated decannulation is routinely managed by the SALT team and the tracheostomy specialist nurses:

  There are four steps to complete decannulation: any signs of continued cough or respiratory distress indicate that it is not safe to go ahead with that weaning step – and that there is a need for the swallow and cough to be checked.

  These consist of:
  1. A cuff deflation trial period – for 24 hours – if tolerated.
  2. A gloved finger occlusion test of the tracheostomy tube for a few minutes – with airflow checked for – through the nose and mouth, and auscultation of lungs.

     (If the patient remains well with no signs of respiratory distress, then this indicates that adequate airflow is passing from the mouth to the lungs and back, past the occluded stoma.)
  3. The third step is to place a one-way speaking valve with cuff deflation. This opens on inspiration and closes on expiration, diverting air past the vocal cords to allow speech. This may increase the patient's work of breathing, and patient tolerance is initially built up to 4 hours – then left for the whole day – if tolerated, before proceeding with the last step, and

4. Lastly, a decannulation cap is placed – again with cuff deflation to allow airflow. The tracheostomy tube is blocked off – again for at least 4 hours, but better still for the day, before the tube is removed.

Let's change the scenario – How would you manage post-operative intraoral dehiscence of the flap?

- I would have pre-warned the patient regarding the high risk of slow healing in the context of osteoradionecrosis and poor quality of surrounding tissues, and I would manage this expectantly:
  - I will continue with nasogastric feeding for 2 weeks to prevent contamination and infection of the neck by intraoral contents, then
  - Proceed to Radiologically Inserted Gastrostomy (RIG) feeding to allow long-term feeding – if he hasn't healed by then – as keeping it in situ for longer than 2 weeks may risk nasal ulceration at home.
  - I will supplement this with Hyoscine patches to keep his mouth dry and decrease saliva tracking in the neck.

It is now 6 weeks down the line, and the intraoral component is still healing very slowly. What about trying hyperbaric oxygen therapy?

- HBO therapy is controversial as there is no strong evidence to support this, and there are few centres in the United Kingdom to refer to.
- A few small studies have shown an increase in capillary angiogenesis, proliferation of fibroblasts, and collagen synthesis due to an increase in oxygen tension in hypoxic tissue. Despite the limited evidence, I will still consider referring him to a centre if there is one nearby, and the patient is willing to try this. They will assess him for his suitability, and contraindications – such as COPD/ asthma, amongst many others.
- If not, I will hold fire and continue with RIG feeding.
- We have the luxury of more time as there is an absence of a 'post-operative wound healing clock' in this instance, as opposed to a situation where complete healing is required by the time adjuvant radiotherapy is due 6 weeks later.
- So, whilst this is a significant issue from the patient quality of life point of view, post-operative healing can take a little longer without affecting their oncological prognosis, as long as their nutrition is being supported.

FURTHER READING

1. Marx RE. Osteoradionecrosis: a new concept of its pathophysiology. J Oral Maxillofac Surg. 1983;41:283–288.
2. Fujita M, Harada K, Masaki N, Shimizutani K, Kim SW, Fujita N, Sakurai K, Fuchihata H, Inoue T, Kozuka T. MR imaging of osteoradionecrosis of the mandible following radiotherapy for head and neck cancers. Nippon Acta Radiol. 1991;51:892–900.
3. Minn H, Aitasalo K, Happonen R-P. Detection of cancer recurrence in irradiated mandible using positron emission tomography. Eur Arch Otorhinolaryngol. 1993;250:312–315.
4. Chrcanovic BR, Reher P, Sousa AA, Harris M. Osteoradionecrosis of the jaws—a current overview—part 1. Oral and Maxillofac Surg. 2010;14(1):3–16.
5. Coyle MJ, Tyrrell R, Godden A, Hughes CW, Perkins C, Thomas S, Godden D. Replacing tracheostomy with overnight intubation to manage the airway in head and neck oncology patients: towards an improved recovery. Br J Oral Maxillofac Surg. 2013;51:493–496.

Case 2.5

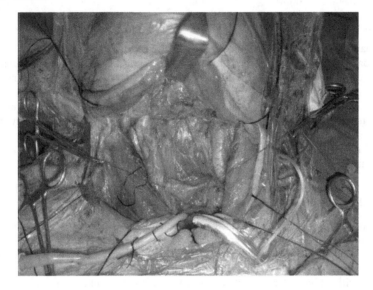

This is an intraoperative photograph of a patient who has had a laryngectomy for radio-recurrent disease. He now requires a tubular pharyngeal reconstruction. To help orientate you, the distal end of the pharynx is marked with stay sutures and artery clips.

What are your aims when reconstructing the laryngopharynx?

These are:

1. a well-healed watertight pharyngeal closure with the absence of leaks,
2. the ability to swallow,
3. adequate voice rehabilitation, and
4. the avoidance of long-term complications such as a stricture, and a pharyngocutaneous fistula.

How would you achieve these aims with your reconstruction through tissue selection and flap design?

- My preference is to use:
  - a thin ALT free flap,
  - the alternative is a free radial forearm flap – if the forearm donor area is adequate, or
  - a free jejunum, but the need for this is now uncommon.
- I prefer the ALT as:
  - It allows a two-layer waterproofing reconstruction.
  - It produces a less wet voice reconstruction than the free jejunum.
  - It is more tolerant to longer ischaemia in the case of unexpected difficulty with the micro anastomosis.
  - In addition, if more than one perforator is present, it allows concomitant reconstruction of the external skin – if required, avoiding the need for two flaps in that scenario.
- I prefer to use a trapezoidal shaped ALT with a flap width of 10 cm, to match the diameter of the native cervical oesophagus of 3 cm. This achieves:
  - an oblique opening at the proximal end of the flap to match the enlarged opening at the base of the tongue, and
  - a distal triangular dart of ALT flap which will be inserted in a myotomy slit in the distal pharynx to reduce ring strictures at the distal end.

DOI: 10.1201/9780429399268-21

However I accept that many other shapes have been described with no evidence of the superiority of any particular one.

- To help minimize a leak, I use a Montgomery salivary bypass tube and inset 'around it' in two layers with an additional waterproofing fascial layer:
    - The first layer consists of suturing the skin edges to the mucosal defect edges with simple interrupted 3.0 vicryl, with care taken to evert the skin against the mucosa, keeping the knots in the lumen.
    - The second layer consists of a continuous suture to ensure there are no gaps.
    - The longitudinal anterolateral thigh seam is placed posteriorly along the prevertebral area to contain leaks, prevent vascular compression, and position the vessels anteriorly for microvascular anastomosis.
    - The flap fascia is then wrapped around the tubed flap to reinforce the suture lines.

The salivary tube is left in place until the first swallow test excludes a leak, usually at 10–14 days post operatively.

You mentioned concomitant reconstruction of the external neck skin. What considerations are important during the inset of this?

It is important to consider the contour of the donor site as a bulky flap can cause problems such as:

- compression of the pedicle,
- problems achieving direct wound closure, especially as the post-radiotherapy neck skin is frequently fibrosed and immobile, and
- possible obstruction of the tracheostomy stoma.

What is your preference for reconstruction of a pharyngeal patch defect?

- My preference is still a thin ALT, as the fascia can be used for waterproofing.
- Failing that, then a radial forearm flap may be used – with a 2 cm rim of extra tissue planned and deepithelialized to be used as a makeshift waterproofing layer. However, this may not be as effective as the ALT fascia waterproofing layer.
- The insetting principles remain the same as that for a tubed flap.

Your ENT resective colleague anticipates they will achieve pharyngeal closure in a radiorecurrent patient. Do you need to still get involved?

- Yes, I do: direct pharyngeal closure in radio-recurrent patients is associated with a higher rate of fistula formation, so I will reinforce the pharyngeal closure with an onlay flap to 'vascularize' the closure layer. This has been shown to reduce the fistula formation.
- My preference is to use a Gracilis free flap in this case, as:
    - the donor site is cheap,
    - it is not overly bulky, and
    - the muscle conforms well to the dead space and helps to contain any small leaks.
- But, disadvantages include a smaller calibre pedicle vessel than an ALT or RFFF.

However, I accept that any other flap is suitable, as the point is to provide an onlay vascularized layer.

When you first meet this patient in clinic, they have a BMI of 16. How would this alter your management?

- This patient is severely malnourished and is at risk of increased complications, such as:
    - poor wound healing (which is even more pertinent, given that this is radiorecurrent disease so healing will already have been affected),
    - infection, and
    - intraoperative complications such as:
        - hypothermia, and
        - increased risk to pressure points, and compression-induced neurapraxias.

- They require an MDT assessment and management to:
  1. Determine the timeline and cause of this: such as dysphagia, cancer cachexia, or other concomitant issues for e.g., alcoholism.
  2. Their nutritional status will be evaluated in detail by the dietician and SALT team as is routine, but in this case, I will also enlist the help of the nutritional team with a specialist gastroenterologist to determine the risk of refeeding syndrome and manage this.
  3. If alcoholism is also an issue, then preoperative admission for detoxification and thiamine replacement is also required.
  4. As is routine in all head and neck cancer patients, their frailty is also assessed, and I am particularly concerned as I anticipate they will score highly for this.
  5. Lastly, if this patient is elderly, then I will also involve the MDT liaison Care of the Elderly physician to help oversee any other comorbidities that may be at play.

Tell me about the nutritional assessment that you mentioned.

- This is usually carried out by the SALT team/dietician within the MDT.
- The two most popular tools are the Subjective Global Assessment (SGA) and Malnutrition Universal Screening Tool (MUST).
- The SGA is a nutritional assessment tool that has been validated for cancer patients.
  - It consists of a history and physical exam tool which considers weight change, dietary intake, GI symptoms, and functional capacity as well as muscle wasting, ankle, and sacral oedema.
  - Scores are then given from Grade A for well-nourished patients to Grade C with severe malnutrition.
  - This has been correlated with hospital stay and rate of complications.
- The MUST is also used in many Trusts despite it not being validated in cancer patients.

Tell me about refeeding syndrome. Why do you need to identify the risk for this?

- This is a potentially fatal metabolic syndrome with shifts in electrolytes, particularly hypophosphatemia amongst others that may occur in patients who receive artificial feeding. This is often unrecognized unless one is on the lookout for it.
- The pathophysiology is due to starvation-induced intracellular loss of phosphate because protein and fat catabolism has occurred rather than carbohydrate metabolism, which can result in rhabdomyolysis, cardiac dysfunction, and death.
- At risk patients include those with a:
  - BMI less than 18.5% (especially less than 16),
  - weight loss of more than 10% in the last 6 months,
  - little or no nutritional intake in the last 5 days,
  - low levels of serum K/PO4/Mg, and
  - a history of alcohol misuse, diabetes and chemotherapy compounding that risk.
- Management consists of slow refeeding with thiamine treatment, and careful rehydration guided by a nutritional team.

You mentioned a frailty assessment. What do you mean by frailty in this context? Please tell me more about this, and why you would specifically assess for this in Head and Neck cancer patients.

- Frailty is a physiologic state in which patients have a decreased ability to recover normal function after a stressful event, such as major surgery – with increasing evidence that this is a predictor of post-operative outcomes in major surgery, including head and neck reconstruction.
- It is thought to reflect physiological age, which is a concept that is gaining traction as being more important than chronological age when treating our increasingly elderly population.
- There are two concepts of frailty models: a physical phenotype and cumulative deficit model.
  - The physical phenotype measures physical strength and daily activity, such as the Rockwood score or the Fried score.
    These are very useful screening tools to recognize those who need more detailed assessment and preoperative optimization.

    – The cumulative deficit model, such as the American College of Surgeons modified frailty index, is validated in head and neck cancer patients but is more time consuming and detailed. This is useful to use in patients highlighted by the Rockwood score as 'at risk'.

How would you manage a leak?

- I will manage an early post-operative leak by requesting the patient remains Nil by Mouth with continued NG patient feeding for a further 2 weeks before checking if the leak has healed with a barium swallow test.
- I will consider inserting a salivary bypass tube if one was not placed at the time of surgery.

    I expect a leak to settle within 4 weeks, to allow radiotherapy 6 weeks postoperatively – if required (unless the tumour is radiorecurrent, as in this case, in which case adjuvant radiotherapy is not required).

This patient presents with a paratracheal pharyngocutaneous fistula a year later and you plan for a reconstruction, but you suspect there are no longer any adequate recipient neck vessels following severe radiotherapy damage. How will you manage this?

- This is a challenging scenario.
- I prefer to save a pectoralis major flap reconstruction as a 'life-boat' for situations where a patient is no longer fit for a free flap, as:
  - they may develop recurrences or future complications that may require further reconstructions.
  - In addition, this bulky pedicled flap may render the parastomal inset more problematic than a thin flap.
- So, if they are still fit enough to undergo free tissue transfer, and this is just a question of a vessel depleted neck, then my preferred option is to use the IMA vessels as recipients, which necessitates a flap with a long pedicle such as a serratus anterior flap. This is my ideal choice as it also provides:
  - a thin flap, to prevent parastomal obstructive problems,
  - and muscle, which I prefer in this instance, especially if there is radiation damage affecting the surrounding skin for inset:
    - As it swells to encourage wound edge contact with the skin that may be friable with poor wound healing potential, as well as filling the tract itself.
    - In addition, the contour will improve further as it undergoes muscle atrophy once healing is achieved.
- I will plan for initial exploration of both sides of the neck prior to flap raising to ensure there are no neck options:
  - If the neck is indeed vessel depleted, then I will dissect the IMA vessels.
  - Once I am satisfied of the adequacy of recipient vessels, then I will raise the flap.
  - If not, then I will proceed with a pectoralis major pedicled flap as a last option.

How would you manage a suspected chyle leak?

- Chyle leaks management is based on their flow rate, be it low or high flow.
- I would suspect a chyle leak if milky drainage fluid is present and confirm this by sending a sample for the presence of chylomicrons whilst ensuring initial management is not delayed while the result is pending.
- A low-flow chyle leak (<1 l/day) is managed with a fat-free diet and Octreotide – which has been shown to decrease the chyle leak persistence by 5 days compared to fat-free diet alone.
- If a high-output leak occurs (>1 l/day), then expeditious surgical treatment is required – preferably with endoscopic clipping of the thoracic duct by my thoracic surgery colleagues to avoid a further neck exploration. If that is not available in my centre, then an open technique will be required – with early exploration before the formation of a proteinaceous capsule:
  - Here, I will identify the leak with NG administration of olive oil on induction. This will allow thoracic duct flow 20 minutes later.
  - I will oversee the area of the leak, then apply a fibrin sealant such as Tisseel,
  - followed by transposition and oversewing of the sternal head of SCM.

    This is followed with a post-operative fat-free diet and Octreotide regime for 5 post-operative days.

What is Octreotide, and how does this help chyle leaks?

This is a synthetic analogue to somatostatin. It decreases the absorption of triglycerides and inhibits splanchnic circulation and gastrointestinal motility, which affect lymph flow.

Tell me – how is voice normally produced, and how would you re-establish voice for this patient?

- In a patient with an intact larynx, the vocal cords enable sound to be produced as they are approximated during exhalation. The mucosal wave of the vocal folds produces a sound that can be varied in pitch and volume. This sound is then manipulated by the upper aerodigestive tract to create voice.
- The larynx is lost in this patient, but there are several ways to re-establish voice:
  - The most common is via a tracheo-oesophageal puncture and speaking valve:
    - Here, air is redirected into the pharynx via the iatrogenic fistula and vibrates the tissues in the reconstructed pharynx to produce sound, which is then manipulated into voice by the upper aerodigestive tract as per normal.
    - If a pharyngeal reconstruction has been used, the tracheo-oesophageal fistula is performed as a 'secondary puncture'. This is where the fistula and insertion of speech valve is delayed for 4–6 weeks to allow for tissue healing.
  - Another option is an electrolarynx – reserved for those who can't get on with the speaking valve, or whilst waiting for valve placement. This has a vibrating head and generates sound as it is held against the neck.
  - Lastly, oesophageal speech can also be used, where patients learn to swallow air into the oesophagus and push it back during expiration to produce speech, but this has been superseded by the other two methods as many patients find this difficult to learn.

What are the long-term consequences of a laryngectomy that you and the patient need to be aware of?

- Apart from the psychological aspect and change in neck appearance,
  1. They will require voice rehabilitation as the larynx is crucial to natural voice production.
  2. The stoma bypasses the function of the upper aerodigestive tract in providing moist warm air for the lungs.
  3. They will lose the ability to Valsalva, necessary to fix their core and strain.
  4. Their sense of smell will be compromised as they cannot inhale through their noses to deliver odours to the olfactory epithelium.
  5. They are at risk of stoma obstruction and aspiration of secretions.
  6. They will be registered as 'neck-breathers' with the local ambulance service, as well as their electricity company as any power cut may be life-threatening if they need the suctioning device.
- In order to manage these changes, they must:
  1. learn to use a speech valve (if one is in place) or an alternative such as an electrolarynx,
  2. meticulously clean the stoma twice a day and remove any crusting,
  3. use external humidification and suctioning, as well as showering bibs,
  4. prevent constipation with regular medication and appropriate diet, and
  5. arrange for smoke alarms to be fitted and to be careful with use-by-dates on food products as they lose their sense of smell.

FURTHER READING

1. Mehanna HM, Moledina JM, Travis J. Refeeding syndrome: what it is, and how to prevent and treat it. BMJ. 2008;336(7659):1495–1498.
2. Talwar B, Donnelly R, Skelly R, Donaldson M. Nutritional management in head and neck cancer: United Kingdom national multidisciplinary guidelines. J Laryngol Otol. 2016;130(S2):S32–S40.
3. Pitts KD, et al. Frailty as a predictor of post-operative outcomes among patients with head and neck cancer. Otolaryngol Head Neck Surg. 2019.
4. Kao HK, Abdelrahman M, Chang KP, et al. Choice of flap affects fistula rate after salvage laryngopharyngectomy. Sci Rep. 2015;5:9180. https://doi.org/10.1038/srep09180

Case 2.6

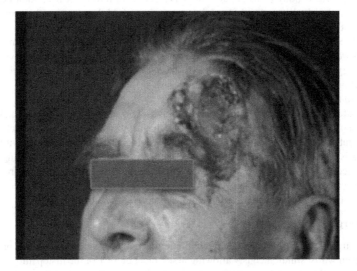

This patient presents to your clinic with the lesion above. Please describe the photograph.

This is the photograph of a male patient with a large, ulcerated lesion involving the left side of his forehead, temple, left brow, and upper lid, with an extension lateral to his left eye.

How will you manage him?

- I will manage him in the context of the skin MDT, with the most important goals being to:
  1. first obtain histological diagnosis,
  2. establish the extent of any invasion with CT/MRI imaging (particularly invasion of bone, the orbit, and perineural involvement), and
  3. determine if this is curable, or if palliative treatment is the goal, and if so, whether the patient is a candidate for either.
- Salient points in the history include:
  - the development timeline of the lesion and the reasons for a possible late presentation if the lesion was slow growing (to establish any cognitive or mental health issues, neglect, or fear of treatment),
  - a history of recurrence – including radiorecurrence,
  - any patient comorbidities such as immunosuppression, and
  - any syndromes predisposing to skin cancer such as Gorlin syndrome.
- Key findings on physical examination include:
  - fixity to underlying bone, and
  - palpable head and neck lymphadenopathy.

The lesion is clinically fixed to underlying bone and biopsies come back as an infiltrative BCC. How will you manage him?

- I will confirm any evidence of bony invasion on CT/MRI and the extent of this:
  - CT is the most accurate method for evaluating bony destruction of the inner and outer tables, and
  - MRI is best to depict marrow involvement of the diploe and to evaluate associated soft tissue invasion including the dura.
  - With regard to the resection:
  - In a medically fit patient with a high-risk surgically resectable tumour, then the ideal treatment is resection with intraoperative margin control such as GA Mohs micrographic surgery – with the understanding that this will only control the peripheral margin, as the deep margin is likely to be bone or periosteum and Mohs is not possible on bone.

DOI: 10.1201/9780429399268-22

- – If the MRI and CT have shown involvement of the periosteum only, then I will excise the periosteum and consider burring suspect areas of bone.
- – If there is frank bony invasion, and the MDT deems him to be fit for a joint neurosurgical resection then I will control the peripheral margin with Mohs micrographic surgery.
- – Alternatively, I will use frozen section control – with the understanding that it is not as accurate as Mohs, as there is random histological sampling of the peripheral margin.

  However, I accept the intraoperative margin control is resource intensive, and if my histology department cannot support this, then I would proceed with GA excision with a 1 cm clinical margin – confirmed on dermoscopy.
- With regard to the reconstruction:
  - – In a patient who is fit for a free flap, then the most important factor to guide my choice of flap is the length of the pedicle as I may need to reach the facial vessels, with long pedicled flaps such as Serratus/LD or ALT being my top choices. I will reconstruct a dural defect with fascia lata.
  - – If this is not surgically resectable, or if the patient is not medically fit or willing to undergo a surgical procedure, then I will suggest radiotherapy (in a non-Gorlin syndrome patient). Treatment with a Hedgehog pathway inhibitor such as Vismodegib was another option in the past, but this is not currently available in the United Kingdom.

What is Mohs surgery?

- This is a surgical and histopathological technique for maintaining continuity and orientation of the specimen whilst simultaneously allowing assessment of 99% of the histopathological margin compared to standard histology which routinely examines less than 1% of the margin.
- It is achieved with staged concentric excision of tissue margins, both circumferential and deep to the tumour, which is rapidly frozen and sectioned horizontally to allow complete microscopic examination. The process is repeated until clear margins are obtained, and this has been shown to substantially decrease recurrence rate of non-melanoma skin cancers.

You mentioned dermoscopy for margin assessment – what is this?

Dermoscopy is a non-invasive method using skin surface microscopy that allows the in-vivo evaluation of colours and microstructures of the epidermis, the dermo-epidermal junction, and the papillary dermis not visible to the naked eye. Certain skin cancers have characteristic appearances: e.g., a BCC such as in this patient may show asymmetrical arborizing vessels, ulceration, and white strand-like crystalline structures.

If that is the case, why didn't you mention its use in the preoperative work up?

- It is useful, in experienced hands, to confirm a clinical diagnosis and avoid unnecessary biopsy of small lesions.
- However, in this case, histological confirmation is needed anyway before planning a possible extensive procedure – but it may still be useful for the clinical assessment of the margin – especially if intraoperative margin assessment is not possible.

You proceed with the free flap option. Which recipient vessels will you use?

- I will first explore the superficial temporal vessels in the pre-auricular region rather than in the temple as the vessels are of larger calibre there. The superficial temporal vein can be of small calibre and tortuous configuration.
- If I am not happy with the quality of the vessels, then I will proceed with an anastomosis of the facial vessels in level I of the neck – if my pedicle is long enough, as again the vessel calibre is larger than along the mandibular border, and this would decrease the risk of flap-related complications.

How would you reconstruct this patient if they were not fit for a free flap, and if the planned resection will leave exposed bone?

I would offer the patient two options:

- One option is to stage the reconstruction to ensure histological confirmation of complete excision with good margins, before using a temporoparietal fascia flap and SSG if the disease has been confirmed not to not involve the anterior aspect of the flap.

- Alternatively, I will use the Crane principle to produce a graftable bed that can then be reconstructed with a simple skin graft. This is achieved using a scalp rotation flap that is left in situ for 6 weeks, then rotated back to the donor site. However, I will warn the patient that this will temporarily transfer hair bearing tissue into the defect, and it will require two episodes of general anaesthesia.

The pathology comes back showing a close deep margin despite resection of periosteum and burring of bone. What now?

Unless there are contraindications – such as Gorlin syndrome or previous radiation to the area, I will suggest adjuvant radiotherapy to the skin MDT.

However, I will be concerned regarding the lacrimal glands, so I will warn the patient regarding the risk of dry red eyes, as well as radiation keratopathy and cataracts.

You mentioned that you would not offer radiotherapy to a patient with Gorlin syndrome. Please tell me more about this syndrome, and why wouldn't you offer radiotherapy to this group.

- Gorlin syndrome is otherwise known as nevoid basal cell carcinoma syndrome, and is a rare autosomal dominant cancer syndrome, associated with mutations in the PTCH1/2 and SUFU genes which affect the hedgehog cell signalling pathway and predispose to the development of multiple BCCs.
- It is diagnosed clinically according to major and minor criteria. Alternatively, genetic testing is used if clinical criteria are equivocal.
- Classical clinical findings include palmar pits and odontogenic cysts.
  - Major criteria include:
    - more than 5 BCCs, or
    - a BCC at age less than 30,
    - mandibular cysts,
    - palmar/plantar pits, and
    - a first degree relative.
  - Minor criteria include:
    - cranial anomalies such as macrocephaly, medulloblastoma, and Cleft lip/palate,
    - vertebral and rib anomalies,
    - hand anomalies such as polydactyly, and
    - ocular anomalies.
- Radiotherapy is contraindicated in this group as the carcinogenic effect of the treatment would place them at high risk of developing further BCCs. Non-surgical treatment in this group was available with a Hedgehog inhibitor such as Vismodegib – however, this is no longer available in the UK at the present time.

FURTHER READING

1. Lear J, Corner C, Dziewulski P, Fife K, Ross GL, Varma S, Harwood CA. Challenges and new horizons in the management of advanced basal cell carcinoma: a UK perspective. Br J Cancer. 2014;111:1476–1481.
2. Apalla Z, Papageorgiou C, Lallas A, Sotiriou E, Lazaridou E, Vakirlis E, Kyrgidis A, Ioannides D. Spotlight on vismodegib in the treatment of basal cell carcinoma: an evidence-based review of its place in therapy. Clin Cosmet Investig Dermatol. 2017;10:171–177.
3. Peris K, Fargnoli MC, Garbe C, Kaufmann R, Bastholt L, Seguin NB, Bataille V, Marmol VD, Dummer R, Harwood CA, Hauschild A, Höller C, Haedersdal M, Malvehy J, Middleton MR, Morton CA, Nagore E, Stratigos AJ, Szeimies RM, Tagliaferri L, Trakatelli M, Zalaudek I, Eggermont A, Grob JJ, European Dermatology Forum (EDF), the European Association of Dermato-Oncology (EADO), the European Organization for Research and Treatment of Cancer (EORTC). Diagnosis and treatment of basal cell carcinoma: European consensus-based interdisciplinary guidelines. Eur J Cancer. 2019 Sep;118:10–34. doi: 10.1016/j.ejca.2019.06.003. Epub 2019 Jul 6. PMID: 31288208.

Case 2.7

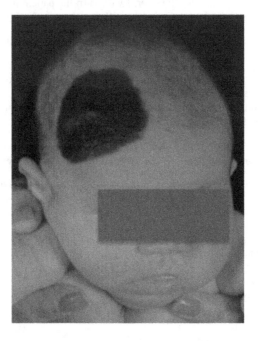

This 3-month-old is referred to you by her GP. Mum is very distressed by the risk that the scalp lesion poses to her baby: she has read online that this carries a risk of melanoma in childhood, and so wants her baby to have this removed as soon as possible to decrease that risk.

How would you manage this scenario?

- This photograph shows a baby with what appears to be a medium-sized congenital melanocytic naevus (CMN) on her anterior scalp, the management of which is widely debated.
- I will first ensure there are no other pigmented naevi, or neurological signs or symptoms, before concentrating on the management of the naevus itself and then counselling the parents.
- The associated lifetime risk of melanoma is much lower than initially reported and is dependent on the size of the lesion and, more importantly, on any evidence of neurocutaneous melanosis.

You mention it being medium sized. What do you mean by this?

These lesions have been categorized by their diameter, with:
- a small naevus less than 1.5 cm,
- a medium naevus between 1.5 and 20 cm, and
- a giant naevus more than 20 cm

Ok, please continue

- I will take a focused history to exclude:
  - other naevi, and
  - symptoms of increased ICP (such as irritability or seizures)
- My examination will exclude:
  - nodules or areas of concern – with dermoscopy if that is the case, as well as
  - clinical signs of raised ICP such as bulging fontanelles.
- I will then organize baseline formal clinical photographs.
- If there are multiple naevi, then I will request a baseline MRI brain and spine with Gadolinium contrast as it gives the opportunity to visualize the characteristic signal for melanin in

DOI: 10.1201/9780429399268-23

neurocutaneous melanosis before myelination takes place at 6 months of age, as well as any other neurological anomaly.

In addition, performing this before 6 months will allow a 'feed and sleep' study with the avoidance of a GA, and its consequent risks of potential developmental delay in infants.

- My indications for routine MRI screening, in the absence of neurology, are:
  - – 20 CMN lesions, irrespective of size,
  - – 2 or more medium lesions, or
  - – a giant congenital naevus.
- If there are any neurological concerns, then I will refer to my paediatric and neurosurgical colleagues for further assessment, in addition to the MRI request.
- If there are any concerning features within the naevus, I will arrange an excision biopsy of the area.
- If there are no other anomalies apart from the lesion in the photograph, then I will inform the parents that accurate estimates of melanoma risk are difficult to obtain and have been historically over-estimated. We do know that the potential risk is related to size. This is considered a medium-sized naevus – which, in addition to small naevi, carries an estimated lifetime risk of melanoma in the region of up to 1%, with most occurring after puberty.

  The risk of melanoma occurring in childhood that they have read about, most probably referred to that of a giant congenital naevus scenario. Here, the lifetime risk of melanoma development is quoted as being in the region of up to 3–5%, with most cases occurring during childhood.

  It is important for them to know that the risk of melanoma represents a generic biological risk unrelated directly to the presence of a specific naevus – so it is not reduced by excision of the lesion as the melanoma may arise in normal skin or other areas such as the CNS, prior to or after excision of the naevus itself.
- So, indications for surgery include:
  1. biopsy of an area suspicious for a potential melanoma,
  2. relieving physical symptoms such as irritation or itching, and
  3. concerns regarding the aesthetic appearance, and parental anxiety.
- Assuming all is correct, then the management of the lesion itself from an aesthetic consideration, does include the option of leaving it alone, as it does not involve an aesthetically sensitive area of the face and many lesions lighten with time – with an improvement in the aesthetic appearance.
- However, if the parents are keen to have it removed, then options include:
  - – serial excision of the lesion,
  - – excision and SSG (preferably from the scalp if possible) – with subsequent serial excision of the graft if required, or
  - – excision and tissue expansion-based reconstruction, although I would avoid that option in those less than 2 years to avoid applying pressure on the developing skull.
- If they are considering surgery, I would counsel that:
  - – Surgery has been shown in some studies to have an adverse effect on outcome with the post-operative development of new naevi, and the darkening of residual naevi (if only partial excision was undertaken), which is thought to be due to the activation and migration of nevomelanocytes.
  - – Early surgery may result in:
    1. over-excision of lesions that could potentially lighten over time,
    2. under-excision of lesions that could continue to evolve in surrounding skin, and
    3. a potential GA-related detrimental effect on the neurodevelopment of infants, so this should be avoided – certainly before 1 year of age, and preferably before 2 years of age – if it is not necessary to proceed at that point.
- I will educate the parents to raise the alarm if they notice red flags such as new nodules, changes in the skin lesion, or symptoms of raised ICP.

I can understand how neurocutaneous melanosis may increase the risk of CNS Malignant Melanoma. But how does it increase the risk of skin Malignant Melanoma in general?

It is unknown why. Postulated theories include that:
- it may be an indicator of a higher burden of mutated cells in the body as a whole,

- the in-utero somatic mutation happened at a particularly crucial stage of development, in those with complex congenital neurological disease, or
- those with abnormal MRIs have other genetic risk factors predisposing both to congenital neurological disease and malignancy.

The parents ask about the possibility of treating it with Laser, again as they read about it online. What would you advise?

- Laser treatment of this lesion is controversial, and I personally wouldn't advise it:
  - The tissue changes resulting from laser photothermolysis of CMNs may result in difficulty with monitoring for signs of malignant transformation in pigmented cells left behind in the deeper dermal layers.
  - In addition, I expect that it may render dermoscopy of any future nodule, unreliable.
  - Furthermore, I am not convinced it would improve the aesthetic appearance either.
- Laser may be beneficial for management of unwanted residual hair following excision, but I don't consider it a good modality for primary treatment of the lesion itself. However, I am aware that this is debated and is used by some of my colleagues in other centres and other countries.

You mentioned tissue expansion – please tell me about that.

- This is the progressive recruitment of tissue of a specific quantity and quality – such as a particular colour, texture, hair-bearing, or sensate skin, with relatively minimal donor site defect and morbidity – albeit with a potentially significant aesthetic deformity during the expansion process.
- The effects are due to the phenomenon of:
  - mechanical creep when the tissue is acutely stretched – which accounts for most of the tissue gain, and
  - physiological creep when it is chronically stretched.
  - Histological changes of mechanical creep include:
    - straightening of collagen fibres and realignment parallel to one another along the vector of force,
    - micro-fragmentation of the elastic fibres, and
    - displacement of water from the ground substance.
      This is the basis of the phenomenon of stress relaxation seen intraoperatively, whereby the force required to maintain tissue elongation decreases over time.
  - The histological changes caused by physiological creep are due to stretch-induced signal transduction pathways promoting:
    - Epidermal proliferation – promoted by decreased contact inhibition and cell gap junction disruption. This is maximal at 6–12 weeks post expansion and normalizes at 6 months.
    - Dermal thinning – with realignment of the dermal collagen, fragmentation of the elastin fibres and flattening of the dermal papillae. This normalizes at 2 years.
    - Finally, angiogenesis occurs in a similar fashion to delayed flaps.

What are your general contraindications when considering expansion as a management plan in any patient?

These are physical, psychological, and social. In a paediatric patient, then I will also consider the psychological and social factors concerning the parents.

- Physical factors include infection, an irradiated field, an unstable scar or graft, or suspected malignancy.
  - I avoid expansion in the extremity if possible, and consider it a relative contraindication due to high levels of complications.
  - I also prefer to avoid scalp expansion in those less than 18–24 months, to decrease the potential of applying pressure on the developing skull – with reported complications in those less than 1 year.
- Psychological factors include: a patient or parent who will not tolerate a potential significant aesthetic deformity during the expansion process, which may take several months.

- Social factors include:
  - a patient or parent whose social situation or employment renders them unable to make multiple outpatient visits, or to consider multiple operations.
  - I also prefer to avoid the 'terrible twos' in children, if possible, as they tend to be less cooperative during that time.

The parents choose to go ahead with expansion. Please talk me through your planning – including your preferred timing, technique, and post-operative management.

- As this is essentially an aesthetic procedure, I personally prefer to wait until the child is nearing 3 years of age if the parents agree, as this will:
  - increase baby's blood circulating volume and minimize blood loss-related complications,
  - minimize the risk of neurodevelopmental delay associated with early GAs,
  - decrease the potential pressure effect on the developing skull of an infant, and
  - it would also avoid the 'terrible twos', with poor cooperation.
- If they insist on earlier surgery, then I will offer serial excision or excision and SSG, after the age of 1 year, to avoid the first two factors that I have mentioned.
- My plan will be to consider:
  1. the implant choice,
  2. the expander pocket plane, site, and size, and
  3. the incision site.
     - With regard to implant choice:
       - I will choose a crescent-shaped expander, as it has a high yield tissue gain and its shape is most conducive to scalp advancement. A rectangular implant is an alternative as this shape offers the maximum percentage gain.
       - I will choose a stable rather than a soft base to ensure expansion occurs superficially and minimizes bone change, with a base diameter at least equal to that of the lesion, and preferably 2.5–3 times the defects' width. If the parents agree to two implants, then this will decrease the expansion time and provide a backup if one of them fails.
       - I prefer a remote port in children, as it less distressing for them.
     - With regard to the expander pockets:
       - I will minimize the risk of implant exposure and extrusion by:
         - placing the expander in the subgaleal rather than the subcutaneous plane,
         - ensuring the expander pocket is at least 2 cm away from the incision, and
         - ensuring the pocket size is 1–2 cm larger than the expander on each side to allow overexpansion.
       - I will ensure the planned pockets and the direction of expansion avoid expanding the forehead, as the anterior margin of the lesion is at the level of the anterior hairline.
       - In addition, I will consider the direction of the hair follicles in the planned advancement flap and the adjacent scalp to ensure they correspond.
     - Once I have planned the direction of expansion and pocket size, then the incision site is planned just within the lesion, parallel to the margin, and perpendicular to the axis of expansion.
        This will avoid tension on the scar and allow me to excise the scar as part of the CMN excision later.
     - I will ensure the expander is filled intraoperatively to 20% capacity, to fill the dead space and prevent a seroma on insertion. Colouring this fluid with some Bonney's blue ink will help identify the correct chamber for expansion in the future.
     - I will wait for 3 weeks before starting post-operative expansion to allow the scar tissue to withstand the tension. The process of expansion will occur at weekly intervals until the skin blanches or the baby is in discomfort.
     - Once the desired tissue gain is achieved, I will then stop expansion and plan for removal 3 weeks after that.
     - At the time of surgery, the expander is over-expanded even further to allow for further stress relaxation, prior to removal of the implant. I will score the capsule perpendicular to the direction of advancement to increase flap mobilization.

How do you know when to stop expanding?

- If the base diameter of the expander is equal to the diameter of the lesion, then I will stop once the dome length is about 3.5× the diameter of the melanocytic lesion if I am using one expander:
  - This is because the theoretical tissue expansion is equal to the dome length minus the base diameter of the expander.
  - In fact, the real tissue gain is only about 1/3 of the calculated tissue gain (it's 32%).
  - I therefore need to inflate the expander to achieve a dome length 3× the diameter of the lesion in order 'to gain one diameter', and I then inflate further to 3.5× to ensure I am not short of tissue and the closure is not under tension.
- I will alter this accordingly if I am using more than one implant.
  For example: I will stop once the dome lengths are about 2–2.5× the diameter of the lesion if I am using two implants, calculated by assuming I need to expand each dome by 1.5× the diameter of the lesion in order to gain half a diameter each (0.5 × 3), and then I inflate further to 2–2.5x the diameter to ensure I am not short of tissue.

How would you manage an exposed expander?

- If it is clinically infected then I will remove the expander, wash the capsule, and allow the wound to heal, before reinserting another expander 3 months later and continuing with expansion in the future.
- If it is simply exposed and at the end of the expansion, then:
  - I will close the wound and continue with the expansion to complete it with antibiotic cover, or
  - remove it if there is sufficient tissue or it is not critical to attain the planned expansion.
- If it is exposed in the beginning of expansion, then I will remove it and reinsert it 3 months later once the scar is stable and the tissues have settled.

Following excision of this pigmented lesion, would you routinely monitor this patient?

- With regard to the skin lesion, then no, I won't routinely monitor this child. There is no evidence to suggest that clinical monitoring makes any difference to outcome.
- With regard to the CNS risk:
  - I won't routinely monitor the child if the baseline MRI were normal.
  - However, if the MRI shows any anomaly, then they would be managed in conjunction with my neurosurgical MDT colleagues who would make that decision based on the anomaly.
- The parents would be advised to return if:
  - the child forms any new pigmented lesions, as their lifetime risk of melanoma is not reduced or
  - they develop any neurological symptoms.

Ok. Let's consider another scenario where the parents bring the baby back to see you, prior to any excision, with a small area of thickening in the middle of the lesion. What now?

- I will aim to exclude malignant transformation by:
  - examining the thickened area dermatoscopically,
  - palpating the cervical lymph nodes,
  - obtaining new photographs, and
  - carrying out an urgent biopsy to exclude malignancy.
- A histopathological diagnosis of melanoma needs to be confirmed by two histopathologists as melanocytic lesions are more difficult to diagnose at this age. For this reason, I will manage this patient within the regional paediatric oncology board, in addition to the skin MDT.
- If the histology is positive, then, in addition to the standard management for a melanoma, I would also request:
  - a brain MRI with contrast – to exclude any change from the baseline MRI, and
  - NRAS and BRAF genotyping, as there have been very small animal studies showing MEK inhibitor use for NRAS mutation-positive patients to relieve the signs and symptoms of leptomeningeal disease – if this is present also.

What features of dermoscopy would you see in a CMN, and which features would make you worried about a potential melanoma?

- The commonest dermatoscopic findings for CMN include:
  - haloed and target globules, and
  - blotches and perifollicular hypopigmentation.
- Those concerning for melanoma include:
  - a 'blue-white veil', which is an irregular area of confluent blue pigment with a ground glass haze as if the image is out of focus,
  - multiple brown dots,
  - radial streaming,
  - scar-like depigmentation due to areas of melanoma regression, and
  - peripheral black dots and globules.

Ok. Let's consider a different scenario – what would you do if the parents report a seizure and increasing irritability? She has been admitted under the paediatric team. Now what?

A seizure, in the absence of a febrile illness, is concerning for CNS disease so I would request another brain and whole spine MRI with gadolinium contrast and involve my neurosurgical colleagues.

The MRI is reported as normal, but her symptoms continue. What now?

I will continue to involve the paediatric and neurosurgical team within the MDT and suggest a repeat MRI 2 weeks later as I am aware that leptomeningeal disease may not be radiologically detectable in the early stage.

FURTHER READING

1. Kinsler VA, O'Hare P, Bulstrode N, Calonje JE, Chong WK, Hargrave D, Jacques T, Lomas D, Sebire NJ, Slater O. Melanoma in congenital melanocytic naevi. Br J Dermatol. 2017 May;176(5):1131–1143.
2. Waelchli R, Aylett SE, Atherton D, Thompson DJ, Chong WK, Kinsler VA. Classification of neurological abnormalities in children with congenital melanocytic naevus syndrome identifies magnetic resonance imaging as the best predictor of clinical outcome. Br J Dermatol. 2015;173:739–750.
3. Kinsler VA, Aylett SE, Coley SC, Chong WK, Atherton DJ. Central nervous system imaging and congenital melanocytic naevi. Arch Dis Childhood. 2001;84:152–155.
4. Price HN. Congenital melanocytic nevi: update in genetics and management. Curr Opin Pediatr. 2016 Aug;28(4):476–482.
5. Arad E, Zuker RM. The shifting paradigm in the management of giant congenital melanocytic nevi: review and clinical applications. Plast Reconstr Surg. 2014 Feb;133(2):367–376.
6. Navarro-Fernandez IN, Mahabal GD. (2022). Congenital Nevus. [Updated 2021 Aug 9]. In: StatPearls [Internet]. StatPearls Publishing, Treasure Island, FL. Available from: https://www.ncbi.nlm.nih.gov/books/NBK559270/
7. Braun TL, Hamilton KL, Monson LA, Buchanan EP, Hollier LH Jr. Tissue expansion in children. Semin Plast Surg. 2016;30(4):155–161.

Case 2.8

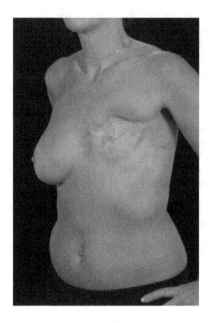

Please describe this photograph.

This is a photograph of a lady who has had a right-sided mastectomy with a lateral longitudinal scar and a split skin graft. I cannot see any radiotherapy tattoo marks.

It is unusual to resurface a mastectomy pocket with a skin graft, so I suspect that the patient may have had a delayed reconstruction (as the resultant defect is elliptical) which may have failed, and a split skin graft was used to close the wound temporarily.

This lady has just moved to your catchment area and would like to consider her options. What is your general approach in the management of a patient seeking a delayed breast reconstruction?

- My reconstructive aims following a mastectomy include:
    1. achieving breast symmetry by replacement of breast volume, and skin – if required – to match the contralateral breast,
    2. addressing the contralateral breast – if required by the patient, and
    3. reconstruction of the nipple-areolar complex – if required.
- I will start with a focused history and examination to establish her oncological and patient-specific factors.
    - Salient oncological treatment factors include:
        - any previous radiotherapy treatment, and
        - the exclusion of recurrence.
    - Patient-specific factors include her wishes regarding:
        - symmetry within or outwith a bra,
        - the contralateral breast,
        - whether she has firm preconceptions regarding autologous or non-autologous-based reconstruction, and
        - her attitude to scarring, the length of surgery, and recovery time.
- This is followed by assessment of:
    1. her BMI, comorbidities, and fitness for surgery,
    2. the contralateral breast (regarding current volume, shape, and quality of the soft tissue envelope),

DOI: 10.1201/9780429399268-24

3. the recipient site and any available donor sites,
4. any significant constraints which may affect her donor site options – be it occupational, due to specific hobbies, or family commitments, and
5. the causes of any previously failed treatment, and her suitability for further treatment.

How would these affect your plan?

- Regarding her oncological treatment factors:
  - I will delay treatment for 1 year following the last radiotherapy dose to allow the tissues and recipient vessels to recover.
  - I will also ensure I exclude a recurrence prior to reconstruction.

What about chemotherapy and predicted survival? Would these affect your plan in this case?

- Chemotherapy treatment is relevant in a patient who is due an immediate reconstruction but not so in a delayed setting, as inflammatory changes take effect 6 weeks post chemotherapy and last for 6 months.
- With regard to predicted survival, this will not affect my plan if the patient is fit for surgery, as it is not uncommon to perform DIEP reconstructions in the setting of stable metastatic disease if this is recommended by the MDT.

Why do you have a cut-off for BMI? And how would you manage this lady who presents for reconstruction, had her BMI been greater than 30?

There is evidence of increased donor site complications such as abdominal dehiscence in those with a BMI of greater than 30.

In a delayed setting such as this, I will encourage her to lose weight, supported by the breast reconstruction specialist nurse, who will put her in touch with weight management programmes that are financially subsidized by the NHS.

What would you do if she is unsuccessful and severely distressed by her mastectomy scar?

- I will organize an MDT planning meeting to determine the overall benefits and risks of surgery.
- If the high BMI is an isolated risk, and the mastectomy scar is causing her severe psychological distress, then I may decide to proceed with the following surgical adaptations, such as:
  - minimal undermining of the abdominal tissue,
  - conservative resection to ensure absolute tension-free closure of the abdominoplasty with minimal flexion of the hip, and
  - the use of incisional negative pressure dressing.
- But I would much prefer to wait until she decreases her risk herself with supervised weight loss.

Ok, please continue.

- With regard to recipient site assessment:
  - I will assess for skin quality and any radiation damage, which, if significant, will affect any planned expansion or dissection of recipient vessels.
  - I will then assess for the amount of skin required to achieve symmetry, by first measuring the clavicular-to-IMF distance on the meridian of the contralateral breast to be matched, and then subtracting the measurement on the breast to be reconstructed.
  - I will check for pectoralis major and anterior axillary fold preservation, and
  - check for the function of latissimus dorsi, as its' innervation is a good indication for the probability of thoracodorsal vessel preservation.
  - I will complete my examination by considering the maximum skin dimensions that can be harvested from the following donor sites in order of preference (if not contraindicated):
    - the abdomen for a DIEP – if it hasn't already been used in this case,
    - the medial thigh for a TUG/PAP flap, and
    - the lower back for the LD flap or a possible lumbar artery flap.
- I will advise her that a purely implant-based reconstruction is not be a recommended option here, especially in the context of a skin graft closure and the possibility of radiotherapy.

Tell me – Would you discount a DIEP in a patient with a previous laparotomy?

- Not necessarily, but I would alter my surgical approach if I decide to go ahead.
- To help me make that decision, I will first establish:
  - the type of laparotomy (be it midline/paramedian, etc.),
  - the length of time that has elapsed since then to determine the expected scarring, and
  - perforator availability with a CTA.
- If I do decide to go ahead, I will:
  - avoid the side with the scar if the scar is not midline,
  - minimize any undermining, and
  - consider the use of a prolene mesh if the scar extends below the umbilicus – within the DIEP territory, to decrease the risk of herniation – as the muscles would have already been manipulated at the previous procedure.

You mentioned radiation damage earlier. What is radiotherapy exactly, and how does it work?

- Radiotherapy is the therapeutic use of ionizing radiation for the primary, adjuvant, or palliative treatment of mostly malignant disorders.
- Electrons, neutrons, or protons are accelerated by microwaves in a linear accelerator, then hit tungsten to produce high-energy X-rays.
- These X-rays deliver photons, which interact with tissue molecules to cause ionization, releasing electrons.
- The resultant injury can be direct or indirect:
  - direct injury causes DNA damage, which subsequently prevents mitosis of the cell.
  - Indirect injury occurs when the released electrons produce secondary damage by the production of oxygen-free radicals and hence is oxygen-dependent.

What are the possible effects of radiation damage that you've talked about?

- The acute effects on the skin include:
  - erythema,
  - tanning, and
  - desquamation.
- Chronic effects are caused by microvascular changes or stem cell depletion.
  - The most serious of which include:
    - osteoradionecrosis
    - cardiac damage, and
    - secondary malignancy.
  - Other chronic effects include:
    - endarteritis obliterans with damage to the endothelial vascular lining,
    - neuropathy,
    - lymphoedema, and
    - cutaneous effects (such as telangiectasia, ulceration, loss of hair, sweat and sebaceous gland function).

How are these sequelae reduced?

By using the principle of fractionation and hyper fractionation:

- Fractionation is the practice of dividing the total dose and administering it over a period of time to allow recovery of normal tissue and the oxygenation of hypoxic areas (to encourage further indirect injury to the tumour cells).
- Hyper fractionation uses smaller daily doses over the conventional treatment time. This theoretically allows dose escalation with a similar tumour response and reduced late tissue damage.

Let's reconsider this lady with a failed DIEP flap following radiotherapy. What will you offer her?

- Repeat surgery is a significant undertaking for the patient in terms of recovery, so I will first discuss the option of a prosthesis if she were open to that.
  - However, I am mindful of the fact that irradiated skin is at risk of breakdown, which may be further irritated by a prosthesis, particularly in the summer months.
  - In addition, the psychosocial effect cannot be underestimated as daily activities may be severely affected by a prosthesis moving or falling out.
- With regard to her surgical options:
  - I will offer her another free flap if the cause of the previous failure was known and avoidable (such as technical error), as a free flap will give her the best aesthetic result. If she agrees to this, then I will go through the donor sites that I have discussed before.
  - If the cause of the flap failure was unknown, I would consider another free flap in a physiologically optimized patient.
  - However, if the flap failure was unavoidable (such as a previously unknown coagulopathy that cannot be corrected), then I will not offer further surgery.

You proceed with another free flap. Which recipient vessels will you use? The internal mammary vessels were used last time.

- My first choice is to try and use the internal mammary vessels again by dissecting the internal mammary vessels in a higher space than previously used – unless the second interspace was used before, in which case:
- I will proceed with my second choice of thoracodorsal vessels. However, they may have been damaged or seriously scarred during an axillary clearance, in which case:
- My third option is to use the thoracoacromial vessels.

Why are the IMA vessels your first recipient choice, and why would you attempt to use them again?

- They offer numerous advantages, such as:
  1. the anastomosis allows zone 1 of the flap to be placed in the medial aspect of the breast, where the tissue is most needed,
  2. they lie within the mastectomy field so a separate incision is not required,
  3. a shorter pedicle is required than with a thoracodorsal anastomosis, and
  4. the IMA is more superficial and more accessible than operating in a deeper field, such as with the thoracodorsal vessels.

Why don't you use preoperative imaging to view these vessels, rather than have to make an intraoperative decision? You have mentioned using that earlier to investigate the DIEP post laparotomy.

The difference here is that an MRA or CTA is not currently sensitive enough to detect the suitability of the recipient vessels, as it would not pick up scarring for example. It is used to preoperatively assess for IMA size in patients with chest anomalies such as pectus patients, but it is not reliable enough in this case.

You mentioned your order of preference for recipient vessels. What if all three were unsuitable? What's next?

I would use vein grafts to reach the transverse cervical vessels or the contralateral IMAs. However, using the contralateral vessels would result in a synmastia, so the patient would have to be preoperatively counselled regarding that.

You mentioned avoidable and unavoidable causes of free-flap failure. What are the causes of free-flap failure in general?

These can be classified into preoperative, intraoperative, and post-operative factors.

- Preoperative factors include:
  - poor choice of patient (such as a known coagulopathy) and
  - poor flap choice (e.g., too bulky causing compression of pedicle).

- Intraoperative factors include:
  - technical error to the pedicle during flap raising, preparation of vessels, or during the microsurgery,
  - flap or pedicle inset with kinking or twisting of the pedicle, and
  - poor intraoperative anaesthesia – hypothermia, hypovolaemia, and vasoconstriction.
- Post-operative factors include:
  - hypothermia, hypovolaemia, and vasoconstriction, and
  - external pedicle compression, such as from tight dressings, a swollen flap, or a misplaced drain.

You mentioned analyzing the CTA. Please tell me about the perforating patterns of the DIEA.

- This has been described by Moon and Taylor with three types:
  - Type 1 is a single main vessel which releases perforators.
  - Type 2 consists of two branches which go on to release perforators. This is the most common.
  - Type 3 is a trifurcation of the vessel.
- This information is valuable as the second or third branch in a type 2 or 3 may be used in a bipedicled flap, or to optimize circulation (e.g., in a large flap, or an SIEA-dominant flap or if the venous drainage is insufficient).

How would you approach the reconstruction of a patient with a quadrantectomy?

- Planning factors for a breast-conserving option include:
  - the overall size of the breast,
  - affected quadrant, and
  - any radiotherapy.
- For a large breast with enough remaining tissue, a breast reduction technique may be sufficient- with modification of the pedicle based on the affected quadrant.
- In a small breast, this would not be applicable, so I would need to decide whether I need to bring in fresh skin, fat, or both:
  - If both are required such as with post-radiotherapy poor skin quality, and/or volume loss that is distorting the nipple, then I will use:
    - local perforator flaps such as a lateral or medial intercostal artery perforator flap (LICAP/ MICAP), or
    - a small latissimus dorsi flap in the case of a high medial distortion (following a medial upper quadrantectomy).
  - If only fat is required and a fat transfer is considered, then I would need to be mindful that the fat take is lower in a post-radiotherapy setting.

Case 2.9

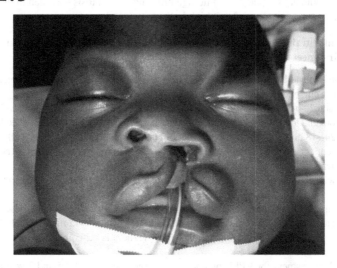

Please describe this photograph.

- This is the photograph of an intubated infant with a left sided complete cleft lip and alveolus and associated nasal deformity.
- With regard to the lip, I can see:
  - discontinuity of the skin and soft tissue of the upper lip,
  - vertical soft tissue deficiency of the lip, and
  - abnormal attachment of the lip musculature into the alar base and nasal spine.

Cleft lip features I would also expect to see are:
  - a cleft in the alveolus at the site of the subsequent canine tooth eruption, and
  - a defect in the hard palate anterior to the incisive foramen.
- The visible features of a cleft nasal deformity include:
  - deviation of the nasal spine, columella, and caudal septum away from the cleft side,
  - separation of the domes of the alar cartilages at the tip (creating a wide tip), and
  - retrodisplacement of the nasal base on the cleft side.

Other features I would expect to see consist of:
  - dislocation of the upper lateral nasal cartilage from the lower lateral on the cleft side,
  - a kink in the lateral crus of the lower lateral cartilage on the cleft side, and
  - flattening and displacement of the nasal bone on the cleft side.

What is the embryological origin of the cleft lip and palate?

- The cleft lip is a failure of fusion of the maxillary prominence (derived from the first branchial arch) and the medial nasal prominence (derived from the central frontonasal prominence), which normally occurs in the 7th embryological week of development.
- A cleft palate is due to failure of fusion of the lateral palatal shelves:
  - These initially project downwards from the maxillary prominences into the oral cavity on either side of the tongue at the 7th week.
  - They then elevate into a horizontal position in a matter of hours in the following week, followed by fusion with one another and the nasal septum from anterior to posterior.
- The exact mechanism for the initiation of palatal elevation is unknown, but theories include:
  - the hydration of glycosaminoglycans,
  - a change in the connective tissue involving the inhibitors of metalloproteinases (TIMPs), and

DOI: 10.1201/9780429399268-25

- a mechanical component due to tongue depression – as a result of head elevation in the 8th week and foetal swallowing.

   This would help explain how micrognathia and glossoptosis – as seen in the Pierre Robin sequence – force the tongue to sit high in the mouth and prevent adequate palatal elevation.

How would you inform the parents regarding the proposed treatment plan and timeline for their child, when you first meet them?

- I would have expected the parents to have already been informed of their treatment plan by the cleft specialist nurse, either at:
   - the prenatal 20-week scan, at a subsequent 4D scan – at which time they would have been informed of the potential for a cleft palate and what to expect – including the impact on feeding, or
   - within 24–48 hours after birth – with feeding assessment and advice, as well as a paediatric assessment for associated anomalies such as cardiac anomalies and an offer for a genetic assessment.
- However, I will go through the timeline of treatment again when I first meet them, by informing them that:
   - A cleft lip repair is timed at 3 months, with or without a McComb nasal dissection.
   - A cleft palate repair – if required – is planned for the age of 9–12 months including intravelar veloplasty in addition to grommets insertion – if there is otitis media with hearing loss >55 dB compared to the better ear.
   - A speech assessment for VPI is planned for between the ages of 2.5 and 5 years – if present – then this will necessitate a:
      - palate re-repair,
      - palate lengthening,
      - pharyngoplasty, or
      - pharyngeal flap.
   - Secondary lip or nasal tip deformities are addressed at school age (around age 5).
   - An alveolar bone graft is placed prior to canine eruption, at about age 8–10.
   - A septorhinoplasty is performed at puberty – if required.
   - Lastly, maxillary advancement and mandibular surgery are planned at the time of skeletal maturity – if required.

You haven't mentioned presurgical orthopaedics. What is this?

- Presurgical orthopaedics, which refers to the passive or dynamic manipulation of the infant's alveolar segments prior to a lip repair, is controversial:
   - Its objective is to facilitate the primary lip repair by narrowing the cleft, but there is a great burden of care – with at least 3 months of daily care required at home, and in the case of dynamic devices – weekly adjustments by an orthodontist.
   - In addition, in the case of passive devices, there is some RCT evidence to show that these do not achieve sustained improvement in alveolar alignment, and worse still, there is evidence to show a detrimental effect on growth in the case of dynamic devices, even though there may be some aesthetic improvement in the repair following their use – especially in wide clefts.

Is this timeline accepted throughout the world?

- No, there is debate regarding:
   - the timing of surgery, and
   - the techniques that are used.
- With regard to the timing of repairs, there is a paucity of prospective randomized trials so there is little firm evidence as to the optimum timing: we do know that delayed palatal repairs result in improved midfacial growth, but this is at the expense of poor speech development due to palatal incompetence. It is generally accepted in the UK that palatal repair should have occurred by 13 months, to prevent an impact on speech. However, the findings of the TOPS trial will give us definitive information as this multicentre RCT aims to determine the impact of timing of palatal repair on speech – with some groups performing surgery from 6 months onwards.

- An accepted conventional timing of lip repair is when the child attains the 'three 10s': 10 weeks of age, a Hb of 10 g/gl, and a weight of 10 lb.

  Other centres advocate neonatal repair within 48 hours of birth, but this has now fallen out of favour as:
  - it has been shown to damage mother-baby bonding with no evidence of improved surgical outcome,
  - it is difficult to pre-operatively diagnose any associated conditions,
  - there are technical difficulties due to the small size of the structures to be repaired, and
  - the logistical organization of surgical teams can be difficult to achieve in a timely fashion.
- With regard to techniques, there are a multitude of established cleft lip and palate repairs, as well as procedures to address the cleft nose and velopharyngeal incompetence – each with their advantages and disadvantages, and little definitive evidence as to the superiority of one over the others in terms of long-term outcomes, hence the continued wide variation in practice.

Mum asks why her child has this abnormality. She is worried that this is her fault and asks about the chances of any future children being affected also. How would you manage this?

- I would start by stating that it is important for her to know that no one is to blame.
- A cleft lip, with or without a cleft palate, is the most common facial difference – with an incidence of 1/700 live births, so three babies are born with a cleft every day in the United Kingdom.
- There is marked racial heterogeneity, with the incidence in children of Asian origin twice that of those of Caucasian origin, who, in turn, have double the incidence of those of Afro-Caribbean origin.
- The causes are multifactorial – with:
  - a known familial association, as well as
  - an association with certain environmental factors such as alcohol, anticonvulsants, possibly folic acid deficiency, tobacco, and retinoic acid.

    There is a current large national cohort 'Cleft Collective Study' led by the University of Bristol to determine how environmental factors interact with genetics, amongst other end points.
- I will let her know that the statistics I will go through are based on multiple studies of different populations, so they represent observations and cannot be used for accurate predictions – for which genetic testing is required.

  Nevertheless, I will go through the average figures for her general information:
  - The relative risk of a child having a cleft lip and palate, with no history in the family is in the region of 0.1%.
  - If no parents are affected, and there is one affected sibling, the relative risk for the next child being affected is in the region of 4%.
  - If a parent alone is affected with no siblings, the risk for the next child is in the region of 2–8%.
  - But if two children are involved, the risk for the third is in the region of 9%.
  - If one parent and one child are involved, the risk for a future child is in the region of 17%.
- Lastly, I will put them in touch with the nurse specialist for support and the UK Cleft Lip and Palate Association (CLAPA) for family support and information.

Please describe the anatomy of a cleft palate deformity, and how you would rectify that in a cleft palate repair.

- A cleft palate may be:
  - complete,
  - incomplete, or
  - submucous
    and
  - unilateral or
  - bilateral.
- The tensor and levator veli palatini, both central to the velopharyngeal sphincter, have anomalous insertions – with:
  - an abnormal attachment of the aponeurosis of the tensor veli palatini along the bony margins of the cleft, as opposed to the posterior border of the hard palate, and

- – Levator veli palatini is attached into the aponeurosis of tensor veli palatini and is cleft, thus interrupting its function as a muscular sling.
- The aim of a cleft palate repair is to achieve:
  - – a three-layer closure of the palate – including the nasal mucosa, muscle and oral mucosa,
  - – lengthening of the palate,
  - – restoration of the muscle sling across the soft palate, and
  - – ensuring minimal dissection and disturbance of the greater and lesser palatine vessels to avoid growth disturbance.
- Vomerine flaps would have been used to close the hard palate at the time of the lip repair.
- My favoured cleft repair technique is:
  - – The Von Langenbeck technique – which consists of a midline adhesion with bipedicled oral mucoperiosteal flaps – created with releasing incisions lateral to the neurovascular bundles to allow closure of the oral layer.
  - – This is combined with an intravelar veloplasty by dissecting out the abnormal musculature and recreating the normal muscle sling of the soft palate.
    I am aware of other centres favouring a Furlow repair instead of an intravelar veloplasty as they cite advantages of additional lengthening of the soft palate, with some evidence of a lower fistula rate. However, speech results have been shown to be equal with both techniques, despite the disadvantage of failure to achieve the anatomical repositioning of the intravelar veloplasty.

Mum rings the cleft specialist nurse post-operatively to say she has noticed a 'hole' in her baby's palate. How would you manage this?

- I suspect that the baby has either developed a post-operative fistula or the 'hole' represents the unrepaired alveolar cleft, that mum may not have noticed before.
- Management a new fistula will depend on its location – be it the hard or soft palate and any associated symptoms. I will arrange to see them both in clinic for assessment and, in the meantime, ask the nurse to establish if there are signs of:
  - – possible infection – such as poor feeding and pyrexia, in which case oral antibiotics are needed expeditiously,
  - – regurgitation (with fluid or solid food), or
  - – hypernasality.
- As per my original treatment timeline, I will manage the unrepaired alveolar cleft with an alveolar bone graft just prior to the eruption of the canine teeth.
- With regard to a post-operative fistula, I will observe a small asymptomatic fistula and reserve surgery for a symptomatic one:
  - – If surgery is required, then my aim is to achieve two-layer closure with a local turnover mucosal flap or vomerine flap, whilst avoiding overlapping oral and nasal suture lines to minimize recurrence.
  - – If local tissue is not sufficient, or scarred, then my next options include:
    - a buccinator flap, or
    - a FAMM flap if there is an alveolar gap.
    - My last option is a tongue flap.

You mentioned alveolar bone grafting of the cleft alveolus at aged 8–10, how do you perform that, and why wait so long?

Early grafting has been shown to affect midfacial growth, and specifically waiting for the ideal time just prior to the eruption of the canine has been shown to result in optimum restoration of alveolar bone height.

In most instances, the bone is harvested from the cancellous bone of the iliac crest, but I am aware that others harvest this from the tibial plateau. The graft is packed into a repaired gingival pocket in the alveolar cleft to help support the alar base.

How would you repair this cleft lip?

I use the Fisher technique: this has evolved from the Tennison-Randall and Millard techniques, with the most important advantage being scar placement along the junction between aesthetic subunits – along the philtral column on the cleft side, as opposed to using a back cut and breaching the philtral column in a Millard repair.

In addition, it shares the advantages of other techniques, such as:

- addressing the length discrepancy between the cleft and non-cleft side,
- addressing the discrepancy in the height of the dry vermillion – with the Nordhoff triangle, which is also a feature of many other repairs,
- creating a natural reconstruction of the alar base, by rotating it upwards and inwards on the cleft side, and
- allowing the muscle to be repaired accurately.

Please draw this and talk me through your markings

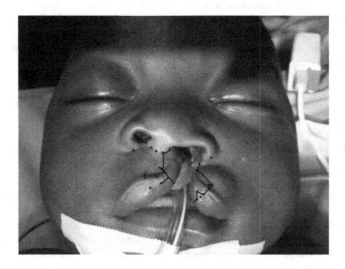

I will start with my markings on the medial lip element, then proceed to the nasal markings, and finally the lateral lip elements:

1. I first mark the midline at the columellar base, followed by
2. the height of the non-cleft philtral column at the columellar base. This is mirrored to mark the height of the cleft philtral column and would normally use a calliper for this.
3. I mark the trough of the cupid's bow and the peak of cupid's bow on the non-cleft side.
4. Next, I will measure the distance between these points and transpose this to create the other peak of cupid's bow.
5. I then mark the white roll-cutaneous junctions at each cupid bow peak, followed by
6. a proposed cutaneous back cut: this point is 1–2 mm from the cleft side peak of cupid's bow and is oriented perpendicularly to the philtral column and will receive a small cutaneous triangle from the lateral lip element to lengthen the cleft side aspect of the medial lip element if that is necessary.
7. I then mark the wet-dry border on the vermillion. This is perpendicular to each point that was marked on the white roll.
8. I mark a vermillion back cut, which will receive a vermillion triangle from the lateral lip – if the height of the dry vermillion is inadequate.
9. I then mark each alar base. In the operating room, the lateral lip side alar base can be manually rotated in to ensure symmetric marking.
10. Next, I mark the distinctive convexity of the non-cleft nostril sill.
11. Now I mark a symmetric point on the nasal floor to the cleft. This will be the site of closure of the nasal floor. The aim of this is to produce a sill of the same width, and a nasal aperture of the same size and shape. This marking can be manipulated if there is insufficient tissue to obtain a symmetric nasal floor.

12. The total lip height is measured on the non-cleft side from the columellar base to the white roll – with the lip at rest.
13. I next measure the greater lip height on the cleft side of the medial lip element, whilst elevating the cleft nostril with a Ragnall retractor to move the dome to the correct position – to give a true length.
14. The lesser lip height is calculated by subtracting ('the greater lip height +1 mm') from the total lip height element.
15. The lateral lip element markings will be more variable from the medial lip to accommodate for differences in lateral lip height.
16. I then mark Noordhoff's point – which is the point with the greatest vermillion height with a full thickness white roll. I then double check that the point I have marked should have a normal white roll and a near normal vermillion thickness to avoid central vermillion deficiency.
17. I then mark the white roll just above this.
18. I measure the non-cleft nasal floor width from prior marks, before marking the same width from the cleft side alar base to the nasal floor.
19. I measure the cleft side nasal sill width with a calliper to use this measurement to locate a point on the lateral lip element.
20. I mark the base of the cutaneous triangle from the previous measurements of total/greater/lesser lip height.
21. This triangle will be connected to the point that I have previously marked. And this distance will match the cleft side philtral column.
22. I mark the wet-dry border on the cleft side, and
23. I then mark an isosceles triangle of vermillion to fit into the previously designed back cut.

You mentioned other available techniques. What are these?

The Millard technique was very popular due to intraoperative adaptability and the relative ease of secondary revision.

It has been labelled a 'cut as you go technique' as it is possible to adjust the lip lengthening intra-operatively, with secondary revision made possible by re-elevation and rerotation of the flaps. However, it has been abandoned by many for the Fisher technique, as a small portion of the scar does cross the philtrum the nasal base.

I am aware of other techniques such as the Rose-Thompson straight line technique, the Tennison-Randall Lower Lip Z plasty technique, and the Skoog Upper and Lower lip Z plasty technique, most of which have now fallen out of favour.

How would you consent the parents for this repair?

There are early risks of wound dehiscence, infection, bleeding, and scar widening.

Over time, scar contractures may lead to vestibular stenosis: narrowing of the nostril sill and shortening of the lip segment with notching of the vermillion, and the creation of a whistle deformity.

I will reassure them that their baby will be back to feeding the way they were before, straight after surgery – if the baby will take it, with the huge variety of bottles available.

I am aware that other units may use elbow splints, but there is no evidence to show this improves results.

How would you manage a whistle deformity?

- In patients where the deficiency is relatively localized, then my first choice is to use a V-Y advancement, with the V in the lip sulcus. This also allows for the correction of the attenuation of orbicularis – if present.
- In those with a deficiency along the whole length of the lip, then I will use a dermal graft. It is simple and can be repeated in the case of resorption. However the disadvantage is that it can be difficult to position them correctly.
- I am aware of the use of laterally based Kapitansky advancement flaps, if there is a discrepancy in the wet dry vermillion; however, the accepted disadvantage is that they leave a lot of scarring along the lip, so I prefer to avoid this.

How does this differ in a bilateral cleft lip repair? What would be your management principle then?

- In a bilateral case, the premaxilla is initially protuberant as its growth is unrestrained, then it may become relatively hypoplastic as the infant grows.
- The principle for repair is the same as in unilateral cleft lip repair: to address the muscular repair and skin repair. There is no consensus on the best technique for repairing bilateral cleft lips – one reason being their relative rarity.
- The cleft may be narrowed with:
  1. Presurgical orthopaedics – but this is controversial as I discussed earlier.
  2. The alternative is a lip adhesion prior to definitive repair (which makes the definitive repair easier –with a decreased risk of muscle dehiscence, but with a disadvantage of an additional GA).
- In very wide deformities, I may consider staged surgery with the repair of one side before the other. The key to any technique is a strong muscle repair along its whole length from the nasal spine to the vermillion edge with no tension.
- The most common technique is the modified Mulliken repair, which is a straight-line repair with premaxillary skin preservation, and midline repair of the muscle that is brought in from the lateral elements. The tension on this midline repair would have been reduced with a previous lip adhesion.
- In order to create a deep sulcus, the wet vermillion from the premaxilla can be used to line the anterior surface of the premaxillary alveolus.
- Alternative techniques include the Millard and Manchester repairs:
  - The Millard repair uses forked flaps from the lateral aspect of the prolabium, which are rotated under the alar bases, but this creates an overly long columella.
  - The Manchester repair uses straight line incisions, but this doesn't repair the muscles at the midline, leaving an empty philtrum and a 'Cheshire cat' smile due to the gap in the orbicularis and the resulting disruption of the pull by the other facial muscles – with alteration in the vector of pull.

How would you address a cleft nose?

- This may be addressed primarily – at the time of lip repair, or secondarily.
- My approach is to consider primary nasal surgery in patients with wide clefts, using a limited McComb technique, and delay the secondary rhinoplasty as much as possible – until nasal growth and midface growth are complete, which is usually by the age of 16.

  At this point, a LeFort I advancement for maxillary hypoplasia can restore normal maxillary projection, before a final rhinoplasty is undertaken.
- However, if there is significant deformity, then I may elect to address the nose earlier by:
  - performing an early tip rhinoplasty at the age of 4–5 to elevate the tip, without affecting growth as the septum is not touched, or
  - a rhinoplasty at preschool age.
- The principle of primary nasal surgery is to use sutures to reposition the caudally rotated lower lateral cartilage – either percutaneously in the case of the McComb technique or via an intranasal incision in the case of the Tajima technique.
  This is controversial as:
  - some believe that this may cause scarring and possible damage to the cartilage, with nostril stenosis at its most severe – especially with the more invasive incisional technique.
  - In addition, some question the relative need for this, as release of the orbicularis muscle and repair of the cleft lip will itself help rectify some of the nasal deformity. This is because Orbicularis oris inserts into the columella on the non-cleft side, creating an unopposed force that pulls the columella and caudal nasal septum to the non-cleft side. On the cleft side, it inserts into the nasal base, retracting it laterally and inferiorly, which is worsened by the poor maxillary skeletal support at the alar base.
  - However, I agree with those who believe that there will be a residual significant deformity without this in patients with wide clefts.

- Regarding the secondary rhinoplasty, I aim to address the following:
  - The alar cartilage on the cleft side, which differs in shape and position and creates a poorly defined nasal tip with less projection.
  - Deviation of the caudal septum in the cleft side nasal airway, which can be significant and results in nasal airway obstruction. In addition, this is compounded by nasal obstruction at the external nasal valve from the introverted alar cartilage.
  - In the case of a bilateral cleft lip patient, there is a greater level of symmetry, but with a much shorter columella, as the medial crurae are splayed very widely. The degree of this is related to the extent of prolabial development, cephalic nasal tip rotation, and cleft severity.

A 4-year old child is referred to you with distinctly hypernasal speech. What do you suspect, and how do you proceed?

- I suspect a submucous cleft palate that may have been missed during routine screening, with hypernasality due to velopharyngeal dysfunction.
- My management plan consists of:
  - a focused history to exclude other cleft palate sequelae such as feeding difficulties and recurrent middle ear effusions,
  - clinical examination for signs of Calnan's triad – consisting of a bifid uvula, a zona pellucida, and a palpable notch in the hard palate – with the understanding that 10% may have an occult presentation, and
  - confirmation with videofluoroscopy, with a flexible nasoendoscopy, if required, to confirm the velopharyngeal closure pattern, and the severity of it.
  - An MRI and EUA may be used to investigate less common situations of persistent uncertainty.
  - Treatment of confirmed velopharyngeal dysfunction – in a symptomatic child like this one – consists of:
    - A Furlow repair in the first instance, with continued speech therapy. (Others may use an intravelar veloplasty instead)
    - A pharyngoplasty or pharyngeal flap is reserved for patients with persistent hypernasality. Posterior pharyngeal wall augmentation (such as with fat or Teflon) is popular elsewhere in the world but carries a catastrophic risk of embolization, so I would shy away from this technique.
- As with the treatment of visible cleft palate defects, there is debate regarding the optimal treatment of submucous clefts:
  - The first debate relates to whether the first line option should be palatal reconstruction or pharyngeal surgery, and
- the second is regarding the exact technique to be used. With regards to the debate of first line palatal versus pharyngeal surgery:
  - Proponents of palatal reconstruction as the first option, such as myself, suggest that normalizing the anatomical abnormality is the first step. This does not compromise the airway, and if hypernasality persists then the option of pharyngeal surgery remains.
  - I understand that other protocols include reserving palatal surgery for patients with small gaps on lateral vidofluoroscopy and pharyngeal surgery for those with larger gaps (with variability with regard to the cut-off point used).
- With regard to the optimal palatal technique:
  - proponents of using the intravelar veloplasty in the first instance rather than a Furlow double opposing Z plasty argue that Furlow repairs result in a levator tip overlap with a potential for asymmetrical movement. However, this has not resulted in any clinically apparent speech deficit.
  - The Furlow repair has the advantage of being technically easier. In addition, it results in lengthening of the palate, and also reduces nasal airflow, as the transverse laxity is used by the Z plasty to obtain the lengthening effect – thus making the palate easier to close.

What are the pharyngeal options for patients with persistent hypernasality, and which will you choose?

- These include:
  - sphincter pharyngoplasties, or
  - posterior pharyngeal flaps.

- There is yet further controversy on the optimal option with no strong evidence regarding the superiority in outcome of either.
- My rationale will depend on the velopharyngeal closure pattern seen on nasoendoscopy and vidofluoroscopy, even though I accept that there is no strong evidence that this makes any difference to results.
  - I will opt for a sphincter pharyngoplasty technique, such as an Orticochea method, in coronal and circular closure situations to preserve palatal mobility.
  - In sagittal closure cases, I will use a posterior pharyngeal flap technique to preserve the lateral pharyngeal wall mobility.

What are the three closure patterns that you referred to?

These are:

1. coronal – where closure is achieved by posterior movement of the soft palate towards to the pharynx,
2. sagittal – where closure is achieved by lateral pharyngeal movement toward the midline, and
3. sphincteric – where closure involves equal contribution from the velum and lateral pharyngeal walls.

FURTHER READING

1. *A surgical tutorial on the markings of the Fisher unilateral cleft lip repair is found on the website of the Cleft Lip and Palate program at the Children's Hospital of Philadelphia:* https://www.chop.edu/pages/fisher-unilateral-cleft-lip-repair-surgical-tutorial-professionals

Case 2.10

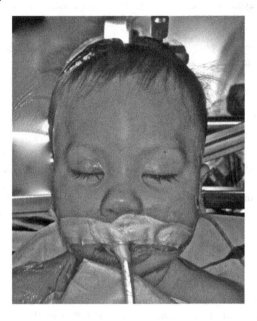

Please describe this photograph.

This is an intraoperative photograph of an intubated infant with the facial features of trigonocephaly, including:

- a metopic ridge,
- bitemporal narrowing, and
- hypotelorism.

What is craniosynostosis?

- This is the premature fusion of one or more cranial sutures, as an isolated anomaly or part of a syndrome. Consequent abnormal cranial growth, described by Virchow's law, occurs predominantly parallel rather than perpendicular to the affected suture, due to the arrest of the normal perpendicular growth at the affected suture site, and the compensatory over expansion at the patent suture sites.

    This leads to abnormal head shapes, facial anomalies, and possible raised intracranial pressure (more commonly in the case of multiple synostoses).

- The aetiopathology includes:
    1. multifactorial factors – as is the case in 80% of patients, such as:
        - mechanical,
        - environmental, and
        - genetic factors.
    2. single-gene mutations – in about 15% of patients with mutations such as FGFR, TWIST, TCF-12, SMAD6, and ERF, and
    3. conditions associated with an increased risk of craniosynostoses, such as:
        - vitamin D deficiency,
        - hypophosphatemia,
        - rickets, and
        - mucopolysaccharidoses.

DOI: 10.1201/9780429399268-26

What are your treatment aims?

- My treatment aims for those with a single synostosis include:
  1. identifying and managing raised ICP, and
  2. addressing a cosmetic deformity to improve psychosocial interactions.
- Patients with complex and often syndromic craniosynostosis may have additional treatment aims to address:
  1. airway compromise,
  2. ocular protection, and
  3. to improve occlusion.

How would you manage this infant if they were brought to clinic?

- I would manage him within the craniofacial MDT – with core members consisting of the craniofacial surgeon, neurosurgeon, psychologist, paediatrician, ophthalmologist, ENT surgeon, orthodontist, speech therapist, geneticist, and specialist nurse.
- A targeted history will establish:
  - the birth history,
  - general health of the infant,
  - any possible familial component,
  - a developmental history,
  - any features of functional compromise, and
  - any aesthetic concerns expressed by the family.
- My examination will establish:
  - the head circumference,
  - the facial and cranial morphology, as well as
  - clinical signs suggestive of ICP, such as a full or tense anterior fontanelle.
- A CT scan with 3D reconstruction is helpful to:
  - confirm the diagnosis and exclude the involvement of another suture or intracranial anomaly,
  - exclude any radiological signs of raised ICP, such as:
    - diffuse copper-beaten appearance,
    - reduced extra-axial space,
    - ventricular effacement, and
    - suture diastasis, as well as
  - aiding in surgical planning.
- Cranial remodelling surgery is offered to address an increase in ICP and/or to address the aesthetic sequelae. It consists of remodelling of the fronto-orbital bandeau and the frontal bone to:
  - remove the metopic prominence,
  - increase the bitemporal width, and
  - increase cranial volume.

How would you proceed if you, or your MDT colleagues, are concerned about the possibility of raised ICP in an infant with a single-suture synostosis, such as this one?

- A baseline ophthalmic review should be performed in the first instance to look for signs of raised pressure – with the understanding that children younger than 8 can have raised ICP with no papilloedema seen on fundoscopy, so direct measurement with an intraparenchymal pressure probe for 24–48 hours will be required to confirm this.
- Although there is controversy regarding the paediatric normal range for ICP, a baseline consistently above 15 mmHg, or more than three abnormal Lundberg waveforms in a 24-hour period, is considered suggestive of significantly raised ICP.
- Therefore, if surgery was already considered by the MDT and agreed to by the parents for aesthetic reasons, and a preoperative CT has excluded any other anomaly that may contribute to a raised ICP, then cranio-remodelling surgery will treat a raised ICP – if present. In this case, invasive ICP monitoring is unlikely to further contribute to clinical management, so would not be indicated.

- However, if surgery was not going to be offered for aesthetic reasons, e.g., if the aesthetic sequelae were very mild, or if surgery was not agreed to by the parents for purely aesthetic reasons, then the measurement of ICP is indicated.

Why does fundoscopy have a lower sensitivity for the detection of raised ICP in young children compared to adults?

It has been postulated that this may be due to:

1. a greater compliance of unfused sutures in the immature cranium, possibly buffering the effects of increased ICP on the optic nerve, and
2. reduced communication of subarachnoid spaces with the optic nerve sheath in infants may reduce the clinical evidence.

Case 2.11

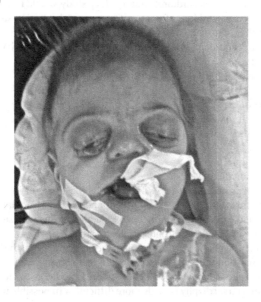

Please describe this photograph

This is an intraoperative photograph of an infant placed on a warming blanket with turribrachycephaly, downslanting palpebral fissures, lagophthalmos, and exorbitism. I note a tracheostomy and possible lateral tarsorrhaphies.

This patient has Pfeiffer syndrome. Please tell me more about this

- This is an autosomal dominant syndrome with FGFR2 mutation on chromosome 2 with an incidence of 1:100,000 live births. A minority of patients with less severe phenotype have FGFR1 mutation.
- It manifests as
  - a turribrachycephaly with bicoronal synostoses, or
  - as a Kleeblattschadel or cloverleaf with numerous synostoses, in 25%.
- Intracranial anomalies include hydrocephalus and Chiari malformation.
- Orbital anomalies include exorbitism, hypertelorism, downslanting palpebral fissures, and strabismus.
- Midface anomalies include midface hypoplasia with a low nasal bridge.
- Classically, they have broad thumbs and halluces.

What is FGFR and how does the mutation of this contribute to these phenotypes?

FGFR signalling plays an important role in numerous biological processes, including bone development and homeostasis by controlling the differentiation of mesenchymal and neuroectodermal cells. Mutations in FGFR 1, 2, and 3 results in unregulated FGF signalling and premature suture closure.

Tell me – How would you approach the management of this patient from birth?

- This patient should be managed in a craniofacial centre within an MDT consisting of a craniofacial surgeon, neurosurgeon, oral surgeon/orthodontist, ENT surgeon, ophthalmologist, speech therapist, paediatrician, geneticist, child psychologist, and specialist nurse.
- In this specific case, the most immediate goals are to:
  1. manage the airway,
  2. manage the eyes, and
  3. manage the ICP risk.

DOI: 10.1201/9780429399268-27

- Longer term goals include normalizing their head shape and appearance with multiple operations during their lifetime.
- With regard to the airway risk, a cardiorespiratory sleep study should be performed to screen for obstructive sleep apnoea, as children often manifest airway obstruction subacutely with episode of hypoventilation rather than acute obstruction, that is more common in adults.

  This may be due to central apnoea in syndromic infants, or due to airway obstruction at any of the following sites:
  - the underdeveloped midface resulting in airflow obstruction
    - within the nose,
    - at the level of the palate and tongue base, as well as
  - anomalies of the larynx and trachea
  Surgical options include:
  - a tracheostomy or
  - a monobloc procedure.
- With regard to managing their eyes:
  - Globe subluxation is an emergency with the potential to result in permanent vision loss. I would manage this with liberal and frequent application of ocular lubricants as well as training parents and carers on the immediate reduction of this with sterile warm wet gauze.
  - Orbital volume is corrected with frontofacial surgery.
  - A tarsorrhaphy may be considered, as is seen in the photograph, but the indications for this are debated, as it may result in increased pressure on the globe, as well as the residual potential for subluxation despite reducing the palpebral width. In addition, reducing the subluxed globe in the presence of a tarsorrhaphy is made more difficult or impossible without surgical release of the tarsorrhaphy.
- With regard to the ICP risk, a neurosurgical opinion should be part of the MDT management as this may be elevated in syndromic patients due to:
  - multi-sutural synostoses and cephalocranial disproportion, or due to
  - additional intracranial pathologies (such as obstructive hydrocephalus from aqueductal stenosis or a Chiari malformation).

    If the raised ICP is purely due to the cephalocranial disproportion, then the treatment is to increase the cranial volume. In young infants, with small circulating volumes of 70–80 ml/kg, this is best achieved with posterior vault expansion surgery, as it is less morbid than cranial remodelling, with a lower risk of hypovolaemia from even small amounts of blood loss. This allows a temporary increase in cranial volume until the infant is older and able to safely undergo cranial vault remodelling.
- If there are no acute concerns to address, then the overall plan is:
  1. Posterior vault expansion to address cephalocranial disproportion and raised ICP at 6–12 months.
  2. Fronto-orbital remodelling at age 12–18 months to address the brachycephaly and increase the orbital volume.
  3. A lefort III procedure is then offered to advance the midface and further improve the airway and aesthetics – usually at early school age.
  4. Otherwise, a Monobloc may be considered to achieve the advantages of the fronto-orbital remodelling and lefort III midface advancement, in either:
     - an infant or toddler for primarily functional reasons – particularly if there are repeated globe subluxations which threaten sight, or
     - it may be offered from pre-secondary school through adolescence for primarily aesthetic reasons.
  5. Finally, Orthognathic surgery is offered at skeletal maturity.
- However, I am aware of wide variation of practice in the management of syndromic patients in different craniofacial centres, both in the United Kingdom and internationally – with considerable debate regarding the indications for and timings of:
  - tarsorrhaphies,
  - tracheostomies,
  - Monoblocs, and
  - the types of posterior expansion procedures, amongst many other considerations.

This child has a tracheostomy, as per the photograph.

Please tell me your indications for this, as well as your understanding of the considerations regarding the airway management of a syndromic craniosysnostotic child with obstructive sleep apnoea.

- My indications for a tracheostomy in this scenario include:
  - establishing an airway when other treatments have failed (such as a NPA, CPAP, and intubation) and
  - the post-operative airway management in patients with residual significant obstructive sleep apnoea following frontofacial surgery.
- However, whilst a tracheostomy is able to completely relieve the airway obstruction, there are significant associated morbidities that should be considered in the discussions with the family, including:
  - the need for patients to be monitored 24 hours a day as there is a risk of accidental decannulation or obstruction (particularly in infants who require a very small tracheostomy),
  - the need for secretions to be managed throughout the day, with increased burden of care,
  - an increased risk of chest infections, and
  - the potential of becoming tracheostomy-dependent, with failure of decannulation.
- For this reason, some centres prefer a monobloc advancement as a first-line option to address the airway, with additional benefits of simultaneously obtaining ocular protection and treating the cephalocranial disproportion-as it advances the forehead, orbit and midface as one unit. This may avoid the need for a tracheostomy altogether or at least allow a more likely successful decannulation if it has already been performed.
- However, parents need to be made aware that:
  - Even though frontofacial surgery is safely carried out in high volume centres, it remains a major surgical procedure, especially in infants with smaller circulating volumes.
  - In addition, a monobloc procedure carries a risk of meningitis due to nasocranial communication.
  - Lastly, early frontofacial surgery carries a higher risk for the need for revision surgery later on, with subsequent surgery being more difficult and associated with an increased risk of complications.

    It is for this reason, that many other centres prefer to defer frontofacial surgery as much as possible, if it is safe to do so from an ocular point of view.

How does a monobloc achieve ocular protection?

It advances the orbital rim as part of the monobloc segment and carries the lids forwards to cover and protect the ocular surface.

You mentioned a Lefort III midfacial advancement earlier. Please talk me through that.

- A bicoronal incision is performed.
- Osteotomies are performed through:
  - the zygomatic arch,
  - the frontozygomatic suture,
  - floor of the orbit,
  - nasofrontal suture, and
  - finally, by completing the cuts with a pterygomaxillary disjunction.

    For small advances (up to 10 mm), the new position can be maintained with bone grafts but cranial distractors (which may be internal or external) are generally used for patients requiring larger advancements, as it:
  1. decreases the risk of morbidity from large dead spaces such as bleeding and infection, and
  2. reduces the relapse seen in large advances from static techniques, by overcoming the natural soft tissue resistance by means of gradual stretching and accommodation, generating new soft tissue simultaneously with skeletal augmentation. However, high patient compliance is required, and a second smaller procedure is required to remove the distractor at the completion of treatment.

What are the possible complications of a Lefort III advancement with distraction?

- Complications following a Lefort III advancement include:
  - skull base fractures with intracranial bleeding,
  - zygomaticomaxillary junction fractures,
  - visual loss after retro-orbital haemorrhage,
  - strabismus,
  - anosmia,
  - CSF leaks and dural tears, and
  - infraorbital nerve injury.
- With regards to complications following distraction, these include:
  - frame migration,
  - intracranial migration of the fixation pins,
  - pin site infection and loosening, and
  - asymmetrical advancement.

Please talk me through a monobloc procedure. What are the pros and cons of performing it, versus staging a fronto-orbital advancement with a delayed Lefort III?

- The monobloc procedure moves the entire forehead with the face and is similar to the combination of a fronto-orbital advancement with a Lefort III advancement. This results in a skull base defect which is reconstructed with a pericranial flap to reduce the risk of meningitis from nasocranial communication.
- The staged approach (Fronto-orbital advancement first, then Lefort III) maintains separation of the cranial cavity from the nasal cavity but requires two large procedures.
- Monobloc osteotomies are undertaken in the following order:
  - frontal craniotomy and division of the zygomatic arch
  - circumorbital osteotomies
  - completion of anterior skull base cut across the midline
  - pterygomaxillary osteotomy
  - separation of the nasal septum from the skull base, and
  - downfracture of the frontofacial segment
- This will achieve an advancement of about 1 cm, with distraction used to achieve further augmentation as necessary.
- An anteriorly based pericranial flap is preserved and used later in the anterior cranial fossa floor reconstruction to address the nasocranial communication

A Chiari malformation. What is that?

A Chiari 1 malformation occurs when the one or both cerebellar tonsils descend through the foramen magnum. Treatment should be considered if symptomatic or associated with a syringomyelia. In children with raised ICP due to cephalocranial disproportion, teams may often consider posterior vault expansion, and if this is not successful, then progress to a foramen magnum decompression.

Case 2.12

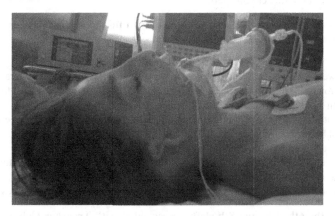

Please describe this photograph

This is the intraoperative photograph of an intubated child with the typical appearance of Treacher Collins syndrome, including zygomatic hypoplasia, a dorsal hump, and a lobular type microtia. I suspect atresia of the external auditory canal but this is not clear in the photograph.

I note the absence of a tracheostomy, which suggests that he does not currently have severe maxillary or mandibular hypoplasia causing severe airway compromise.

What is Treacher Collins syndrome?

- This is a facial cleft 6–8 syndrome which may be autosomal dominant, or sporadic – with a variable phenotype in 1:50,000 births.
- It is caused by a mutation in chromosome 5, mostly of the TCOF1 gene or more rarely the POLR1D or POLR1C genes – which encode for Treacle protein, and subsequent p53-dependent neuroepithelial apoptosis and neural crest hypoplasia.
- Typical features include:
  - eye anomalies such as:
    - downslanting palpebral fissures,
    - a quadrilateral palpebral fissure, and
    - lower eyelid colobomas,
  - ear anomalies such as bilateral microtia, with or without middle/inner ear malformations,
  - hypoplasia of the midface, with or without cleft palate, and
  - hypoplasia of the mandible.

Please talk me through your understanding of facial clefts

- These can affect all layers of the face with a soft tissue defect that does not always correspond with the bony abnormality.
- The exact pathology may be due to:
  - failure of the facial prominences to fuse,
  - lack of mesodermal penetration, or
  - intrauterine compression by amniotic bands.
- They are classified by Tessier into Clefts number 0–30, with a cleft 0, 14, and 30 corresponding to midline clefts of the superior, mid, and lower face, respectively.
- Facial clefts numbered 1–7 are inferior to the orbit, with each subsequent cleft being more lateral than the last, starting with cleft 1 – as a paramedian cleft – and cleft 7 – extending from the lateral aspect of the mouth and curving upwards to the lateral canthus.

DOI: 10.1201/9780429399268-28

- Cranial clefts numbered 8–14 are superior to the orbit, with each subsequent cleft being more median than the last, starting with cleft number 8 – running above the lateral canthus and cleft number 14 – as a midline cranial cleft.

You've mentioned the failure of the facial prominences to fuse as a possible cause of a facial cleft. What is the embryology of facial development?

- Development of the face occurs between the 3rd and 8th week of gestation.
- In the 3rd week, the neural folds fuse to form a neural tube: the cranial neural tube forms a central frontonasal prominence and six paired branchial arches – each of which form a cartilage precursor, an artery, nerve, muscle, and skeletal structure:
    - The frontonasal prominence is destined to form the forehead, nose, and the central upper lip.
    - The first branchial arch develops the maxillary and mandibular prominences, which form the midface and lower face respectively.
        - The maxillary prominence will form the cheeks, maxillae, and lateral upper lips.
        - The mandibular prominences become the lower lip, chin, and mandible.
    - The second branchial arch forms the facial nerve and muscles of facial expression.

You've mentioned the 6th, 7th, and 8th clefts – associated with Treacher Collins. What are their phenotypes?

- Cleft number 6 passes between the maxilla and zygoma and may be associated with a coloboma of the lateral lower eyelid.
- Cleft number 7 runs between the zygoma and the temporal bone. It may extend medially across the cheek into the lateral aspect of the mouth – and may result in macrostomia.
- Cleft number 8 passes outwards from above the lateral canthus. It extends between the zygoma and the temporal bone into the greater wing of the sphenoid.

What is the usual treatment timeline?

- At birth, the priority is the airway, the eyes, and feeding:
    - Obstructive Sleep Apnoea is assessed for using a cardiorespiratory sleep study (called a polysomnogram), and flexible nasoendoscopy can be useful in determining the level of obstruction, which may be multiple.
    - It is managed with prone positioning if mild, progressing to the use of a NPA, CPAP, mandibular distraction, and finally a tracheostomy.
    - If the globe is not sufficiently protected, a tarsorrhaphy or lower lid reconstruction may be required.
    - Enteral feeding may be required via an NG or gastrostomy tube, if there is significant feeding difficulty secondary to maxillary and mandibular hypoplasia.
- In infancy, the focus is on a cleft palate repair, if required, and the management of hearing loss:
    - A cleft palate repair is performed at around 1 year of age – with a preoperative sleep study with imitated closure, to rule out potential post-operative respiratory distress.
    - The use of a soft band hearing device for conductive hearing loss may also be commenced.
- In childhood, the focus is on addressing the anomalies of the:
    - eyelids,
    - zygoma,
    - mandibular hypoplasia, and
    - optimizing hearing and considering external ear reconstruction.
- Finally orthognathic and orthodontic treatment as well as a septorhinoplasty are delayed until adolescence.

What hearing restoration options are you aware of?

These include:

- educational support,
- conventional air conduction hearing aids,

- bone conduction hearing aids, and
- implantable hearing aid devices.

What is a BAHA?

Bone anchored hearing devices (BAHA) are an established treatment for conductive hearing loss, for single sided deafness in children.

There are two broad categories of devices:

- Firstly, the traditional technique uses a titanium osseointegrated implant into the skull bone, onto which an external audio processor is clipped. This is effective in children, but is associated with:
  - implant loss due to failure of osseointegration or trauma, and
  - recurrent skin inflammation.
- A second type of device has been developed which involves the placement of a subcutaneous magnet that transduces vibration from an externally worn processor. This reduces the amount of skin inflammation although skin necrosis has been reported.

You've mentioned osseointegration – what is that?

- This is the formation of a direct interface between an implant and bone without intervening soft tissue, with a histological appearance of a functional ankylosis. The process involves:
  1. an initial incorporation with interlocking between the bone and the implant body, followed by
  2. biological fixation through continuous bone apposition and remodelling towards the implant.
- Titanium was first used in this process described by Branemark, as it is:
  - highly biocompatible,
  - it lacks an inflammatory response in the peri-implant tissues,
  - it has an oxide layer which protects against corrosion, as well as
  - porous surfaces that increase the tensile strength of the bond via bone ingrowth.

Tell me about middle ear implants. How are these different to BAHAs?

These are an option for hearing rehabilitation in children with atresia, which may be used in addition to autologous ear reconstruction. Such devices have both internal and external components – as for transcutaneous BAHAs – but the internal component produces mechanical vibrations, which stimulates the middle ear directly, causing it to vibrate.

You mention that this is a lobular type microtia. Which classification is that based on?

- The Nagata classification divides microtias based on the remnants present into
  - lobular type,
  - conchal type,
  - small conchal type,
  - atypical microtia, and
  - anotia.

What other classifications are you aware of?

There are several others that have been described, such as the Tanzer classification and Weerda classifications, but these are used less commonly in clinical practice.

Tell me, what is the embryology of ear formation?

Answered in Case 3.6.

What about formation of the inner ear?

- This starts in the 4th week and has a different embryological origin to the external ear. This is why hearing loss tends to be conductive rather than a mixed picture of conductive and sensorineural loss.
- Two otic placodes appear as thickenings lateral to the hindbrain that invaginate to form a pit, then close to form a cyst-which then forms the utricle, saccule, semi-circular canals, and cochlea.

- The bony labyrinth is formed from the mesenchyme surrounding the inner ear.
- An invagination of the first branchial groove, called the tubo-tympanic recess, forms the auditory tube and tympanic cavity.
- Finally: Meckel's cartilage, from the first arch, forms the malleus and incus, and Reichert's cartilage forms the stapes.

How would you manage a patient with microtia?

- Patients with microtia and aural atresia have a complex craniofacial condition that may impact all aspects of their lives. It is essential that patients and their families have access to specialized microtia teams with colleagues from ENT, audiology, and psychology, in addition to ear reconstruction surgeons.
- My initial assessment includes:
  - consideration of a renal ultrasound scan, as there is some evidence to suggest an increased frequency of renal structural anomalies associated with external ear anomalies,
  - baseline clinical photographs,
  - age-appropriate audiological assessments, and
  - referrals as appropriate to the geneticist, psychologist, and paediatrician.
- I will liaise with my ENT colleague regarding the optimal timing for placement of a definitive bone anchored device. This may be prior to auricular reconstruction from age 4 onwards, or post auricular reconstruction.
  - Most ear reconstruction surgeons prefer for this to occur post auricular reconstruction to avoid operating in a scarred bed, and I would encourage that – where possible.
  - However, if it occurs prior to auricular reconstruction, then it needs to be placed 6.5–7 cm posterior to the expected position of the external auditory meatus, to allow sufficient space for subsequent ear reconstruction, and to ensure the surrounding blood supply is not compromised.
- With regard to the auricular reconstruction, I will discuss the timing and possible management options:
  - Regarding the timing, I will defer this until about 10 years of age, as this allows:
    - a sufficiently mature patient to weigh up the pros and cons of surgery and make a personal, informed decision,
    - sufficient thoracic cartilage to permit the use of autologous costal cartilage for any reconstruction, and
    - an almost fully grown contralateral unaffected ear, in cases of unilateral microtia.
    - In addition, it predates the pubertal growth spurt when the costal cartilage may hollow.
  - Options include:
    - doing nothing,
    - the use of an external adhesive prosthesis,
    - the use of an internal prosthesis (such as a Medpor porous polyethylene implant), and
    - autologous reconstruction using costal cartilage.
    - Finally, I am aware that tissue engineering may become a reality in the next 5–10 years with teams around the world attempting to culture autologous cartilage onto an ex-vivo ear shaped scaffold.
  - Doing nothing is an important option, as reconstruction should not be undertaken lightly. Many patients are very proud of their un-reconstructed ears and individuals should not be coerced into surgery either by clinicians, or by their families. These patients can be kept under regular review.
  - Prostheses offer an excellent aesthetic alternative for:
    - Patients with poor local tissue (from burns, trauma, or radiation) or
    - Those who are unfit for/or who do not wish to undergo a major reconstructive procedure.
  - Whilst Medpor implants offer an aesthetic result, they risk infection, extrusion, and subsequent scarring. A temporo-parietal fascial flap and skin graft is required to provide vascularized coverage.
    Autologous reconstructions were originally introduced by Tanzer, then subsequently modified by Brent, Nagata, and Firmin. It remains the best long-term reconstructive option.

However, disadvantages include:
- donor site morbidity and residual chest wall deformity,
- the need for staged procedures, and
- potential skin necrosis resulting in downgrading of the aesthetic result.
- Finally, I will give the patient and family information about patient support groups such as Microtia UK and Changing Faces.

Which autologous technique would you use? Please talk me through it.

- I will use the Firmin technique for autologous reconstruction, with two stages starting at about the age of 10. This is a modification of both Brent's four stage and Nagata's two stage techniques – with the goals to:
  - create a harmonious and life-like 3D structural framework, and
  - successfully adapt the skin to it.
- The first stage consists of:
  1. determining the correct location and orientation of the ear and skin pocket (using templates and/or the contralateral ear as a guide),
  2. removing aberrant cartilaginous remnants (except for the tragus and pretragus – if present), and developing a viable skin pocket for the framework,
  3. creating the framework most commonly from the 6–9th ribs (my preference is to use the right side to avoid possible inadvertent iatrogenic cardiac injury, but I am aware that some teams prefer using ipsilateral and others prefer using contralateral ribs),
  4. placing the framework in the skin pocket, and
  continuous suction drainage for 3–5 days to allow good adaption of the skin to the framework.
- The framework consists of:
  - the base,
  - antihelix,
  - helix,
  - tragus/antitragus – if present – and
  - projection pieces.
- The projection pieces may be placed in the first stage if the overlying skin is compliant and the height of the framework does not place the skin flaps under tension – which would compromise flap vascularization.
- Otherwise, they are saved for the second stage, and can be banked under the thoracic skin at the rib donor site.
- Placement options for projection pieces include:
  - as a connecting strut deep to the root of the helix and tragus – to increase stability of the construct and improve the 3D contour,
  - deep to the antihelix – to increase the height of the posterior wall of the concha – and
  - deep to the lobule – to compensate for a hypotrophic mastoid.
- The second stage is undertaken 6 months later to allow good adaptation of the skin to the underlying framework. It consists of:
  - elevation of the framework with a projection block, and
  - creation of the retro-auricular sulcus, with either:
    - an SSG from the scalp, for adequate colour match – if a small projection is needed, or
    - if more projection is needed, then:
      - a mastoid fascia flap and SSG, or
      - a superficial temporoparietal fascia flap and SSG.

How would you choose where to place the ear in patients with anotia?

- Ear placement is based on:
  1. the distance from the root of the helix to the orbit,
  2. the distance from the lobule to the oral commissure, and
  3. the angle determined by the axis of the ear to the nasal dorsum.
  These are measured on the normal side if there is one or that of a parent in patients with bilateral anotia.

- Alternatively, specific acetate templates (such as those described by Nagata and Magritz) can be used with various ear sizes. These are sized and aligned based on the positions of the eyebrow and alar of the nose on the unaffected side.

What complications would you counsel the parents and child for?

- Acute complications consist of:
  - infection,
  - haematoma,
  - skin loss, and
  - donor site complications such as:
    - atelectasis,
    - pneumothorax,
    - chest wall deformity, and
    - hypertrophic scar – which may become significant in girls with respect to the inframammary fold.
- Long term complications include:
  - cartilage resorption, and
  - final size discrepancy in 50% of patients.

How would you address the maxillary hypoplasia that is evident in the photograph?

- This does not cause severe airway distress as the child does not have a tracheostomy, so correction is indicated to support the lower eyelids and improve the aesthetics.
- I will propose lipofilling to increase soft tissue volume to support the lid and optimize the tissue thickness, prior to zygomatic reconstruction with bone grafts or implants – if required.

What would you suspect if this patient also had bilateral radial deficiency of their upper limbs?

I will suspect Nager syndrome, which is a pre-axial acrofacial dysostosis. It is autosomal dominant with facial features similar to Treacher Collins syndrome, but with preaxial limb deformities such as radial deficiency, and less commonly other hand anomalies such as hand syndactyly and camptodactyly.

Please talk me through your understanding of radial deficiency and its management principles.

- This is hypoplasia or aplasia of the pre-axial structures of the upper limb resulting in radial deviation of the wrist, with treatment options based on:
  - the patient's age,
  - the severity of the deformity, and
  - the degree of functional deficit.
- It is most frequently associated with syndromes such as:
  - Holt-Oram – which involves cardiac anomalies,
  - VACTERL – which involves Vertebral, Anal, Cardiac, TracheoEsophageal fistula, and Renal and Lower extremity anomalies,
  - TAR – involving Thrombocytopaenia as well as an Absent Radius,
  - Fanconi anaemia, and
  - Nager syndrome – as in this case.
- Because of that, my management will start with referring any child with radial deficiency to the paediatric team to exclude cardiac, renal, pulmonary, and haematological abnormalities before addressing the limb anomaly.
- I will then clinically and radiographically assess for the degree of:
  - hypoplasia or aplasia of the upper limb as a whole,
  - radial angulation of the hand,
  - hypoplasia of the thumb,
  - function of the elbow – as it may be affected by humeroulnar synostosis, and
  - function of the wrist and hand.

- Treatment options include:
  - Conservative management with splinting and physiotherapy at birth. This may avoid surgery if patients develop and maintain good function, despite a hypoplastic radius.
  - Surgical options include
    - centralization or radialization of the ulna from 6 months onwards, with or without distraction lengthening of the radius – unless surgery is contraindicated, such as in patients with absent elbow movement, who rely on radial deviation of the wrist to allow hand-to-mouth reach.
    - Thumb hypoplasia is managed with pollicization.

What do you mean by centralization and radialization of the ulna?

- Centralization is an option in patients with good elbow movement and involves wrist distraction followed by repositioning of the third metacarpal over the ulna. Radial deviation is counteracted with a closing wedge osteotomy of the ulna and ulnar carpus, and ulnar tendon transfers of FCR, ECRB and ECRL.
- Radialization is reserved for those with reduced movement at the elbow level and involves wrist distraction followed by repositioning of the scaphoid and second metacarpal over the ulna. Again, radial deviation is counteracted by FCR tendon transfer to FCU.

Case 2.13

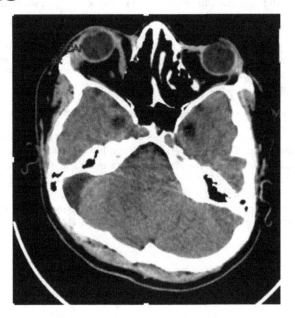

Please describe this image.

This is a coronal cut of a CT head of a child with a positional plagiocephaly.

The head shape assumes a parallelogram configuration with:

- frontal bossing ipsilateral to the occipital flattening, and
- bilateral equal eye-to-ear distance with:
  - anterior ear displacement on the occipital flattened side, and
  - posteriorly ear displacement on the occipital bossing side.

I would expect the cheek position to be prominent on the side of occipital flattening but I am unable to see that on this cut.

How would you manage this child? The parents are extremely worried and arranged for their baby to be scanned abroad where they lived until very recently. Mum is distressed that her daughter's head shape is being commented on at mum and baby groups. She has read a popular 'new Mum's blog' discussing how helmet therapy helped a child's head shape, and they are prepared to 'go private' to obtain this. What would you advise?

- I will reassure them that this is not a craniosynostosis, but a common deformation with no functional consequence, that occurs in up to 50% of infants due to external forces such as:
  - supine positioning – from the 'back to sleep campaign' to decrease the risk of sudden infant death syndrome, and
  - rotational forces, due to:
    - torticollis most commonly and
    - more rarely visual defects.
- Management will include:
  - treating any torticollis or neck stiffness early with physiotherapy,
  - 'tummy time' – to allow baby to spend time lying on their front whilst awake, supervised, and playing,
  - the use of a sling or a front carrier to reduce the amount of time baby spends lying on a firm flat surface, and

DOI: 10.1201/9780429399268-29

- modifying parental lap 'nursing' position to promote contact with the less flattened side of the parental chest.
- However, I will stress that all babies, including those with positional plagiocephaly, must be laid to sleep on their back. Sleeping in positions other than this is associated with an increased risk of sudden infant death syndrome. For the same reason, no pillows or props should be used to change a baby's sleeping position.
- I will also inform them that head shapes usually improve to socially acceptable stages when the child can sit unsupported with time, once the offending external force is removed, but that I cannot guarantee that she will not be left with a possible residual deformity.
- Regarding Helmet therapy, this involves wearing a customized helmet for 23 hours a day with space to allow the flattened area to remould. This requires regular monitoring with serial adjustments, with the risk of pressure injuries. This is not funded by the NHS, as there is no strong evidence to show any significant difference in head shape at 2 years in those who have had this treatment compared to those who haven't.

How does that differ from a craniosynostotic plagiocephaly? How would you manage the infant in that situation?

- Plagiocephaly is due to the premature fusion of the coronal or lambdoid sutures.
- Anterior plagiocephaly presents with restricted ipsilateral growth because of the premature fusion of the ipsilateral coronal suture – so I would expect:
  - ipsilateral frontal flattening and temporal fossa convexity,
  - a recessed supraorbital, lateral, and inferior rim producing a shallow orbit,
  - deviation of the root of the nose to the ipsilateral side,
  - a shorter eye-to-ear distance on that side, and
  - a harlequin deformity as a radiological pathognomonic sign – due to the lack of descent of the greater wing of the ipsilateral sphenoid.
- A posterior plagiocephaly presents with:
  - ipsilateral occipital flattening,
  - ipsilateral mastoid bossing, and
  - contralateral parietal bossing, with
  - typically little facial scoliosis or asymmetry.
- I will manage them within the craniofacial MDT with core members consisting of the craniofacial surgeon, neurosurgeon, psychologist, paediatrician, ophthalmologist, ENT surgeon, orthodontist, speech therapist, geneticist, and specialist nurse.
- A targeted history will establish:
  - the birth history,
  - general health of the infant,
  - any possible familial component,
  - a developmental history,
  - any features of functional compromise, and
  - any aesthetic concerns expressed by the family.
- My examination will establish:
  - the head circumference,
  - the facial and cranial morphology, as well as
  - clinical signs suggestive of ICP, such as a full or tense anterior fontanelle.
- A CT scan with 3D reconstruction is helpful to:
  - confirm the diagnosis and exclude the involvement of another suture or intracranial anomaly,
  - exclude radiological signs of raised ICP, such as:
    - diffuse copper-beaten appearance,
    - reduced extra-axial space,
    - ventricular effacement, and
    - suture diastasis, as well as
  - aiding in surgical planning.
- Cranial remodelling surgery is offered to address an increase in ICP and/or to address the aesthetic sequelae.

Which surgical procedure would you propose to normalize the appearance of a patient with an anterior plagiocephaly?

I will propose:

- a frontal craniotomy,
- fronto-orbital advancement,
- repositioning of the frontal bar, and
- recontouring of the frontal bone.

When would you do this, and why?

I will defer it until 12–18 months of age. This is ideal as it:

- avoid the complications of neonatal surgery such as the risk of blood loss in very low circulating volumes as well as general anaesthetic complications, and
- the bones are still malleable at this age, and there is less compensatory growth and asymmetry.

FURTHER READING

1. NICE Guidance [NG127]. (2019) Suspected Neurological Conditions: Recognition and Referral.
2. Wilbrand JF, Wilbrand M, Malik CY, Howaldt HP, Streckbein P, Schaaf H, Kerkmann H. Complications in helmet therapy. J Craniomaxillofac Surg. 2012 Jun;40(4):341–346. doi: 10.1016/j.jcms.2011.05.007. Epub 2011 Jul 8. PMID: 21741852.
3. Kmietowicz Z. Expensive helmets do not correct skull flattening in babies. BMJ. 2014;348:g3066. PMID: 24791750.
4. Tamber MS, et al. Congress of neurological surgeons systematic review and evidence-based guideline on the role of cranial molding orthosis (helmet) therapy for patients with positional plagiocephaly. Neurosurgery. 2016 Nov;79(5): E632–E633. PMID: 27776089.
5. van Wijk RM, van Vlimmeren LA, Groothuis-Oudshoorn CG, Van der Ploeg CP, Ijzerman MJ, Boere-Boonekamp MM. Helmet therapy in infants with positional skull deformation: randomised controlled trial. BMJ. 2014 May 1;348:g2741. doi: 10.1136/bmj.g2741. PMID: 24784879; PMCID: PMC4006966.

Case 2.14

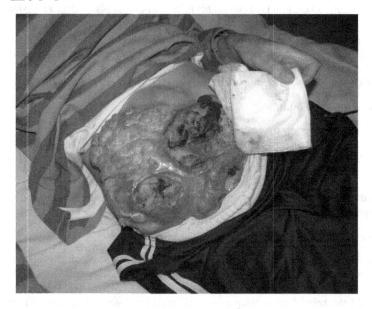

This patient presents to your clinic with the above lesion. He has had problems with IV drug dependency and has been homeless for many years. This has only come to light when he showed it to a doctor from the local needle exchange programme. How would you proceed?

- This patient presents with a significant lesion of the anterior abdominal wall. The visible area affects at least the left half of the anterior abdominal wall, and possibly even the groin and pubic areas.
- My primary concern is that this is malignant – unless proven otherwise – and my plan will be to:
  - establish histological diagnosis,
  - establish the extent of disease, and
  - manage this patient within a skin MDT to determine the optimal plan – whether that is curative or palliative.
- My focused history will determine:
  - the onset of the lesion – which will give me an idea regarding its clinical progression, and the reason for the possible delay in presentation – particularly mental health disease. I anticipate from the history that I may need to involve the mental health and social care teams.
  - Their comorbidity, smoking, and alcohol history will establish their WHO and frailty scores to determine if this patient is fit for a possible major surgical procedure.
- My examination will establish:
  - the clinical extent of the lesion, and
  - palpable inguinal lymph nodes.
- I will establish an urgent histological diagnosis with outpatient clinic incisional biopsies at the junction of the tumour and normal skin margin – perpendicular to the lateral margin, as this is where viable representative tumour is most likely to be present for histological assessment (as opposed to a biopsy of the centre of the tumour with a high risk of sampling necrotic tissue).
- I will request an urgent MRI of the abdomen, and a CT of the chest/abdomen/pelvis to:
  - determine whether this is surgically resectable, and
  - exclude regional and distant spread.
- Lastly, given his history, I will obtain his consent to test for hepatitis C/B, HIV, and TB for his own and staff protection, if his infectious status is not known already.

DOI: 10.1201/9780429399268-30

So, it transpires that this is an SCC that has spread to his chest, liver, and thoracolumbar spine. How will you proceed? He is now complaining of severe pain, and it is extremely malodorous.

This is stage IV disease, so the aim is to control his pain and possibly also induce remission.

- I will suggest palliative radiotherapy to the skin MDT.
- The MDT oncologist may also suggest concomitant immunotherapy such as Cemiplimab, which is a PD-1 systemic checkpoint inhibitor.
- Charcoal dressings may also help with the odour until then.

What is a PD-1 checkpoint inhibitor?

This is a type of immune therapy treatment.

PD-1 is a checkpoint protein on T cells. It acts as a type of 'off switch' by inactivating T cells when they bind to other cells using this protein – including cancer cells. So, inhibiting this process boosts the immune response.

Let us change the scenario: the lesion is shown to involve the full thickness of the abdominal wall and involves the right inguinal nodes only.

The FNA of the nodes comes back as an SCC. What now?

- This is a challenging situation as the lesion is theoretically and anatomically resectable.
- I need to first establish the patient level of fitness within the MDT, before a joint decision is made regarding the possibility of curative treatment.
- I will enlist the help of my colleagues in anaesthesia and general surgery to help determine his fitness, as it will likely involve a subtotal resection of the anterior abdominal wall, the reconstruction of this, and an inguinal dissection. We would need to establish his cardiorespiratory reserve, exercise tolerance, albumin level, and POSSUM score.
- If we deem him to be suitable as an MDT, then I will present the option to him with the understanding that he is likely to have a protracted hospital stay with the risks of
  - post-operative respiratory compromise with atelectasis/pneumonia,
  - flap loss – if used,
  - abdominal sepsis and the development of fistulae,
  - DVT/PE, and
  - death.
- The alternative would be the possible option of palliative chemoradiotherapy (if the oncologists had given the green light for that).

What about the reconstruction: what would that involve?

- In a patient who is fit for a free flap, I will use an acellular dermis to reconstruct the abdominal fascia and bilateral ALTs, or a large free LD, or likely – a combination of those.
- I would prefer an ALT reconstruction, if possible, to decrease further chest wall morbidity, as his respiratory compromise is already at risk following a morbid abdominal procedure.
- If the patient is not fit for a major reconstruction, then this can be staged with an SSG to graftable areas – including the peritoneum. However, this will leave the patient with a significant abdominal wall weakness, which can be revised later with a flap reconstruction when the patient has had more time to be further optimized.

How do you perform an inguinal dissection?

I will ensure:

- supine positioning with hip abduction on a vein board,
- a lazy S incision from the anterior superior iliac spine to the medial thigh,
- development of lateral and medial flaps just above the superficial fascial plane from the medial border of Gracilis to the lateral border of sartorius muscle– whilst avoiding the lateral femoral cutaneous nerve,

- ligation of the saphenous vein tributaries,
- the fatty node-bearing tissue is swept cephalad to the saphenofemoral junction, with ligation and division of the saphenous vein (and oversewing of the femoral end),
- retraction of the inguinal ligament to expose the femoral canal, and
- removal of nodal tissue.

What if the scan also showed involved pelvic nodes – how would you proceed?

I will ensure an MDT assessment to ensure he is fit for a pelvic node dissection, even more so if the open – as opposed to an endoscopic – approach is used.

How would you perform an open pelvic node dissection in this man?

I will perform this in conjunction with my general surgery, vascular or urology colleagues, depending on my MDT set up, but the principle is to:

- place deep self-retaining retractors such as an Omni-Tract and divide the external oblique aponeurosis,
- displace the spermatic cord medially and divide the inferior epigastric vessels,
- displace the peritoneum medially to expose retroperitoneal structures,
- begin laterally on the pelvic sidewall and sweep nodes and associated tissues medially,
- mobilize the rectum and bladder medially and retract these behind moist packs,
- perform an obturator node dissection by following the obturator nerve and artery,
- obtain haemostasis and reapproximate abdominal wall structures, and
- place closed-suction drains and close in layers.

Case 2.15

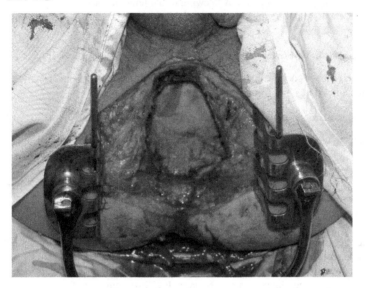

Please describe this photograph.

This is an intraoperative photograph of a patient with a perineal defect, who has likely undergone an abdominoperineal resection or pelvic exenteration.

How would you approach the reconstruction of this patient?

I will plan the reconstruction within a colorectal MDT. My aims are to:

- close the resultant dead space,
- provide vascularized tissue to a likely irradiated area – if that is the case,
- reconstruct the pelvic floor – if required – and
- provide skin cover – if required.

Why not just close the defect directly once the tension from the retractors is removed?

There is strong evidence to support the use of immediate flap reconstruction for patients such as this, with improved wound healing and a decreased risk of pelvic sepsis, as well as herniation of pelvic organs.

What is your flap of choice in this instance?

- This is dependent on the structures that needs to be reconstructed-whether that is:
    - the pelvic floor, or
    - just the external skin, or
    - both
- My go to flap of choice is the IGAP flap because:
    - it is a large flap that provides both volume and skin,
    - it has consistent anatomy so is technically easy to raise, and
    - it has an acceptable donor site.
- If reconstruction of both the pelvic floor and external skin is required, then I will use bilateral IGAPs to achieve this. If only one is required, then a unilateral IGAP will suffice.

    I will reserve a VRAM flap as a backup if the IGAP is not available, e.g., following severe skin involvement either from an extensive resection or previous radiotherapy.

DOI: 10.1201/9780429399268-31

Whilst it is the classical workhorse flap for perineal reconstruction – with bulk and reliable anatomy, it is not my first choice as:

- I prefer to leave the abdominal wall donor site untouched as much as possible, in case my colorectal colleagues need to fashion a urostomy or move a stoma to the contralateral side in the future, and
- there is an associated donor site morbidity with up to 25% of patients left with an abdominal bulge or a hernia.

- Other options include:
  - bilateral pedicled Gracilis flaps to reconstruct the pelvic floor, and
  - local flap options for skin reconstruction – although the local flap donor site tissue is frequently resected as part of the irradiated field.

Please talk me through how you would proceed with a VRAM flap reconstruction.

I will first establish the side that the colorectal surgeons will need for their neo-stoma. It is usually the left side.

The procedure starts with the patient supine. I prefer to raise the VRAM prior to the laparotomy – to minimize operating in a potentially contaminated field.

- I will raise the rectus muscle with a skin paddle based on the predicted skin requirement and the supraumbilical anterior rectus sheath – whilst preserving the posterior and infraumbilical rectus sheathes.
- The deep inferior epigastric vessels are visualized and followed to the external iliac vessels.
- I will then transect the rectus insertion off the pubis using cutting diathermy but ensuring that I preserve the pyramidal component to take the tension off the vessels.
- Once the abdominal resection is complete, I will place the flap in a bag, then rotate the flap 180 degrees to pass it into the pelvis, and then
- incise the peritoneum where the vessels enter it to prevent the vein from kinking along the edge of this.
- I will then close the rectus sheath with a double PDS suture and an onlay mesh to further decrease the risk of an abdominal weakness.

Are you aware of other options to decrease abdominal donor site morbidity following a VRAM?

Yes, these include fascial-sparing VRAMs, and component separation donor site closure has been described.

What is component separation?

This is a procedure popularized by Ramirez to increase the potential for direct closure of the abdomen with possible medial advancement of 3–5 cm per side. It is achieved by division of the external oblique aponeurosis which allows medialization of the rectus/internal oblique/transversus abdominis muscle complex. Release of the rectus muscle from its posterior sheath provides an additional 2 cm of advancement.

Modifications have been described such as:

- an endoscopic-assisted technique, and
- a perforator-sparing technique, where lateral umbilical dissection is avoided to preserve the periumbilical perforators.

How would you manage this patient if they also needed a vaginal reconstruction?

My option would be to use a thin ALT or VRAM, which would be coned over a vaginal mould in a complete vaginal reconstruction. If this is not an option – such as in high BMI patients – then I would use a Gracilis flap.

It is important to plan for an additional flap for bulk and perineal skin, in addition to the flap required for vaginal reconstruction. So, for example, I may use an ALT for the perineal skin and a Gracilis for the vaginal reconstruction.

FURTHER READING

1. Witte DYS, van Ramshorst GH, Lapid O, Bouman M-B, Tuynman JB. Flap reconstruction of perineal defects after pelvic exenteration: a systematic description of four choices of surgical reconstruction methods Plastic Reconstr Surg. 2021 Jun;147(6):1420–1435.

Case 2.16

Please draw a cross section of a penis and talk me through your illustration.

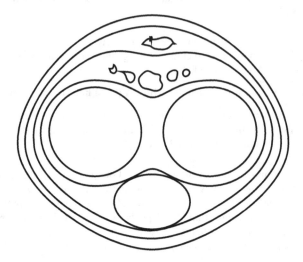

From superficial to deep: Dartos and Buck's fascia are the superficial and deep fascial layers deep to the skin. They are separated by areolar tissue that contains the superficial dorsal vein.

The next layer is the Tunica Albuginea which binds the Corpora cavernosum and Corpus spongiosum together. The deep dorsal vein and both dorsal arteries and nerves lie between the Tunica and deep fascia.

What is hypospadias? And why does it occur?

- This is a congenital condition, which may be familial, and is characterized by the triad of:
  - a proximal meatus on the ventral surface,
  - an incomplete prepuce which may be hooded, and
  - a ventral curvature of the shaft.
- It may also be associated with:
  - urethral valves,
  - paraurethral sinuses, and
  - a flattened glans.
- Proximal hypospadias is associated with:
  - inguinal hernias, and
  - anomalies of the genito urinary tract – including an undescended testis.
- Theories regarding its aetiology include:
  - androgen receptor deficiency,
  - an increase in the levels of environmental oestrogens, and
  - genetic anomalies in syndromic cases, such as chromosome 19 deletion in hand foot genital syndrome.

When you say a ventral curvature of the shaft, do you mean a Chordee?

No, the term chordee is an outdated terminology that has been abandoned by the hypospadias surgical community as it was found to be confusing to patients and parents.

 DOI: 10.1201/9780429399268-32

Penile curvature may occur with or without hypospadias: it is formed by maldevelopment of the corpus spongiosum with consequent fibrotic tethering, regardless of the position of the meatus.

What is the embryology of the development of male genitalia and what is going wrong in hypospadias patients?

- The development of external genitalia occurs in two phases:
    - an early hormone-independent phase (from 5 to 8 weeks of gestation), and
    - a later hormone-dependent stage (in weeks 8–16).
- During the hormone-independent phase, the external genitalia are indistinguishable between males and females.
    - During the 5th week of gestation, mesodermal paired cloacal folds fuse along the midline to form the genital tubercle.
    - These cloacal folds then divide into urogenital folds flanking the urogenital sinus and anal folds posteriorly.
    - Labioscrotal folds then develop on each side of the urogenital folds.
- The hormone-dependent phase of sexual differentiation begins from week 8 onwards, when the gonads have differentiated into testes in XY males.
    - The presence of testosterone produced by the testis causes the genital tubercle to elongate and the urethral groove appears, laterally defined by the urethral folds.
    - The distal portion of the urethral groove terminates in a solid epithelial plate, called the urethral plate.
    - Formation of the urethra starts with canalization of the urethral plate by progressive apoptosis, which is androgen-independent, followed by the androgen-dependent epithelial fusion of the urethral folds along the shaft of the penis from proximal to distal.
    - The genital tubercle then gives rise to the glans and the labioscrotal folds fuse to form the scrotum.
    - Finally, the penile skin, including the foreskin, develops from ectodermal tissue externally covering the entire penile length, and the corporeal bodies arise from mesenchymal condensations.
    - Closure of these structures on the ventral midline gives rise to a ridge of tissue referred to as the median raphe.
- Hypospadias is caused by abnormal or incomplete urethral closure during weeks 11–16 of embryonic development, which may be due to:
    - abnormal formation of the urethral plate,
    - failure of canalization of the urethral plate, or
    - failure of midline fusion of the urethral folds.

How would you manage a baby referred to you with a hypospadias?

- Salient points in the history include:
    - Any family history, if present, then it is important to educate parents regarding the risk of subsequent children having this, with a subsequent risk that is doubled compared to the rest of the population.
    - Witnessed erections, to establish whether they were straight and the direction of urinary stream.
- I will examine the child by:
    - palpating both testes in the scrotum to exclude undescended testes, and
    - feeling for inguinal hernias.
- I will request an upper urinary tract USSS if there is a proximal hypospadias or inguinal hernias.
- Surgical correction depends on the meatal position and the degree of curvature:
    - I would use a two-stage repair for more proximal cases or those with extensive curvature – regardless of the position of the meatus, and
    - a one-stage Snodgrass repair for a very distal hypospadias such as a glandular or coronal hypospadias, with no curvature.

Why would you use a two-stage procedure? Surely one should try and avoid an additional stage if possible?

This produces excellent cosmesis with a slit-like terminal meatus, and is very versatile and applicable to all possibilities – including revisions. So this is my go-to option for all except the most distal cases – unless they are associated with a curvature, in which case I would use a two-stage technique as well.

I reserve one stage techniques for a subcoronal or coronal hypospadias with no associated curvature. This technique has been shown to have a higher revisional rate, with less patient satisfaction in adulthood, if applied to more severe cases – especially with regard to the rate of meatal stenosis. So, if the operation is performed before genital awareness, an extra stage is not detrimental to the patient.

Please talk me through how you would perform a one-stage, and a two-stage repair.

- Prior to any hypospadias repair:
  1. I will intraoperatively assess for a penile curvature using a Horton's test, and release it – if present.
  2. I will also instrument the urethra with Clutton Sounds – until the level of the bladder – to ensure there are no urethral strictures or stenoses. If so, I will enlist the help of my urological colleague for an endoscopic release of this.
- With regard to the one-stage repair:
  1. The first step is glans flap elevation, followed by
  2. urethral plate incision, progressing distally to the level of the corpora cavernosa (which appears bluish).
  3. The neourethra is tubularized over an 8-gauge stent in two layers of 7/0 vicryl, ensuring this is stopped at the midglans level to prevent stenosis.
  4. A ventrally-based waterproofing flap is then raised from the foreskin (to minimize subsequent fistulae), followed by
  5. glans remodelling with 5/0 vicryl and
  6. a prepuceplasty with 6/0 vicryl rapide.
- With regard to a two-stage repair:
  - The first stage consists of splitting the glans longitudinally and using a skin graft to resurface the defect – taken from the inner prepuce if available, otherwise from the buccal mucosa – ensuring I plan for a larger graft to factor in post-operative contraction.
  - The second stage follows the same stages as a one-stage repair now that the first stage has brought enough tissue to enable tabularization, with:
    1. tubularization of the skin graft over an 8-gauge catheter to form the neo-urethra, followed by
    2. a waterproofing flap that is ventrally-based from the foreskin,
    3. glans remodelling, and
    4. a prepuceplasty.

What is a Horton's test? And how do you perform it?

This is an artificial erection test that is performed by placing a tourniquet at the base of the penis and injecting sterile saline into one corpus cavernosum, usually using a blue butterfly needle.

How do you release a curvature that is apparent after the Horton's test?

- This is a controversial topic.
- Penile curvature is arbitrarily termed as a 'mild', 'moderate', and 'severe' curvature with angles of up to 30 degrees in the mild group, 30–60 degree in the moderate group, and 60–90 degrees in the severe group.
- I will preoperatively counsel patients that moderate and severe curvatures are likely to need a graft to release it adequately, with the consequent risk of graft failure.
- I will counsel patients with a mild curvature that there is the option of a Nesbit dorsal plication to fully release the curvature. This avoids a graft but does result in penile shortening by a few mms. If they do not accept this, then the alternative is the potential need for a skin graft.
- Patient dissatisfaction has been shown to result with any clinically detectable curvature, which is usually about 5 degrees.

- With regard to the surgical release:
  1. I will catheterize the patient in the first instance to prevent accidental damage to the urethra, then,
  2. partially deglove the penis to access the ventral surface and dissect and excise any inelastic tissue I encounter until the level of the corpora cavernosum is reached.
  3. I will then check the effectiveness of my release by repeating a Horton's test.
  4. If it is not fully released, then I repeat the process.
  5. If it remains curved despite this, then:
     - I will proceed with dorsal plication in the mild group – if they have accepted the consequence of this, or
     - the alternative is a ventral release by incising the tunica albuginea that surround the corpora, with grafting of the defect.

When would you perform this?

- I will perform the first stage at 1 year (because there is evidence of developmental sequelae with general anaesthesia prior to 1 year), with the second stage at 18–24 months.
- I aim to complete surgery before the age of 24 months and avoid the 'terrible twos' period when they will be much less cooperative.

What are the risks and possible complications of hypospadias correction?

- Early complications include:
  - swelling,
  - accidental catheter displacement,
  - pressure on the repair,
  - infection,
  - haematoma – with potential skin necrosis,
  - wound dehiscence, and
  - graft loss.
- Late complications include:
  - a fistula,
  - urethral stricture,
  - persistent UTIs – usually secondary to stenosis,
  - meatal stenosis (which is more common in one stage repairs),
  - psychological dissatisfaction with the aesthetic result of 'penile difference', and
  - recurrence of curvature.

How would you manage a fistula?

- I will wait for 1 year, as some will resolve conservatively.
- If this persists, then I will proceed with a fistula repair that consists of a 3-layer repair with non-aligned suture lines and a waterproofing layer.

How would you manage a urethral stricture?

- The first step is to diagnose it: the patient will present clinically with symptoms of frequency and repeated infections.
- Investigations include:
  1. ultrasound of the bladder and kidneys – with expected secondary hypertrophy of the bladder and renal cortical thinning in the case of a urethral stricture, and
  2. urine flowmetry – which is expected to show an abnormal flow rate curve and a residual volume due to the outflow obstruction.
- It is important to note that some patients will have mild obstruction visible on flowmetry but will be asymptomatic and these patients do not need an operation.
- Treatment
  - consists initially of urethral dilation,
  - but many will eventually require a urethroplasty.

FURTHER READING

1. Li Y, Sinclair A, Cao M, Shen J, Choudhry S, Botta S, Cunha G, Baskin L. Canalization of the urethral plate precedes fusion of the urethral folds during male penile urethral development: the double zipper hypothesis. The Journal of Urology. 2015;193(4):1353–1359. https://doi.org/10.1016/j.juro.2014.09.108
2. Blaschko SD, Cunha GR, Baskin LS. Molecular mechanisms of external genitalia development. Differentiation. 2012;84:261–268
3. Bouty A, Ayers KL, Pask A, Heloury Y, Sinclair AH. The genetic and environmental factors underlying hypospadias. Sex Dev. 2015;9(5):239–259. doi:10.1159/000441988
4. Talab SS, Cambareri GM, Hanna MK. Outcome of surgical management of urethral stricture following hypospadias repair. J Pediatr Urol. 2019 Aug;15(4):354.e1–354.e6.

Case 2.17

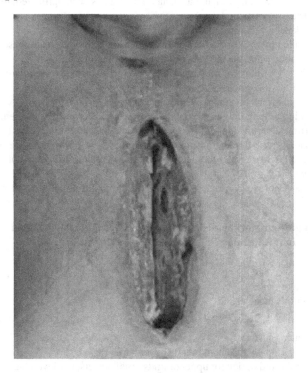

This 55-year-old gentleman develops a deep sternal wound infection and mediastinitis following a CABG procedure. This is managed with excision of devitalized soft tissue and systemic antibiotics.

What are your reconstructive goals in managing sternal defects in general?

I aim to achieve:

- stable soft tissue cover,
- protection of any vital structures,
- obliteration of any dead space, and
- stabilization of the thoracic skeleton:
    - if there is dissociation between the left and right sides of the chest wall, or
    - if the size of the unreconstructed skeletal defect would lead to paroxysmal movement during breathing.

How would you proceed in this case?

This is a potentially life-threatening complication that should be managed in combination with the cardiothoracic team.
- Prior to planning a reconstruction, I will first ensure that any residual infection has been completely eradicated, and any remaining potentially infected metalwork such as sternal wires have been removed – with confirmatory evidence from the patient's clinical picture, microbiology, and imaging.
- Next, I will establish the following salient points from the patient history and cardiothoracic team:
    - their general fitness, including their nutritional state,
    - whether the CABG has been successful, and
    - whether the internal thoracic arteries have been harvested.

DOI: 10.1201/9780429399268-33

- I will use an interim negative pressure dressing to control fluid discharge, reduce bacterial load, and reduce wound oedema whilst the patient is being optimized.
- Once sepsis is controlled and the patient's general health has been optimized, then I will proceed with planning the reconstruction.
- With regard to skeletal reconstruction:
  - I will be guided by the cardiothoracic team and intensive care team, based on the patient's chest wall stability and the mechanics of their ventilation.
  - As a principle, I will aim to keep any use of foreign material to a minimum.
- With regard to soft tissue reconstruction:
  I will plan for a latissimus dorsi myocutaneous flap:
  - including a large, long oblique skin paddle over the lower portion of the muscle – with the long axis from superomedial to inferolateral: this allows the skin paddle to be rotated easily into the defect as the flap is transposed around the chest – with the superomedial tip being inset into the inferior end of the defect, and the inferolateral tip inset into the superior end of the defect.
  - I can further improve flap reach by releasing the distal attachment of the muscle to the humerus, if needed.

Please talk me through your workhorse flap options for sternal reconstruction – would you use any of these other options in this instance?

In addition to LD, my other go-to options include:

1. the pectoralis major muscle,
2. the rectus abdominis muscle, and
3. the omental flap.

- The pectoralis major muscle:
  - may be used as an advancement or a turnover flap.
  - This is my preferred option for upper or midsternal defects, but I would not use this option in this case, as the flap does not cover the lower aspect of the sternum reliably.
  - It is a Mathes and Nahai type V flap with a dominant thoracoacromial supply – upon which the advancement flap is based – and a secondary IMA perforator segmental supply – upon which the turnover flap is based.
  - Bilateral advancement flaps provide bulk and sternal stability, and the flap reach can be extended by division of the clavicular attachments and even the humeral insertion (with the acceptance that this last step will distort the anterior axillary fold).
- The rectus abdominus muscle:
  - is a Mathes and Nahai type III flap, with dual supply by the superior and inferior epigastric vessels, with the superior epigastric artery being the continuation of the internal mammary artery.
  - This provides a reliable skin paddle and plenty of bulk to fill any dead space.
  - This may be an option in a patient who has not had an IMA harvest, but it does weaken the abdominal core, so I prefer the LD.
  - I am aware that it is anatomically possible to raise a rectus based on the cardiophrenic branch of the IMA, which anastomoses with intercostal vessels, but this may be less reliable, so I would prefer to avoid that – especially in a situation like this where the stakes for success are high.
- The omental flap:
  - can be based on either gastroepiploic artery, with the right side being dominant.
  - It provides less bulk than muscle flaps and consequently less chest wall stability. In addition, the abdominal donor site may be more morbid – even with laparoscopic harvest – so I reserve it for patients with:
    - sternal defects involving the lower pole,
    - bilateral IMA harvest, and
    - in whom an LD is not a good option.

Tell me – you've mentioned the Mathes and Nahai classification. What is this and why do you use it?

- This is a classification of muscle flaps based on the pattern of their blood supply. It is widely used as it helps predict how to elevate the flap with:
  - the vascular basis of the flap and
  - the predicted arc of rotation or lack of, e.g., in the case of type IV segmentally based flaps.
- Type I flaps are supplied by single vascular pedicles such as tensor fascia lata supplied by the transverse branch of the lateral femoral circumflex artery.
- Type II flaps are supplied by a single dominant pedicle and smaller pedicles – upon which the flap cannot be based, such as the gracilis flap with a dominant supply from the medial femoral circumflex vessels and minor branches from the superficial femoral artery.
- Type III flaps are supplied by two pedicles and can be based on either one – such as gluteus maximus with supply from the superior and inferior gluteal arteries.
- Type IV flaps are supplied by multiple segmental pedicles which make them more troublesome to use for transfer as each pedicle supplies a small portion of the muscle, such as the tibialis anterior with segmental branches from the anterior tibial artery.
- Type V flaps have one dominant vascular pedicle and a secondary pedicle – upon which the flap can also be based, such as the LD – with a dominant thoracodorsal pedicle and secondary intercostal and lumbar perforators.

Let's go back to the same patient: the cardiac surgeon contacts you to say the patient has presented 1 year post operatively in their clinic, with multiple cutaneous fistulae. How do you proceed?

- I suspect chronic osteomyelitis of the sternum.
- I will manage this along with my cardiothoracic colleague and microbiologist within the MDT setting, with preoperative imaging with CT and MRI scans to radiologically confirm the diagnosis and the extent of the disease process.
- If confirmed, then this will need joint plastic and cardiothoracic surgeon excision of necrotic tissue including bone, with bony and surrounding soft tissue biopsies sent for culture-specific antibiotic management.
- This will need to be performed with immediate bypass support available, as the pericardial scarring to the deep surface of the sternum increases the risk of cardiac injuries. We may need the involvement of a bone infection MDT if this is extensive.

Ok – you find that the whole sternum, along with the costochondral junctions, are affected and require excision. What now?

- I will discuss this within the MDT and suggest that the defect will need stabilization to avoid paroxysmal chest wall movement, as well as soft tissue reconstruction of the excised area that has been affected by fistulation.
- As before, I will ensure that infection is eradicated, and the patient is optimized for surgery, and proceed with reconstruction consisting of:
  - Semi-rigid chest wall stabilization provided by a biological mesh such as Permacol, and
  - a soft tissue reconstruction based on the size and location of the defect:
    - If the soft tissue and skin defect is small and the defect is in the upper half of the sternum, then I will use bilateral pectoralis advancement flaps to provide bulk and further increase stability.
    - If it involves the lower half of the sternum, or is large, then I will opt for a free ALT. This will provide bulk and improve stability further.
      - I have elected for a free flap in this instance, as the pedicled options such as the other LD, or rectus muscle will further weaken his core – especially as his chest wall is mechanically unstable.
      - I have chosen the ALT in particular, as I need a bulky flap with a long pedicle to reach recipient thoracoacromial or neck vessels – if the IMAs have been damaged or excised.

What is Permacol? And why have you chosen this option to improve chest wall stability in this case?

- This is a porcine dermal collagen implant, that is commonly used for hernia and abdominal wall repair. It has the advantage of becoming vascularized and hence reduces infection rates and extrusion. There are many other biological meshes on the market with similar characteristics, which would be equally effective in this case.
- Alternative options that have been described include:
    - other semi-rigid fixation options, such as Gentamicin-impregnated polymethylmethacrylate cement sandwiched between synthetic meshes,
    - titanium plates, and
    - bony flaps.
- However, they each bring certain disadvantages, such as:
    - the high risk of extrusion of methyl-methacrylate,
    - the potential for chronic infection of metalwork and biofilm in an infected environment, and
    - donor site morbidity of autologous skeletal reconstruction such as with a fibula flap.

FURTHER READING

1. Levy AB, Aschermann JA. Sternal wound reconstruction made simple. Plast Reconstr Surg Glob Open. 2019 Nov;7(11):e2488.
2. Bakri K, Mardini S, Evans KK, Carlsen BT, Arnold PG. Workhorse flaps in chest wall reconstruction: the pectoralis major, latissimus dorsi and rectus abdominis flaps. Semin Plast Surg. 2011;25(1):43–54.

VIVA III

Case 3.1

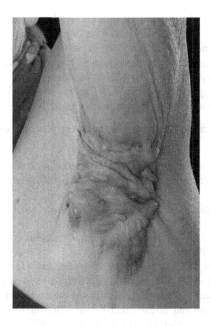

This patient presents to you in clinic with a longstanding lesion. Please describe this photograph.

This is the photograph of a patient's left axilla showing signs of hidradenitis suppurativa (HS) with nodules, sinuses and severe scarring that is consistent with Hurley Stage III disease, in a patient who appears to be of higher BMI.

What is hidradenitis suppurativa?

- This is a chronic relapsing inflammatory disorder of the folliculo-pilosebaceous units of the intertriginous areas – such as the axillae, groins, and submammary areas – that is clinically defined by recurrent inflamed nodules in the first instance, followed by sinus tracts, fistulae and scarring in more severe cases – as is classified by the Hurley Stage I-III Scoring System.
- Whilst the pathogenesis of this disease has not entirely been established, the historical theory of infectious disease of apocrine sweat glands has now been replaced by dysregulation of skin immunity around hair follicles in intertriginous regions, with elevated levels of cytokines such as Interleukins-1/7/10, TNF, and Toll-like receptor signalling.
  1. The initial pathogenic event is now thought to involve perifollicular inflammation leading to hyperkeratosis and occlusion of hair follicles in the predilection areas.
  2. Subsequent rupture of the dilated follicle and extrusion of sebum and debris into the dermis initiates an inflammatory response resulting in the formation of painful inflamed nodules (the culture of which are predominantly sterile or show only commensal skin flora.)
  3. Sustained inflammation in the area results in the formation of fistulae and sinus tracts, which creates a favourable environment for biofilm formation, secondary bacterial colonization, and suppuration.
- Common predisposing factors include
  1. smoking, and
  2. obesity.
- Rarer causes include
  1. mutations in gamma-secretase genes in familial cases, and
  2. syndromes, such as PASH and PAPASH.

DOI: 10.1201/9780429399268-35

- There is also an association with Diabetes and PCOS, but no causal link has been found.
- Smoking is thought to worsen the disorder through stimulation of epidermal hyperplasia and inflammation.
- Obesity is thought to contribute by stimulating a low-grade pro-inflammatory environment.
- Genetic mutations in NCSTN, PSENEN, and PSEN1 gamma-secretase genes lead to abnormal epidermal proliferation and differentiation. Secretase is an enzyme that has an integral role in cutaneous biology and is responsible for the intramembranous cleavage of transmembrane proteins.
- Syndromic HS (such as PASH and PAPASH syndromes) is characterized by a more severe phenotype and recurrent episodes of pyrexia – coexisting with pyoderma gangrenosum and acne in the case of PASH, and additionally pyogenic arthritis in the case of PAPASH syndrome.

You mention the Hurley Scoring System: what is that? Are you aware of any other classification or scoring systems available?

- The Hurley Scoring System is the most commonly used clinical scoring system, in which:
  - Mild disease (Hurley Stage I) is characterized by isolated nodules and/or abscesses without permanent lesions.
  - Moderate disease (HS II) is defined by widely separated recurrent nodules and or abscesses with sinus tracts and scarring.
  - Severe disease (HS III) is determined by multiple interconnected sinus tracts, abscesses, and scarring affecting an entire anatomical area.
- It is a simple system that is useful in daily clinical practice, but it is not dynamic, nor sufficient for monitoring the response to medical treatment – unlike other systems such as:
  - the modified Sartorius Scoring – which is based on the lesion type and count, number of anatomical regions involved, and distance between two relevant lesions, or
  - the Hidradenitis Suppurativa Clinical Response score (HiSCR) – which evaluates the acute phase outcome of patients who are specifically treated with Adalimumab.
- However, in contrast to the Hurley Scoring system, the modified Sartorius system is more time consuming to use, and difficult to interpret with limited applicability in severe diseases stages where lesions are confluent.
- In addition, two other research systems exist, including the HS Physicians Global Assessment and HS Clinical Response systems, but these are not relevant in routine clinical practice.

How will you manage this patient?

- As per the guidelines produced by the British and North American Associations of dermatology, I will identify:
  - any additional areas affected and the severity of disease in these,
  - any predisposing factors – including confirmation of the high BMI suspected from the photograph – as addressing these conditions may improve the disease course,
  - how this affects their quality of life (e.g., pain, suppuration with the need for dressings, psychological distress, inability to continue their work, and effect on interpersonal relationships), and
  - a familial history – for consideration for genetic testing.
- In a patient who is fit for a general anaesthetic, with Hurley Stage III disease – as this photograph demonstrates, and a high BMI: I would suggest a joint MDT approach with my dermatology colleague to discuss:
  1. If this patient is a candidate for neoadjuvant Adalimumab prior to surgical excision to attempt to decrease the disease burden (with adjuvant therapy resumed once wound healing is complete) – especially if more than one area satisfy Hurley Stage III disease, and/or if the patient has other inflammatory syndromes.
  2. Surgical excision and reconstruction with a heavily quilted SSG and a dermal replacement such as Matriderm, that is splinted with a negative pressure dressing for the 1st week. The alternative is a flap option such as a pedicled TAP flap to avoid a skin graft in the axilla but this would only be suitable in a slim patient who is not on Adalimumab.
     - Of note, I would stop any Adalimumab treatment for 2 weeks both before and after surgery to prevent severe wound healing delay, but warn the patient that their wound healing may be delayed anyway by their previous biologic therapy.

    – If the disease affects both axillae equally, then I would stage the excision to allow for patient hygiene, according to patient choice.
3. Lastly, to decrease the risk of recurrence and future flare-ups, I would also encourage the patient to:
   – routinely use chlorhexidine washes, and
   – decrease any modifiable risk factors, such as:
     ▪ smoking,
     ▪ a high BMI,
     ▪ uncontrolled Diabetes, and
     ▪ untreated PCOS or inflammatory conditions.

What is Adalimumab? And what is the evidence for its use in HS?

This is an IgG1 antibody specific for TNF-alpha that limits the promotion of inflammation. It is recommended by NICE to treat active Hurley Stage II and III disease in adults, who have not responded to conventional systemic therapy.

Why do you prefer the skin graft option in the first instance? Will you not risk shoulder problems with graft contraction?

- This is my preferred option, in the first instance, as I believe that this would offer the best of both worlds:
  – it is a simple technique,
  – the artificial dermal layer improves the pliability and result of the graft, and
  – if the patient has delayed wound healing due to Adalimumab immunosuppression, then they would have had a 'cheap donor site' and the wound can be treated conservatively (with or without negative pressure therapy) to achieve wound closure.

    In practice, patients with good quality skin grafts – especially with added dermal replacements – that are placed with the shoulder in abduction and external rotation to maximize the defect prior to grafting, rarely have subsequent shoulder problems which limit their activities. In the rare instance that they do develop a reduced ROM, the graft can always be replaced later with a flap.
- I would reserve the regional flap option, such as a pedicled TAP flap, in:
  1. a slim patient, who does not want to consider the skin graft option (to avoid the transfer of bulky tissue to the axilla in a heavier patient, which will require numerous liposuction sessions), and
  2. who is also not at risk of wound healing problems caused by Adalimumab (so as not to have a transferred flap that is 'floating in the breeze' due to delayed wound healing), or
  3. in the rare event of a patient with joint mobility issues following their skin graft.

How would you reconstruct a patient with bilateral inguinal Hurley stage III disease?

My preference is for SSG and Matriderm as before with bilateral simultaneous excision and reconstruction, with an alternative for bilateral ALTs if the patient is slim and is not at risk of wound healing problems caused by Adalimumab.

What is Matriderm? Why choose it over another dermal replacement, such as Integra?

Matriderm is a highly porous membrane composed of a 3D coupled bovine dermal collagen and ligamentous elastin that can be used as a single stage procedure along with the SSG placement.

    Prior to the introduction of single-layer Integra, its advantage was a one-step procedure, and as a result remains a popular choice but there is no evidence for any superiority of outcome with any one dermal replacement over another.

How would you manage a patient with mild disease?

- As before, this patient would be jointly managed with my dermatology colleague within the HS MDT, with the aim to reduce the burden of disease and the management of any acute symptomatic lesions.

- Most of these patients would have been managed by their GP or dermatologist prior to referral but if they haven't, then I will advise:
  - cessation of smoking,
  - weight reduction – if applicable,
  - the use of antiseptic washes such as Hibiscrub,
  - a referral to their gynaecologist if there is a suspicion of PCOS, and
  - a referral to their GP for consideration of Metformin if they are obese or have metabolic syndrome.
- With regard to short flare-ups, I would recommend topical Clindamycin (but not beyond 3 months as longer courses have been shown to lead to antibiotic resistance).
- Multiple recurrent flare-ups would warrant oral Tetracycline for at least 6 months.

FURTHER READING

1. Alikhan A, Sayed C, Alavi A, Alhusayen R, Brassard A, Burkhart C, Crowell K, Eisen DB, Gottlieb AB, Hamzavi I, Hazen PG, Jaleel T, Kimball AB, Kirby J, Lowes MA, Micheletti R, Miller A, Naik HB, Orgill D, Poulin Y. North American clinical management guidelines for hidradenitis suppurativa: A publication from the United States and Canadian Hidradenitis Suppurativa Foundations: Part I: Diagnosis, evaluation, and the use of complementary and procedural management. J Am Acad Dermatol. 2019 Jul;81(1):76–90.
2. Saunte DML, Jemec GBE. Hidradenitis suppurativa. JAMA, 2017;318(20):2019.
3. Blok JL, Spoo JR, Leeman FWJ, Jonkman MF, Horváth B. Skin-Tissue-sparing Excision with Electrosurgical Peeling (STEEP): A surgical treatment option for severe hidradenitis suppurativa Hurley stage II/III. J Eur Acad Dermatol Venereol. 2015 Feb;29(2):379–382.
4. Vinkel C. Hidradenitis suppurativa: causes, features, and current treatments. J Clin Aesthet Dermatol. 2018;11(10):17–23.
5. Kimball AB, Sobell JM, Zouboulis CC, Gu Y, Williams DA, Sundaram M, Teixeira HD, Jemec GB. HiSCR (Hidradenitis Suppurativa Clinical Response): A novel clinical endpoint to evaluate therapeutic outcomes in patients with hidradenitis suppurativa from the placebo-controlled portion of a phase 2 adalimumab study. J Eur Acad Dermatol Venereol. 2016 Jun;30(6):989–994.

Case 3.2

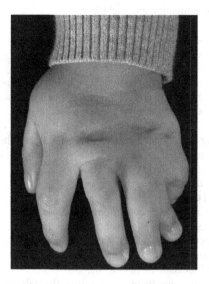

This infant is brought to your clinic. Please describe this photograph.

This photograph shows an infant with a synpolydactyly affecting the post-axial aspect of the left ring finger, with a possible element of proximal syndactyly that would need to be confirmed radiographically. I cannot see any skin creases on the dorsum of the ring finger so I would be concerned about the development of joints in this digit.

In addition, I cannot comment on whether the little finger is fully and normally formed.

What is the embryology of the hand? And what is the embryological insult in this case?

- Embryological development of the hand begins in the 4th week of gestation in a highly orchestrated temporal and spatial fashion, by relying on interactions between three known signalling centres and a host of transcription factors, secreted proteins, and receptors, to ensure differentiation of the upper limb in three axes.
  The three primary signalling centres consist of:
  1. the Apical Ectodermal Ridge (AER),
  2. the Zone of Polarizing Activity (ZPA), and
  3. the Wingless type signalling centre (WNT).
- The AER is a specialized region of the ectoderm that condenses over the developing limb bud and mediates proximal-to-distal orientation by expressing several signalling molecules in the fibroblast growth factor family such as FGF-2, 4, and 8.
- The ZPA exists within the posterior limb bud and determines:
  - the AP radio-ulnar axis, via secretion of the Sonic Hedgehog protein, and
  - proximal-to-distal growth, by inducing FGF-4 expression in the AER via a positive feedback mechanism, which ensures proportional growth along both axes.
- The WNT signalling centre resides in the dorsal ectoderm and determines the dorsal differentiation pathway via the secretion of LMX-1. A complementary protein called Engrailed-1 exists in the ventral portion of the limb and is responsible for the ventral differentiation pathway.
- The three signalling centres act on transcription factors within the cells in the developing limb bud. One of the most important factors is the HOX protein family, and in this case of synpolydactyly, the underlying aetiology is most likely HOX D13 mutation, inherited in an autosomal dominant fashion.

DOI: 10.1201/9780429399268-36

How would you manage this patient?

- I will manage this child within an MDT in a congenital hand referral centre.
- My focused history and examination will include
  - a family history,
  - whether the other hand is affected also, and
  - whether the child uses their hand, and if so – how.
- I will request a genetic consultation, as polysyndactyly of the ring finger has been linked to a mutation of the HOX D13 gene on chromosome 2, with implications for future offspring.
- I will also request a radiograph to determine a syndactylous component and the extent of any bony involvement – such as a duplicated or bifid metacarpal or phalanx, or a shared joint, to create a surgical plan.
- With regards to the timing of the procedure – I will aim for 12 months of age, as this is considered a safe anaesthetic age in most tertiary paediatric hospitals with an experienced anaesthetist.
- With regard to the surgical procedure, the goals are to:
  - ablate the duplicated digit, and
  - augment the retained digit.
- There is no prescribed operation, so reconstruction is tailored to the specific characteristics of the anomaly, but I would adhere to principles such as:
  - using zigzag incisions to minimize post-operative contracture, which are cheated towards the extra digit to maximize available skin for closure,
  - the centralization and rebalancing of tendons,
  - the reconstruction of collateral ligaments to restore the stability of involved joints,
  - the narrowing of a widened proximal articular surface if a joint is involved, and
  - the use of osteotomies to correct angular deformities of the metacarpal or phalanges if required.
- I would also counsel the parents for the high rate of revision for contractures or angular deformity.

FURTHER READING

1. Comer GC, Potter M, Ladd AL. Polydactyly of the hand. J Am Acad Orthop Surg. 2018;26(3):75–82. doi:10.5435/jaaos-d-16-00139
2. Farrugia MC, Calleja-Agius J. Polydactyly: a review. Neonatal Netw. 2016;35(3):135–142. doi:10.1891/0730-0832.35.3.135
3. Watt AJ, Chung KC. Duplication. Hand Clinics. 2009;25(2):215–227.

Case 3.3

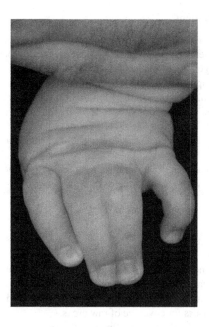

Please describe this photograph.

This is the photograph of an infant's hand with a complete syndactyly of the left, middle, and ring fingers which are the most commonly affected digits. I cannot see the thumb, so I am not sure if it is normally developed or not.

What is syndactyly?

- This is a congenital hand anomaly that was historically classified as 'embryonic failure of differentiation' according to Swanson's classification and is now classified as 'malformation unspecified axis' according to the OMT classification.
- It occurs in 1 in every 2000 births, and is twice as common in males than in females, with the most affected interspace being the middle-ring interspace in non-syndromic patients, as shown in this case.
- It is bilateral in half of the patients and is usually sporadic, although it can be familial with autosomal dominant inheritance, or 'complicated' such as in those with Poland sequence or Apert syndrome.
- Syndactyly may be classified based on whether it is:
  - simple or complex – depending on whether bony and cartilaginous structures are affected as well as soft tissues, or
  - complete or incomplete – with controversy regarding the definition of a complete syndactyly as to whether it includes the fusion of both adjacent nails or digital fusion to the level of the DIPJ.

What is the embryogenic insult in this case?

- Normally, webbing between the digits undergoes apoptosis during the 6th to 8th weeks of gestation in a distal to proximal direction, mediated by cytokines such as BMPs, which override the activity of FGFs.
- Here, the embryogenic insult involves a three-step pathway with:
  1. suppression of BMP-signalling or activation of WNT-signalling, leading to
  2. overexpression of FGF-8 in the AER, which in turn leads to

DOI: 10.1201/9780429399268-37

3. suppression of retinoic acid in the interdigital spaces, which leads to
4. suppression of both apoptosis and ECM degradation.

How would you manage this patient?

- After establishing whether the thumb is involved, I will confirm whether this is an isolated third-web syndactyly, or whether it is complicated by the presence of other syndromic associations.
- With regard to the management of the hand itself:
  - I will obtain radiographs to establish whether this is simple or complex.
  - As this does not involve border digits, I will wait until the age of 1 year before surgery to minimize anaesthetic complications.
  - The goals of this are:
    - separation of the digits with tension-free closure – to allow independent digital movement, and
    - creation of an anatomically normal web space – with reduced chances for web creep.
- I will counsel the parents with regard to the risks of:
  - web creep,
  - flexion contracture,
  - graft loss,
  - graft pigmentation, and
  - problematic scarring.
- In the case of a simple syndactyly, my preferred technique would be to use:
  - a proximal dorsal local flap to create the proximal web space,
  - interdigitated ulnar-and radial-based mirror image Z flaps, and
  - full-thickness skin grafts for coverage of raw areas.
- For a complex syndactyly, the management plan is the same, except that I will ensure that any bones and joints are adequately covered with skin flaps, as opposed to skin grafts.
- With regard to managing the synonychia, I will use a Buck-Gramcko stiletto flap to optimize tip fullness and contour.
- Post-operatively, I will check the fingertips for adequate perfusion and arrange a dressing change in 2 weeks.

Are there any contraindications to the surgical release of a syndactyly?

Yes, general contraindications include:

1. systemic comorbidity which would increase the risk of a general anaesthetic,
2. a very mild incomplete anomaly that does not impair function,
3. a very severe complex syndactyly that risks further functional impairment with attempted separation, such as in the case of synpolydactyly, where there is often abnormal vasculature, and
4. lastly, the presence of a very hypoplastic digit that is dependent on the syndactylized digit for function, so that separation would render it functionless.

What is your rationale and algorithm for the timing of surgery?

This is somewhat controversial:

Earlier surgery is more technically challenging with smaller structures and increased anaesthetic concerns; however, delayed surgery may affect hand function especially if border digits are involved.

- In patients with complex syndactyly that affects border digits: surgery is expedited to 6–9 months of age, as postponing this to a later stage may result in asymmetric growth with angulation of joints.
- Otherwise, surgery is delayed until 12 months of age. This allows for a decreased anaesthetic risk and a reasonable compromise with larger structures. I would give priority to releasing a first-web syndactyly with recovery completed before 18 months at the latest – as thumb prehension is crucial for hand function.
- If multiple digits are involved, I would stage separation of the digits to avoid surgery on both sides of fingers.

What would you do for bilateral symmetrical anomalies?

I will plan for simultaneous surgery in non-ambulatory infants of 1 year of age.

What are the principles of syndactyly release?

These include:

1. the creation of a new web space sloping at 45 degrees from dorsal to palmar with a free transverse distal edge, and
2. the distal release of digits by interdigitating fasciocutaneous flaps and full-thickness skin grafts to resurface the interdigital space. I will avoid visible scars on the dorsum/volar aspect as much as possible as well as longitudinal scars crossing joints to avoid scar contractures.

Please draw the syndactyly releasing incision lines for me on the illustration provided, and talk me through your planning:

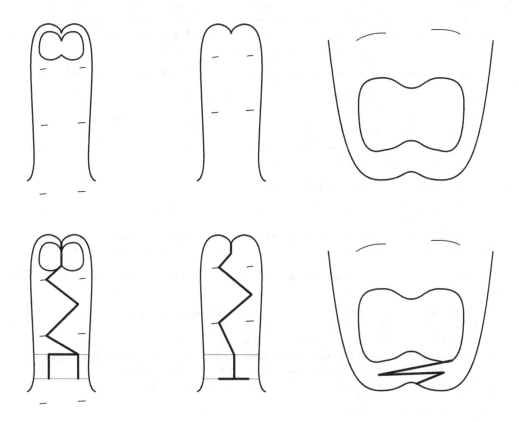

1. I first divide the distance between the MCPJ and the PIPJ into thirds (marked as a thin line at the level of the proximal phalanx).
2. I then place the planning incision for the dorsal flap between the proximal third and the distal 2/3 of this. The width of the flap does not cross the midline of the digits.
3. The zigzag flaps are marked with apexes at the midlines of the DIPJ and PIPJ joint creases, as well as the midline of the midpoint of the middle phalanx.
4. The volar surface is marked with a T-shaped flap at the base to accommodate the dorsal flap into the new web crease.
5. The volar zigzag flaps are mirror images of the dorsal ones.

6. The fingertip is divided with Buck-Gramcko triangular flaps, planned by connecting the pulp midline with one lateral aspect of the distal nail plate and the other pulp midline to the distal volar incision point.

You mention using full-thickness skin grafts. Are there any other options to avoid that?

Yes – modifications of the Bauer dorsal flap by Giele and Niranjan, to recruit more skin have been described – but I reserve them for incomplete cases up to the level of the PIPJ, as there is a particular soft-tissue deficit in complete syndactylies. Beyond that, the local tissue deficit is too great for adequate circumferential coverage without the use of skin grafts.

Why would one want to avoid skin grafts?

They may become hyperpigmented or hairy with time. Also graft loss may result in hypertrophic scars.

You mentioned the OMT classification replacing the Swanson classification. Why was it adopted by the International Federation of Societies of the Hand as a replacement for the Swanson classification?

The Oberg-Manske-Tonkin classification separates malformations from deformations and dysplasias, based on the embryological insult rather than the morphological classification in Swanson's classification.

It has been shown to have high intraobserver reliability – especially amongst senior consultants – which allows updates as our knowledge of embryology and genetics is improved.

You've mentioned the possible syndromic associations of syndactyly. What do you mean by that?

Syndactyly can rarely be associated with certain syndromes such as:

- Poland syndrome, which is classically associated with symbrachydactyly and the absence of the sternal portion of pectoralis major, as well as
- Apert syndrome, which is associated with bilateral multiple complex syndactylies with symphalangism and craniofacial features.

Would you manage an Apert hand any differently?

1. Here, the thumb is frequently involved, so management would involve creating a first web space as a matter of urgency.
2. In addition, the digital interphalangeal joints are functionless; therefore, the need for the usual zigzag incisions does not apply here so I would use a straight-line incision with skin grafts.

You mentioned the possibility of thumb hypoplasia earlier. What is your management algorithm if that were the case?

- I would first exclude syndromic causes of radial longitudinal deficiencies such as Holt-Oram, VATTERR, and TAR syndromes, as well as Fanconi anaemia.
- I would then use the modified Blauth classification to determine the treatment required.
- The most important sign is the presence and stability of the CMCJ, which differentiates a Type 3A from a Type 3B, and necessitates a pollicization in Type 3B to Type 5, whereas
- Type 1 is treated conservatively or may require thumb lengthening, and
- Type 2 to Type 3A require
  - stabilization of the MCPJ,
  - first web space release, and
  - opponensplasty.
- If a pollicization is indicated, then it is important to preoperatively check whether the child has a stiff index finger or not, and how they use it preoperatively, as that may affect the result of the pollicization.

What are the types of hypoplastic thumbs that you have mentioned?

- Type I denotes minor hypoplasia – with all anatomical structures present but smaller in size.
- Type II denotes:
  - MCPJ ligamentous instability, and
  - thenar hypoplasia.

- Type III A denotes Type II, as well as:
  - metacarpal hypoplasia,
  - tendon anomalies, and
  - a stable CMCJ.
- Type IIIB denotes Type II, as well as
  - partial metacarpal aplasia,
  - tendon anomalies, and
  - an unstable or absent CMCJ.
- Type IV denotes a floating thumb, with attachment to the hand by the skin and digital neurovascular structures.
- Type V denotes complete absence of the thumb.

How would you perform a pollicization?

1. I would start by creating a first web space by transposition of a dorsal flap from the radial side of the index, followed by
2. interfascicular dissection of the common digital nerve to the index-middle finger web, and
3. resection of the metacarpal head of the index to form the new trapezium and the metacarpal epiphysis to prevent future growth,
4. the remaining metacarpal is then rotated to 160 degrees to allow opposition, and secured at 40 degrees of abduction.
5. The muscle attachments are then repositioned such that:
   - EIP becomes the new EPL,
   - EDC becomes the new APL,
   - the first dorsal interosseous becomes the new APB, and
   - the first palmar interosseous acts as the new adductor.

FURTHER READING

1. Goldfarb CA, Ezaki M, Wall LB, Lam WL, Oberg KC. The oberg-manske-tonkin (OMT) classification of congenital upper extremities: update for 2020. J Hand Surg. 2020; 45(6):542–547.
2. Braun TL, Trost JG, Pederson WC. Semin Plast Surg. 2016 Nov; 30(4):162–170.
3. Al-Qattan MM. A review of the genetics and pathogenesis of syndactyly in humans and experimental animals: a 3-step pathway of pathogenesis. Biomed Res Int. 2019;2019:9652649.

Case 3.4

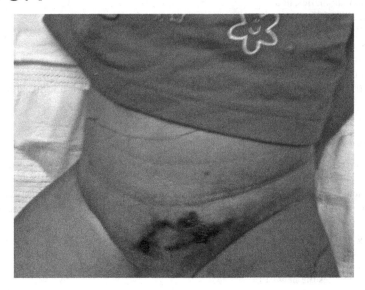

This 2-year-old is referred to your registrar 1 week after contracting chicken pox from her sibling. Mum is worried that the skin around the small blisters in the suprapubic area 'has gone black around a pale area of skin', with surrounding skin erythema that has been marked by the ER doctor.

The patient has entirely normal observations apart from a temperature of 37.6°C and appears generally well in herself – although mum does report that her child's appetite has been reduced in the last 12 hours.

What do you suspect and how do you proceed?

- I am concerned she has necrotizing fasciitis and will manage this with urgent surgical exploration, and debridement if my suspicion is confirmed intraoperatively.
- Whilst this is being arranged, I will ensure the child has urgent IV access and will contact the paediatric, and paediatric ITU teams as appropriate.
- I will also send urgent blood cultures, an urgent Gram-stain of the bullae fluid if possible and start empirical intravenous broad-spectrum antibiotics as per my local hospital protocol. This usually includes Clindamycin, and will then be adjusted as per the intra-operative specimen culture results.

What is necrotizing fasciitis?

- This is a rapidly progressive inflammatory infection of the fascia with relative sparing of muscle and skin tissue.
- As the disease progresses, thrombosis of the cutaneous perforators devascularizes the overlying skin with pain, blistering, ecchymosis, necrosis, and skin anaesthesia as a late sign.
- A systemic inflammatory response caused by the release of toxins then produces the signs of septic shock and multiorgan damage.
- The cause is most commonly polymicrobial, although monomicrobial pathology caused by group A Streptococcus is most commonly associated with cases following Varicella, as in this case. Rarer causes may be clostridial, or fungal.

DOI: 10.1201/9780429399268-38

Are you sure you want to rush to theatre in this scenario and subject her to a potentially unnecessary general anaesthetic? The child appears to be systemically stable. Why not admit her for observation in the first instance?

- I agree that, had she been an adult with stable systemic observations, I would have considered performing a 'finger sweep test' under local anaesthesia, and continued to treat with intravenous antibiotics and observe for any progression if the finger test was negative. However, this is not possible in children, so a general anaesthetic procedure is the only way forward to rule out a potentially fatal condition.
- In addition, I will not wait for her to potentially develop systemic signs, as children have a larger physiologic reserve than adults and will develop signs of shock much later – but once they start to decompensate, they can deteriorate extremely quickly.
- Her systemic observations are relatively normal for the moment, although I note a mild grade pyrexia and anorexia.

I believe these signs, along with the skin changes, and the history of Varicella Zoster, are enough for me to have a high enough index of suspicion and warrant surgical exploration.

What is the finger sweep test?

This is a bedside procedure under local anaesthesia, used mainly as a clinical tool to exclude necrotizing fasciitis in adult patients with equivocal and potentially 'early signs of disease' and allows safe observation of the patient if the test is negative.

A 2-cm incision is made down to the level of the deep fascia with a positive test denoted by a lack of tissue resistance to blunt finger dissection, with or without the characteristic 'dishwater fluid'.

Why not just use a scoring system to guide your decision-making? Are you familiar with any?

- Yes, I am, various scoring systems have been described in the literature, but none of which have been validated to recognize all patients with necrotizing fasciitis, and they have not gained much traction amongst experienced clinicians for the purpose of diagnosis.
- This condition remains one that is diagnosed clinically by those with a high degree of suspicion. Given the possibly fatal consequences of failing to recognize the condition with enough timeliness, I will still surgically explore any patient with suspicious clinical signs regardless of any scoring system score.
- The most popular scoring system is the Laboratory Risk Indicator for Necrotizing Fasciitis (LRINEC). This was developed with six laboratory values including:
  - CRP,
  - total WBC,
  - Hb,
  - Na,
  - creatinine, and
  - blood glucose.

  A score of more than 6 has a positive predictive value of 92%, but it is important to note that 10% of patients with necrotizing fasciitis in the original paper had scores of less than 6. Subsequent validation studies have shown that those with scores of more than 6 do have more severe conditions with a higher rate of death and amputation.
- In addition, this scoring system was not described for the paediatric population, and there have been some papers suggesting a paediatric version which includes a high CRP and low sodium level only.

Why is Clindamycin part of most hospital empirical antibiotic protocols?

Penicillin may not be as effective in this type of infection, as bacteria may reach a stationary phase of growth and stop expressing a critical Penicillin-binding protein.

Clindamycin, on the other hand, is not affected by the stage of bacterial growth and can switch off exotoxin production even in stationary phase organisms, as well as inhibit M-protein synthesis, thus promoting phagocytosis, decreasing toxin production, and preventing septic shock. In addition, it has a broader cover with some anaerobic cover.

What is the M-protein?

This is a protein found on the surface of group A Streptococcus and is responsible for resistance to phagocytosis, and adherence to keratinocytes.

You take her to theatre, and she decompensates as she is transferred to the operating table with multiple advancing edges of disease. How would you proceed now?

- This is a surgical emergency that has become even more time-crucial, and I need assistants. I will ask the theatre runner to contact any of my plastic surgery consultant colleagues who are available as an extra pair of hands would be useful.
- Whilst the patient was being put to sleep:
  1. I would have asked the theatre team to warm the theatre, and
  2. asked the nurses to prepare adrenaline-soaked gauze to help minimize bleeding, and instructed my assistant to dress the excised areas with adrenaline-soaked gauze as I progress with the excision.
- Time is of the essence here: it is essential to rapidly gain control of the advancing edges with a full-thickness incision down to muscle and excision of the diseased fascia and overlying tissue until the advancing edge is excised. I will recognise diseased fascia as dull grey with a lack of resistance to digital pressure, and there may or may not be presence of the classically described 'dishwater fluid'.
- If I am in any doubt, I will excise the tissue until I am certain of the viability of the tissue I encounter.
- Once I have gained control of the advancing edges, I can then assess the tissue at the peripheries for fascial viability with the appearance of glistening white tissue that will withstand tugging with a haemostat.
- Next, I will assess for subcutaneous and dermal viability of the peripheral tissue. I will excise the overlying tissue if there is any concern of subcutaneous disease, such as calcification or liquefaction of fat, or thrombosis of the subdermal venules.
- I will then assess the skin for dermal bleeding and again excise any questionable skin.
- Finally, I will obtain haemostasis – along with my assistant to minimize the time taken, and dress the area with Jelonet, Betadine-soaked gauze, wool, and Crepe.
- She will then be transferred to the paediatric intensive care, with a plan for a second look in the next 24 hours if it is safe to do so.

Complete debridement results in loss of tissue on her abdomen, chest, groin, and the anterior aspect of both thighs affecting a TBSA of 25%. What now?

Once I am satisfied that debridement is complete, I will transfer her to the intensive care for stabilization. If she is safe for transfer, I will discuss her case with my local burns unit, if this is not based in my hospital – for possible transfer, as she now effectively has a similar post-operative defect to a 25% burn that has been debrided.

Your local paediatric burns unit is full, as are many others. The only one available is 200 miles away. Your paediatric intensivists are comfortable managing her. How would you proceed?

I will continue to manage her locally whilst remaining in regular communication with the burn surgery consultants, as a long-distance patient transfer is not appropriate in this case. I will aim to graft her in the next 24 hours if this is safe to do so from an anaesthetic point of view (as long as no further debridements are required) to minimize her fluid losses and minimize her inflammatory response.

Why would grafting minimize her fluid losses and affect her inflammatory response?

This is because:

- The control of fluid loss is one of the functions of the skin, so early grafting will minimize this.
- In addition, an open wound results in inflammation. A wound of this surface area, in addition to the effects of the recent infective insult, would result in a systemic inflammatory response.

You've mentioned the control of fluid loss by the skin. What are the other functions of the skin?

This has protective, regulatory, and special functions.

- Protective functions include:
  - a mechanical barrier to invasion by the stratum corneum, in addition to the control of transepidermal water loss that I have mentioned – with about 100 ml/m^2 of water loss per day,
  - protection against ultraviolet light by Melanocytes, and
  - bactericidal properties of the sebum in the stratum corneum.
- Regulatory functions include:
  - the regulation of body temperature – via regulation of the dermal vascular plexus and sweat gland function.
- Special functions include:
  - sensation via the dermal nerve plexus and the mechanoreceptor function of Merkel cells,
  - immunological surveillance via the antigen-presenting function of Langerhans cells, and
  - lastly, vitamin D synthesis by keratinocytes – from dehydrocholesterol via the assistance of UVB light.

You've mentioned the stratum corneum. Please tell me more about the structure of the skin.

- The skin is composed of two layers, the epidermis and dermis which rest on a panniculus adiposus:
  1. The epidermis is composed of four or five layers of stratified squamous epithelium that is of ectodermal origin but colonized by Melanocytes, Merkel cells-both of neural crest origin, and Langerhans cells-derived from the mesoderm.
     The layers, from deep to superficial, are Stratum:
     - basale,
     - spinosum,
     - granulosum,
     - lucidum – only present in glabrous skin, and
     - corneum.
  2. The dermis accounts for 95% of the skin thickness and is derived primarily from mesoderm. It is formed by the papillary and reticular dermal layers separated by a neurovascular plexus.
     The papillary dermis is superficial and contains more fibroblasts and finer collagen fibres.
     The reticular dermis is deeper and contains fewer fibroblasts with thicker collagen fibres.
- The deepest two epidermal layers are actively proliferating layers that produce Keratinocytes. In addition, Melanocytes, Merkel cells – which are mechanoreceptors, and Langerhans cells – which are T lymphocytes, are also found here.
- Keratinocytes originate in the basal layer.
  - They are responsible for the formation of the water barrier by producing keratin as well as the secretion of lipids.
  - In addition, they also regulate calcium absorption, which is essential to the conversion of cholesterol precursors to form vitamin D.
- Melanocytes produce melanin during the conversion of tyrosine to DOPA by tyrosinase – the secretion of which is stimulated by UVB light.
- Melanin is then packaged into melanosomes and transferred via phagocytosis from Melanocytes to keratinocytes in the deepest two epidermal layers, and also transferred to the more superficial layers in those with Fitzpatrick skin type 5/6.
- As the layers become more superficial, Keratinocytes undergo a maturation process called keratinization, in which their cytoplasm is replaced with keratin as the cell dies and becomes more superficial, until they reach the stratum corneum, where they become Corneocytes. These are nonviable keratinized flattened cells that are evolved for barrier function only.
- The stratum corneum further protects against trauma with a 'brick and mortar' arrangement of keratin linked by disulphide bonds with lipid in between. This insulates against fluid loss and protects against bacterial invasion when lipid is excreted as keratin takes over the cell.

Tell me, is there an alternative to debridement and skin grafting in the management of patients with necrotizing fasciitis? And if so, why haven't you mentioned that in this case?

- Yes, a skin-sparing technique has been described with the aim of decreasing the subsequent reconstructive burden. This is based on the principle that some of the healthy skin at the periphery of the diseased fascia may be salvageable, as it will survive on collateral circulation even if the underlying fascia is excised.
- It is based on a model that is specific to necrotizing fasciitis, akin to Jackson's zones of burn injury, whereby:
    1. Zone 1 includes the epicentre of disease with haemorrhagic bullae, fixed staining, and frank dermal gangrene.
    2. Zone 2 includes the transitional area with signs of erythema that can be potentially salvaged if the infection is rapidly controlled.
    3. Zone 3 is healthy uninvolved tissue.
- This technique involves fascial excision, with the overlying dead skin in Zone 1.
- With regard to Zone 2, a full-thickness incision is made down to muscle – extending into Zone 3 to excise the affected fascia and examine the overlying skin and subcutaneous tissue viability.
- If the skin and subcutaneous fat is healthy, then it is preserved.
- Any uncertainty will result in continued excision of the skin and subcutaneous tissue in that area until completely healthy tissue is encountered.

However, I will not use this technique in this case as a rapid technique is essential in a decompensating child – with the acceptance that there is a potentially greater need for reconstruction.

You've mentioned simple skin grafting. Are there any other methods of reconstruction available?

Yes, the use of dermal replacements such as one stage Integra and Matriderm to improve durability and pliability can be considered if resources allow and no contraindications are present, such as secondary infection. Flap reconstruction may be required over areas that aren't graftable such as tendons – although it is unlikely to be applicable here.

FURTHER READING

1. Wong C-H, Yam AK-T, Tan AB-H, Song C. Approach to debridement in necrotizing fasciitis. Am J Surg. 2008;196(3):e19–e24.
2. Rüfenacht MS, Montaruli E, Chappuis E, Posfay-Barbe KM, La Scala GC. Skin-sparing débridement for necrotizing fasciitis in children. Plastic Reconstr Surg. 2016;138(3):489e–497e.

Case 3.5

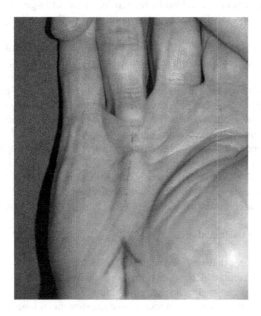

Please describe the photograph.

This is a photograph of the palmar aspect of a patient's right hand, with what appears to be a pretendinous Dupuytrens cord affecting the fourth ray.

What is Dupuytrens' disease?

- It is a benign fibroproliferative condition characterized by contraction of the palmar or digital fascia resulting in pits, nodules, and cords.
- It most commonly affects the ulnar rays of the hand in elderly men of Caucasian descent – with an increasing genetic association to mutations on chromosomes 6, 11, and 16.
- In some patients, it has also been found to be associated with factors such as:
  - smoking,
  - excessive alcohol intake,
  - repeated injuries,
  - diabetes, and
  - epilepsy
- Dupuytren's diathesis is a more aggressive presentation with earlier disease, more rapid progression, and increased recurrence after treatment. It is more common in:
  - males,
  - those with early onset disease,
  - bilateral and/or radial involvement,
  - those with a positive family history, and
  - those with ectopic disease (such as Garrod's pads affecting the dorsal PIPJ, Peyronie's disease affecting the penis, and Ledderhose disease affecting the plantar aspect of the foot).

What is the pathophysiology involved? And how does that relate to normal palmar fascial anatomy?

- The pathophysiological process involves proliferative, involutional, and residual stages.
  - The proliferative stage is characterized by the formation of a nodule with a high fibrinolytic activity leading to progressive differentiation of fibroblasts into myofibroblasts, along with a high percentage of type III collagen.

DOI: 10.1201/9780429399268-39

- – The involutional stage is characterized by the reduction of myofibroblasts, with concentration of the remaining cells along tissue constraint lines.
  - – The residual stage is characterized by the reinforcement of large amounts of type I collagen and further reduction of myofibroblast numbers, as the condition progresses with the development of mature cords.
- There are several theories regarding the cause of the initial myofibroblast proliferation such as:
  - – ischaemia-induced proliferation – e.g., caused by repetitive injuries, and
  - – abnormal TGF – Beta 1 and 2 activities, resulting in the accumulation of:
    - ▪ beta Catenin – which is involved in the mechanotransduction of myofibroblasts, amongst other regulatory roles of gene transcription and cell-to-cell adhesion, and
    - ▪ periostin – a protein which regulates actin proliferation and the transformation of fibroblasts into myofibroblasts.
      Androgen is thought to play a role in this process as androgen receptors have been identified in Dupuytrens nodules.
- With regard to normal palmar fascial anatomy, the palmar aponeurosis is made up of longitudinal, transverse, and vertical layers – from superficial to deep.
  Distally, the longitudinal fibres themselves split into three layers and insert into:
  - – the skin,
  - – the lateral digital sheet, and
  - – the flexor sheath
- Normal fascial structures that are relevant are as follows:
  1. The natatory ligament, which passes transversely across the web space.
     Contracture of this causes a web space contracture.
  2. The pretendinous band, which is thickening of the superficial longitudinal fibres.
     Contracture of this forms the pretendinous cord, which itself causes contracture of the MCPJ.
  3. The spiral band, which is normal thickening of the fascia from the pretendinous band to the natatory ligament.
  4. The lateral digital sheet, which runs from the natatory ligament along the lateral aspect of the neurovascular bundle.
  5. Grayson's ligament, which is fascial thickening between the flexor sheath and the skin volar to the neurovascular bundle, at the level of the proximal and middle phalanges (as opposed to Cleland's ligament which is the mirror structure dorsal to the neurovascular bundle and is not involved in Dupuytrens disease).
     The spiral cord is formed by the pretendinous cord, spiral cord, lateral cord, and Grayson's ligament. It contributes to contractures of the MCPJ and PIPJ, and displaces the neurovascular bundle superficially and to the midline of the digit – exposing it to potential iatrogenic injury.

How will you manage a patient with Dupuytrens' disease?

- I will take a focused history to determine:
  1. the effect of the disease on their activities of daily living or quality of life – to determine if any intervention is required at all,
  2. their general medical history – to note for factors associated with Dupuytrens, and more importantly to determine fitness for possible surgery, and
  3. any evidence of Dupuytren's diathesis – to counsel regarding a higher chance of recurrence and aggressive progression.
- My examination will determine:
  1. the extent of the disease:
     - ▪ in the palm and digit,
     - ▪ the presence and extent of any contractures of the MCPJ and PIPJ,
     - ▪ any skin involvement, and
     - ▪ any ectopic disease.
  2. any preoperative numbness or vascular insufficiency, and
  3. any signs of poor outcome after contracture release, such as:
     - ▪ a Boutonniere deformity, or
     - ▪ ligamentous and capsular PIPJ contracture (rather than contracture due to the cord).

In addition, I will perform a Hueston tabletop test as a quick screen: if is negative, then this patient is not for treatment, unless they have an isolated painful palmar nodule that may benefit from a steroid injection.

- My threshold to offer open surgery is:
    - an MCPJ contracture of more than 30 degrees, and
    - any symptomatic PIPJ contracture that meets my CCG funding criteria.
- I will manage their expectations by:
    - making it clear that there is no cure for the disease and that recurrence is common – even more so if there is evidence of diathesis, and
    - informing them of any preoperative signs of poor outcome – if present.
- I will manage patients with symptomatic palmar disease who do not meet the threshold for open surgery with a discussion regarding:
    1. conservative measures such as activity modification, and
    2. percutaneous fasciotomy.

How would you assess for the true contracture of the PIPJ?

I will measure this by flexing the MCPJ and reassessing the PIPJ contracture in this position. This will give me a better idea of the likelihood of achieving a full PIPJ release – which is more likely if less than 40 degrees.

The patient has done some research online and asks about collagenase injections.

- I will inform them that this is an enzyme produced by Clostridium histolyticum that is licensed for percutaneous injection of isolated palpable cords but is no longer available in the UK market.
- For their general information, and if they are considering travelling for this:
    It is injected in the palmar palpable cord then the patient is brought back 24 hours later to manually extend the digit and break the cord, followed by nocturnal splinting for 3 months.
    Risks include tenderness of the injection of the injection site, swelling and bruising which can be extensive, skin tears, and tendon rupture.

Ok, what will you offer this patient?

- Assuming this is primary disease, I will offer a needle fasciotomy as it appears to be an isolated simple contracture of the MCPJ.
    I will explain that there is a recurrence rate of at least 50%, but that does not preclude a repeat needle fasciotomy, or a decision to convert to more invasive surgery if the disease recurs.
- If this were recurrent disease, I would explain that there is a trade-off between a quick treatment with a short recovery but a higher recurrence rate – such as a repeat needle fasciotomy, versus a fasciectomy with a longer recovery period and time off work, but lower recurrence rates.

Tell me about the other surgical options that are available to treat Dupuytren's disease in general.

The general options are fasciotomy, fasciectomy, and dermofasciectomy.

- Fasciotomy, as discussed, may be open or percutaneous (needle fasciotomy) – and is associated with higher recurrence rates.
- Fasciectomy may be limited (with resection limited to diseased fascia) or radical (with resection of all fasciae, both diseased and normal). Radical fasciectomies are historical procedures as they increase morbidity with no improvement in recurrence rates.
- Dermofasciectomy with skin grafting includes resection of diseased fascia and overlying involved skin. My indications for this are skin involvement, and recurrent cases.

How would you design your skin incisions?

- I prefer to use a Skoog approach, which consists of a midline straight-line incision broken up by Z-plasties. This allows me flexibility to place Z-plasties where required after the resection, especially after skin resection.

- However, I am aware of other options – such as:
  - Brunner zigzag incisions, and
  - Palmen incisions, which incorporate multiple Y-V plasties.

How would you manage a residual PIPJ contracture at the end of the fasciectomy?

- This is controversial with considerable debate regarding periarticular ligamentous release procedures – with a high rate of recurrence and salvage procedures.
- I will counsel the patient that release procedures are a reasonable first option – as long as they accept a high rate of recurrence. If they agree, then I will release the collateral ligaments, then the checkrein ligaments if required.

  A volar capsulotomy was classically described as part of this procedure, but this is rarely required, as it is possible for the hand therapists to address this non-surgically.
- I would offer a salvage procedure if there were a functionally restrictive recurrent contracture following a dermofasciectomy. This includes:
  1. fusion of the PIPJ joint in a more functional position, or
  2. amputation in selected severe cases – e.g., for fixed severe combined contractures of the MCP and PIPJ causing ulceration of the palm.

How would you manage a patient who develops late post-operative pain, swelling, and stiffness?

- I suspect that the patient has developed complex regional pain syndrome (CRPS).
- This is a chronic pain condition that is classified into two types based on whether a nerve injury is involved or not and is characterized by:
  - allodynia,
  - hyperalgesia, and
  - at least one symptom and sign according to the Budapest criteria – such as:
    - vasomotor changes with differences in skin temperature of more than 1°C, or differences in skin colouration between different sides of the body,
    - sudomotor changes with asymmetry in swelling or sweating, and
    - motor or trophic changes with decreased movement or changes affecting the hair, skin, or nails.
- I will manage this with:
  - early recognition,
  - analgesia, and
  - hand therapy.
- Analgesia management consists of:
  - simple analgesia,
  - local anaesthetic patches, and
  - Gabapentin, followed by
  - referral to the pain team if that is not successful: with eventual consideration of ganglion blocks.
- Hand therapy includes an early graduated exercise program with desensitization exercises and mirror visual feedback.
- Lastly, there is some evidence that vitamin C improves outcomes, and I will suggest 500 mg for 50 days.

Let's consider another scenario: You release a severe contracture, and the finger remains white after tourniquet release. How would you manage that?

- The causes of this are either:
  - systemic vasoconstriction, or
  - a digital artery injury, or
  - digital artery spasm.
1. I will first check that the patient is systemically warm and well-filled – and confirm this with my anaesthetic colleague.
2. I will then explore the digital arteries within the palm and affected finger to ascertain whether these are intact. If not, then I will proceed with repair of the digital artery with a vein graft if required.

3. If there is no injury seen, then I will assume it may be due to spasm – so:
   - I will allow the finger to sit in a semi-flexed position to avoid tension on the vessels which may have contracted due to the longstanding deformity,
   - apply topical Verapamil, and
   - cover the finger with warm swabs that are regularly changed for 15 minutes.
4. If there is no improvement, then I will consider:
   - 5% Lignocaine patches post operatively, and
   - I will discuss a proximal sympathetic block with the anaesthetist – if not already undertaken as part of the procedure's anaesthesia. This gives excellent analgesia and minimizes peripheral vasoconstriction.

What would you do if your senior trainee calls you to say they have performed a dermofasciectomy and release of a contracted A2 pulley, but have been left with an exposed flexor tendon?

- This is a difficult situation and is best avoided, if possible, by careful planning of:
  - the skin excision,
  - skin flaps, and
  - the site of any flexor sheath release.
- However, if this has occurred, then skin grafts cannot be applied directly to bare tendon.
- The first option is to surgically examine the finger to see if this can be converted into a graftable situation – with possible advancement of local tendon sheath or skin advancement – if the breach in the flexor sheath is small.
- If this is not possible, then I will have to consider a flap – such as a cross finger flap.
- If the patient is asleep, then I will simply dress the finger and wake them. I will fulfil my duty of candour with a full and frank conversation with them to obtain consent for this.
- However, if the patient is awake and willing to have this conversation, then I will proceed to do so to avoid a return to theatre, but I will also ask for a second opinion from a fellow consultant colleague, as this is good practice in an elective scenario with an unexpected on-table complication.

What would you do if you discover that you have divided the nerve during your dissection?

- I would have previously ensured that a theatre microsurgery set, and magnification are available, as with any elective hand surgery list.
- This is a recognized complication that happens infrequently, and I would have counselled the patient about this risk, as part of their informed consent.
- This is sharp division of the nerve and so I expect direct repair will be possible with standard microsurgical techniques using 10/0 ethilon and a microscope.
- I will ensure that I complete my duty of candour discussion post-operatively and document this.
- I will personally follow this patient up – as will all complications – but also to ensure they do not develop a neuroma-in-continuity with localized tenderness overlying it.
- I expect some recovery of sensation – but this will depend on the patient's age and comorbidities.
- Lastly, as with any complication, I will discuss this at the next departmental morbidity and mortality meeting.

How will this nerve repair heal?

- Following the initial cellular response to injury:
  - Wallerian degeneration occurs, followed by
  - regeneration
- The cellular response to injury includes:
  - An influx of sodium and calcium ions along a concentration gradient resulting in depolarization. This generates a change in gene expression, switching the neuron from its signal transmission to regenerative status – with a change in molecular synthesis from neurotransmitters to cytoskeleton and growth-associated proteins.
  - Loss of axonal contact induces the dedifferentiation of Schwann cells from a myelinating to a growth-promoting and cytokine-secreting phenotype, which then recruit macrophages.

- Wallerian Degeneration occurs in the distal segment, with retrograde extension to the most proximal node of Ranvier.

  This consists of axonal degradation by proteases and phagocytosis of the debris – and with it – axon growth inhibitors at the site of injury, which then promotes a pro-regenerative environment in the distal axonal stump.
- Regeneration then occurs with a proximal growth cone that appears after 1 month and guides the regenerating axons at a rate of about 1 mm/day – along:
  1. neurotrophic factor gradients – such as that of nerve growth factor, brain-derived neurotrophic factor, and TFG-b1 amongst many others, as well as
  2. neurotropic contact guidance – along the bands of Büngner, formed by dedifferentiated Schwann cells that are organized along the basal laminar scaffold, and
  3. pruning of growth cones that do not reach the correct target.

     This may be impeded by scar tissue formed by fibroblasts in the epineurium, perineurium, or endoneurium, and the development of multiple branched axonal terminals to form a neuroma.

You are asked to see a patient in dressings clinic with skin flap necrosis of the operated digit. How would you manage this?

- I will first assess for infection and collections, that may require IV antibiotics and or surgical drainage.
- In the absence of these, most patients can be dealt with non-surgically with simple non-adherent dressings and regular review to allow demarcation and granulation.
- If a joint or tendon is exposed, then I will consider local or regional flaps, such as a cross finger flap.

FURTHER READING

1. Michou L, Lermusiaux JL, Teyssedou JP, Bardin T, Beaudreuil J, Petit-Teixeira E. Genetics of Dupuytren's disease. Joint Bone Spine. 2012 Jan;79(1):7–12.

Case 3.6

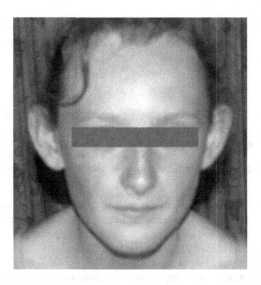

Please describe this photograph.

This is the photograph of a young girl with bilateral prominent ears, with unfolded antihelical folds and what I assume are deep conchal bowls, but I would have to see other views to confirm that.

What is the embryology of ear formation?

- The external ear is formed from the first and second branchial arches starting in the 6th week of gestation.
- The first branchial arch forms the first 3 hillocks, which form the upper third of the ear – including:
    - the tragus,
    - the root of the helix,
    - the cymba,
    - concha, and
    - the superior helix.
- The second branchial arch forms the lower two-thirds of the ear – including:
    - the antihelix,
    - antitragus,
    - lobule, and
    - concha cavum.
- The ear is fully formed by 4 months of gestation but initially located caudal to its normal position and lies in a horizontal plane, hence the caudal position in some patients with microtia and some developmental anomalies.
- As the face develops, it rotates clockwise and moves to a more cephalic position.

At what age would you offer surgery to correct this?

- I will offer surgery to a child who asks for it themselves, rather than their parents. This is usually for those aged 6–7 and upwards, when the ear is nearly fully developed, and they have started school (and with it, the potential distress caused by their classmates' teasing).
- In some cases, if the child is very distressed by their appearance, and is likely to be cooperative with the post-operative instructions, then I may offer it to a 5-year-old.

DOI: 10.1201/9780429399268-40

How would you assess her ears pre-operatively?

I will assess for:

1. any asymmetry in the size, vertical position, and axis of the ear (to pre-operatively point this out to the patient and parents, and warn them regarding the risk of residual post-operative asymmetry),
2. the degree of antihelical folding,
3. the depth of the conchal bowl,
4. any deformity of the lobule,
5. the spring of the auricular cartilage,
6. any other anomalies such as a Stahl's ear or Darwin's tubercle, as well as
7. their Fitzpatrick skin type, as patients with darker skin types may be predisposed to problematic scarring, combined with ear surgery, which itself is a higher risk location.

What are your goals for surgery, and what techniques would you use to achieve this?

- My goals include:
  1. correction of the superior third prominence of the ear aiming to achieve an ideal projection of 21 degrees from the lateral border of the head (with a normal range from 21 to 30 degrees)
  2. correction of the middle and lower portions – such that the helix is visible beyond the antihelix and the helical rim projects laterally beyond the lobule,
  3. a smooth and regular contour of the helix,
  4. symmetry between both ears – regarding correctable aspects (to within 3 mm), and
  5. the treatment of Darwin's tubercle – if present
- Regarding my chosen techniques:
  - I use Mustarde scapho-conchal sutures to correct a poorly defined antihelical fold.
  - I use the suture-based Furnas setback technique to correct conchal excess. In patients with particularly deep conchal bowls, where this is not sufficient, then I will also excise a crescent of conchal cartilage.
  - I use a modified fishtail excision, such as that described by Wood-Smith, to correct a prominent lobule.

So how do you perform the procedure?

1. I mark a linear incision just above the post-auricular sulcus, ensuring that:
   - the superior extent stops short of the root of the helix, to prevent visibility of the scar from the front, and
   - the inferior extent allows access to the concha, or lobule if required.
2. The cartilage is then exposed until the helical rim is reached, ensuring I do not extend the dissection beyond that on to the anterior aspect. I then expose the post-auricular muscles and ligaments as well as the mastoid fascia.
3. I ensure meticulous haemostasis is achieved at this point, as diathermy around the Mustarde sutures placed in the next step may weaken them.
4. I then mark the position of three to four mattress sutures with a Methylene-dipped 25-gauge needle on either side of the anti-helical fold to recreate this. I use clear 4/0 Prolene sutures to place the mattress sutures as per the tattooed marks, ensuring I do not pierce the anterior skin. I then tension the sutures to achieve a smooth line.
5. With regard to the middle third, I divide the post-auricular muscles using bipolar dissection to decrease the risk of subsequent bleeding. I then use one or two 4/0 clear Prolene mattress sutures between the posterior aspect of the concha and the mastoid fascia and periosteum, again ensuring I do not pierce the anterior skin.
6. If the lobule is prominent, I correct this with a fishtail pattern excision.
   - I first extend the inferior skin incision by marking a V extension, with the apex of the V at the most prominent point of the lobule.
   - I then mark a mirror image on the mastoid skin, by pressing the lobule on the skin before the ink dries to form the fishtail pattern that is excised.
7. Subcutaneous haemostasis is then repeated before skin closure.

Do you know of any other techniques?

Yes, anterior and posterior scoring techniques have been described. Whilst scoring techniques can produce excellent results, they have been associated with higher complication rates such as haematomas, as well as anterior skin necrosis with the anterior technique. In addition, the effect of scoring is permanent so there is less room for error – especially when training more junior colleagues.

Why did you use a suture-based technique?

- It produces a good shape in my hands,
- it is associated with a lower complication rate compared to other techniques, and
- It allows for intraoperative adjustment which is very useful, especially when training junior colleagues.

Do you know of any non-surgical treatments for prominent ears?

- Non-operative moulding techniques are best initiated in the first 72 hours of life, or as soon as possible – by taking advantage of cartilage malleability due to circulating maternal hormones.
- There are custom-made or commercially available splints such as Earbuddy™ or EarWell™, as well as taping and gluing techniques.

What information would you give her and her parents pre-operatively?

- I will point out any anomalies that would remain following the correction, and go through the operation in simple terms (based on her age):
  She appears to be at least a pre-teen in this photograph, so she would understand the following: 'the shape of the ear is formed by cartilage and covered by a skin envelope, like a hand in a glove. To shape the cartilage, we first lift the skin up, then use stitches to hold the cartilage in the new shape, before redraping the skin back in place'.
- I will go through the risks with her and her parents, which include:
  - haematoma, with the need for another procedure required to evacuate this,
  - infection, which must be treated promptly to avoid the risk of chondritis,
  - recurrence of prominence,
  - residual asymmetry,
  - a problematic scar, including a Keloid scar, and
  - lastly, contour irregularities, which are unusual with this technique but not impossible.
- I will advise her to avoid contact sport for 6 weeks, and to wear a tennis band at night for 6 weeks.

Do you use a head bandage after surgery?

Yes, I do – but I am aware that this is debated. Any type of coverage is really a 'psychological dressing': most surgeons would use a variation of this for up to 1 week to avoid patient and parental distress and anxiety due to bruising and swelling in the immediate aftermath.

You see this 14-year-old girl, who presents with her mum in clinic. She is very keen to have a bilateral pinnaplasty as she has been severely bullied in school for many years because of this. Her mother is vehemently against her having anything done as she herself has prominent ears and does not believe that a surgical procedure will improve the bullying, but she has agreed to attend the consultation in the hope that you agree with her. Of note, correction of prominent ears has been pre-approved by the relevant CCG in your area for NHS treatment. How would you proceed?

- This is an uncomfortable situation for all involved.
- Considering the situation purely from the medical point of view, she does have prominent ears and she would benefit from the correction – especially as she has suffered socially because of this. There is some evidence to show that patients experience psychological benefit after otoplasty, such as reduced bullying and improved confidence.
  1. I will first explain what the procedure involves to both mum and her daughter – including the risks, benefits, and the expected post-operative recovery.
  2. I will also obtain a psychologist's opinion, as this may sway mum's opinion and provide more weight and support to potentially go ahead.

3. The next point to establish is Gillick competence:
   - If this does not apply in her case, then the situation is simpler – as the mother is the legal guardian, so I cannot proceed with this operation until she consents. I will approach this by probing the mothers' concerns further over multiple consultations.
   - If Gillick competence does apply, then:
     - from a legal point of view: she may have the capacity to consent, depending on her maturity and ability to understand what is involved. Parents cannot legally override the competent consent of a young person to treatment that is in their best interest – as is potentially the case here. Ultimately, I have a legal duty to respect this child's autonomy.
     - The GMC's 'Good medical practice guidance on the consenting process in 0–18-year-olds' further stresses the importance of carefully assessing her maturity and understanding of the implications of the procedure.
4. However, we have the luxury of time: this is a non-urgent, essentially aesthetic procedure, that is not required from a medical point of view, and is not even approved by all CCGs, even if there may be psychological benefits from it.
5. So, I will make every effort to include and obtain consent from both parents, by doing my utmost to try to bring mum on side, as well as attempting to contact her father to seek his consent also.

Mum does not change her decision, despite numerous consultations. It becomes apparent that she is recently divorced from the father – with an ongoing dispute regarding parenting style. You contact the father separately, as he is the joint legal guardian, and he is strongly in favour of his daughter going ahead with the procedure. What now?

- From a legal and GMC point of view, if Gillick competence applies, then I must respect the child's autonomy. Even though I would – of course – much rather proceed with the agreement of both of her parents, I have a legal obligation to respect the patient's decision.
- I will take advice from my hospital's legal team and my medical director, then set up a mediation process and advocate for the child in this.
- This is an elective aesthetic procedure, albeit with potential psychological benefits for the child, so I would ideally want a resolution both parents are happy with, before proceeding.

You've done all this – Mum is still unhappy. What now?

In that case, if the child and the father want to proceed, there is a case for me to do so but I will first seek:

- a second opinion from a senior consultant colleague,
- further legal advice from my hospital's legal team, as well as
- advice from the medical director, whilst continuing to try and resolve the situation until the time of surgery.

What if she were 6-year-old who was bullied to the point where she was refusing to go to school, how would you proceed then?

- This is an entirely different scenario where Gillick competence does not come into play.
- The legal issues here are:
  1. who has parental responsibility, and
  2. how many parents are required to consent.
- The Children's Act for each devolved UK nation states that the mother has automatic parental responsibility. The father would also – if they were married or if his name was on the birth certificate. As both were married, I assume both have legal responsibility here, but I will confirm that with the hosptial's legal team.
- With regard to the number of parents required to consent, the 'Department of Health's 2009 reference guide to consent' states that one is usually enough – even if the other disagrees, with the exception of a small group of important decisions where both need to consent or a court order sought – such as circumcision or vaccinations. As, this does not apply here, only one parent's consent is required from a legal point of view.

- However, I am still concerned as otoplasty is a cosmetic procedure with purely psychological rather than physical benefits. Ultimately, performing a procedure that some would consider to be unnecessary in an immature minor, where there is parental disagreement is not good medical practice. I suspect this would not stand up to legal scrutiny.
- I will obtain legal advice and expert psychological assessment of the child, and wait until the child is older to have legal gravitas.
- In addition, I will involve the school as the bullying may be addressed there and hopefully stopped, or I will suggest that her parents consider moving her to another school in the meantime, if possible.
- If the situation deteriorates to the point where the child is severely distressed, and no resolution is found, then it may be appropriate to involve her GP and safeguarding services.

FURTHER READING

1. https://www.nhs.uk/conditions/consent-to-treatment/children/
2. https://www.gmc-uk.org/ethical-guidance/ethical-guidance-for-doctors/0-18-years
3. https://www.legislation.gov.uk/ukpga/1989/41/contents
4. https://assets.publishing.service.gov.uk/government/uploads/system/uploads/attachment_data/file/138296/dh_103653__1_.pdf

Case 3.7

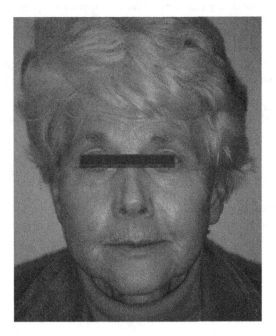

Please describe the effects of ageing on the face.

This affects the skin itself, as well as volume changes in the soft tissue and skeleton.

- The skin becomes thinner, more fragile, and less elastic, with increasing actinic and pigmentation changes with time.
  - Histological changes include:
    1. changes in the collagen composition of the dermis with reduced levels of types I and III collagen,
    2. loss of elastin,
    3. a reduction in glycosaminoglycans,
    4. flattening of the dermoepidermal junction, and
    5. depletion of fibroblasts, Langerhan cells and melanocytes.
  - As the skin thins and loses collagen and elastin, this leads to loss of the dermal capacity to resist the forces of the underlying muscles – with resulting etching in the skin in a pattern corresponding to the underlying muscle contraction. This corresponds to the development of dynamic then static rhytids.
- With regard to soft tissue changes, these include:
  - attenuation of retaining ligaments, with resulting fat pad ptosis,
  - muscle ageing – especially of the upper lip orbicularis – with decrease in muscle thickness, smaller muscle fascicles, and increase in surrounding epimysium. This is visible clinically as an elongated upper lip, and
  - SMAS laxity.
- Bone changes include:
  - a decrease in facial height due to a decrease in the height of the maxilla and mandible, as well as
  - resorption of the pyriform area of the nose, the superomedial and inferolateral aspect of the orbital rim, and the prejowl area of the mandible, which
  - results in a further loss of soft tissue support by placing further strain on the retaining ligaments, which will eventually increase their attenuation further.

DOI: 10.1201/9780429399268-41

How would you assess a patient with an ageing face? Please use her photograph as an example.

- I will first establish her goals and press her regarding her exact concerns.
- Salient points in her history include:
  - smoking,
  - diabetes,
  - hypertension,
  - medication affecting coagulation or wound healing – including over the counter remedies,
  - any allergies, and
  - a history of mental health issues.
- My examination includes an assessment of her skin quality in general, facial movement and sensation, before systematically assessing her face in thirds.
  - Using the photograph as an example: her skin displays fine rhytids affecting most of her face and deep static rhytids in her forehead.
  - In addition, there is mild asymmetry with right side dominance (with the orbit, midface, and mandibular areas affected). This is important to point out to her as this may persist after treatment.
- Regarding the assessment of her face in thirds:
  1. Assessment of the upper third include:
  - the level of her hairline,
  - any forehead ptosis (either compensated or not),
  - forehead rhytids (either dynamic or static),
  - temporal hollowing,
  - eyelid dermatochalasis, and
  - periorbital hollowing – with an A-frame deformity of the upper eyelid and a tear trough deformity of the lower eyelid.
- I cannot see the level of her hairline here, or her temples.
- She does have forehead rhytids with ptosis of the lateral tail of the brow.
- In addition, with regard to the periorbital area, I note dermatochalasis of the upper eyelid despite the area being partly obscured in the photograph.
- There is some volume loss of the lower eyelids with no obvious excess skin. I am unable to comment on the position of the lower eyelid for certain.
  2. Her midface assessment includes looking for:
      - a palpebromalar groove,
      - ptosis of the malar fat pad,
      - circumoral wrinkles,
      - nasolabial folds, and
      - an elongated upper lip.
- All of these features are evident in the photograph.
  3. Assessment of the lower third includes looking for:
      - marionette lines,
      - jowls,
      - submental fat deposits, and
      - platysmal bands, and divarication.
- I note marionette lines, heavy jowls, and can just see platysmal bands – but I would not be able to comment further as the neck is partially hidden by clothing. However, I would establish this clinically.

This lady comes to you seeking facial rejuvenation as her daughter is getting married the following year, and she wants to feel confident on the day. She tells you that she is unhappy with her 'wrinkles' jowls, and her 'jawline'.

How would you proceed?

- Assuming that I establish that she is physically and psychologically fit for an aesthetic procedure, I will inform her that skin quality – including fine rhytids, can be improved with resurfacing treatments, such as:
  1. laser treatment,
  2. retinoic acid,

3. chemical peels, and
4. dermabrasion.
- Dynamic rhytids can be improved with chemodenervation with the understanding that this is temporary, and that static rhytids may also be improved but they will not disappear entirely.
- With regard to the jowling, this can be improved with a facelift:
  - I will explain that the aim of this is to reposition the deeper soft tissue layers – either at the level of the SMAS or subperiosteum – to further support the overlying skin and minimize any skin tension and early recurrence that would occur with a skin-only facelift.
  - I will offer her a SMAS plication lift, as this is an established technique with predictable results. I suspect she may benefit from a neck lift as well as I the superior aspect of anterior platysmal bands, but I would examine her in person to determine that.

She asks about a MACS lift under local anaesthesia, because she is interested in 'the least invasive option' to be on confident on the big day. What are your thoughts?

- This is only a potential option if the anticipated result matches her expectation, and she understands and fully accepts the limitations of the procedure.
- I will warn her that a MACS lift is not a powerful technique to address heavy jowls, so whilst this may be improved, she must accept that:
  - there is a potential risk of residual mild jowling – which may be potentially addressed with some liposuction – if she is intent on this technique, and
  - that the longevity will be reduced compared to other facelift options.

She proceeds with a MACS lift under local anaesthetic. On post-operative review the next morning, you notice she has a facial weakness. What now?

- I will consider that the local anaesthesia might still have an effect. If it persists beyond the timeline for this, then I will have to assume this is a neurapraxia or a neurotmesis.
- I will be open and honest with the patient and inform her of both possibilities, however the likelihood is that this is a neuropraxia as the MACS lift involves a limited dissection that is not sub-SMAS.
- My options are to either re-explore or manage conservatively – which may be considered a controversial area. If the patient agrees, then I will re-explore for two reasons:
  1. if the nerve branch has indeed been cut, then this will give me the opportunity to repair it in the acute stage with a better outcome, and
  2. it also affords the opportunity to give a more certain prognosis if the nerve is visualized directly and found to be intact.

However, I understand that others may manage this conservatively as it is likely to be a neuropraxia, and an exploration would result in another procedure that may be considered by some to be unnecessary.

This is indeed a neurapraxia, which settles in 1 month. She then returns 8 months later with recurrence of her jowling. How will you proceed now?

- I would have extensively counselled her about this risk – both in person in the preoperative consultation, and in my consultation letter.
- I will have an in-depth discussion with her about how she feels about this, and whether she wants another intervention, such as a SMAS face lift, with or without a neck lift.

She decides to go ahead with your advice regarding the next procedure. What now?

- The options are either:
  1. a SMAS plication–type procedure including a neck lift that addresses the platysma with a lateral and/or medial plication, or
  2. a SMAS flap–type procedure: either a high or deep plane, including surgery to platysma.
- My decision-making regarding which facelift type depends on the quality of the SMAS, which I would have assessed during the MACS lift.
  - As per her photograph, I would expect this patient to have a thicker SMAS but I would have confirmed this intraoperatively, so she would be suitable for a SMAS flap procedure if that is the case.

- Given her previous nerve injury, the patient would have to be especially counselled about the risk of this happening again in a further procedure.
- Therefore, my options would be either a high, or deep plane:
  - A high SMAS involves lifting the flap at the level of the zygoma and fixed SMAS, whereas
  - the deep plane involves lifting the SMAS at the junction of the fixed and mobile SMAS.

I prefer the deep plane because it involves a composite lift with less skin undermining and a more direct lift on the area of concern, however there is no consensus in the literature as to which is superior.

How would you reduce the chances of a haematoma? And what are the possible sequelae of this?

- This consists of pre-operative, intra-operative and 'extubation' considerations:
- I preoperatively assess and optimize risk factors such as hypertension and anticoagulation – including over the counter supplements, and I will not proceed with surgery if preoperative optimization is not possible.
- Intraoperative techniques include:
  - adrenaline infiltration – which also facilitates hydro dissection,
  - the use of tranexamic acid – both intravenously and within the infiltration cocktail,
  - meticulous intraoperative haemostasis,
  - the use of fibrin glue, and
  - a haemostatic net in Caucasian patients:
    - this aids in skin redraping and the reduction in the incidence of haematoma and seroma, and is removed 48–72 hours post operatively, to avoid suture marks.
    - I will use a drain if the net is not accepted by the patient or not advisable due to the risk of pigmented suture marks in darker skinned patients. I appreciate that this would not directly decrease the chance of a haematoma but my rationale for its use is to enhance skin redraping and decrease dead space.
- Considerations for the anaesthetist include the avoidance of extremes of blood pressure, and a smooth extubation – if under GA.
- Potential sequelae include:
  1. a potentially life-threatening airway complication if it is of significant size in the neck,
  2. overlying skin necrosis,
  3. contour irregularities of the overlying skin-which may take a long time to resolve, as well as
  4. patient discomfort and distress

Evacuation is indicated for most – unless very small.

You mentioned using tranexamic acid. How does it work?

It has an antifibrinolytic action by reversibly binding lysine receptor sites on plasminogen. This decreases the conversion of plasminogen to plasmin, preventing fibrin degradation.

Its use was first popularized following the beneficial evidence of blood loss reduction in major trauma patients. However, I will be cautious of using it in those with renal disease due to decreased clearance, and it is contraindicated in those with a history of seizures and thromboembolic disease.

Let's go back to this patient. She returns a couple of weeks later with a large cheek swelling. How will you proceed?

- This is either
  - a haematoma,
  - a seroma, or
  - a siloma.
- I will first aspirate it:
  - If it is blood stained and significant, then I will take her back to theatre to wash it out.
  - If it is clear, then I will send it off for amylase to exclude a siloma:
    - If the aspirate is positive for amylase, then I will organize an MR sialogram with contrast, to determine if the parotid duct has been divided (in which case this would need repair).

- ▪ The more likely scenario is that the parotid capsule has been breached either during flap raising or with a suture. I would treat this with aspiration and Botulinum Toxin, and then anticholinergic medication.
- ▪ If it is a seroma, then I would counsel her that she may need repeat aspiration.

You've mentioned neck lifts. Please talk me through your assessment for this and your treatment algorithm.

- My assessment includes recognizing the factors which contribute to ageing of the jaw line, and submental volume and laxity, including:
  - the skin,
  - fat volume and location,
  - platysmal laxity and bands, and
  - submandibular gland ptosis.
- The approach to the neck is dependent on the structures affected and the severity. This is either:
  1. purely lateral, or
  2. anterior, or
  3. both.
     - An anterior neck lift requires a submental incision. It is suitable for younger patients with submental fat excess and reasonable skin quality.
     - A lateral neck lift is usually undertaken in conjunction with a face lift and allows for plication and/or lifting of the platysma in the lateral aspect.
     - The combined anterior and lateral approach is used for corset platysmaplasty and division of medial bands along with excess fat removal – if required.
     - Some patients may be suitable for liposuction of the submental area, but this would only address the subcutaneous fat rather than the preplatysmal fat, which requires an open excision approach.
     - Lastly, there is the option for a direct neck lift in patients who are elderly, or otherwise unfit for extensive surgery, or have significant excess skin post weight loss, and will accept the resultant scar.

FURTHER READING

1. Coleman SR., Grover R. The anatomy of the aging face: volume loss and changes in 3-dimensional topography. Aesthetic Surg J. 2006 Jan;26(1_Supplement):S4–S9.
2. Auersvald A, Auersvald LA. Hemostatic net in rhytidoplasty: an efficient and safe method for preventing hematoma in 405 consecutive patients. Aesthetic Plast Surg. 2014 Feb;38(1):1–9.
3. Grover R, Jones BM, Waterhouse N. The prevention of haematoma following rhytidectomy: a review of 1078 consecutive facelifts. Br J Plastic Surg. 2001;54(6):481–486.
4. Mendelson B, Wong C.(2018) Facelift: Facial Anatomy and Aging. In: Rubin J, Neligan P (eds.) Plastic Surgery: Volume 2: Aesthetic Surgery, 4th ed. Elsevier, pp.79–111.

Case 3.8

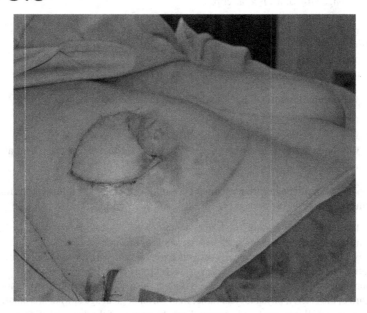

Please describe this photograph.

- This is an intra-operative photograph of a female patient who appears to have had a flap reconstruction of her right breast.
- The skin paddle is superolateral to her native nipple areolar complex, which would indicate that:
  - she has either had a nipple-sparing mastectomy, or
  - that only part of her native breast was removed – such as a lumpectomy or quandrantectomy.

This patient has undergone a DIEP flap reconstruction. Tell me – how does a microvascular anastomosis heal?

- Following completion of the anastomosis, platelets cover endothelial breaches immediately, and disappear between the 1st day and 3rd day provided that collagen within the media is not exposed.
- A pseudo-intima forms over the first 5 days, with
- a new endothelial layer within the first 1–2 weeks.

So, which factors would increase the risk of anastomotic thrombosis?

Prothrombotic factors are any that will increase the risk of platelet aggregation, and/or turbulence – which itself will increase the risk of platelet aggregation – with the consequent release of ADP and thromboxane, and activation of the coagulation cascade.

- I would divide these into three categories:
  1. patient factors,
  2. intra-operative factors (including surgical technique and anaesthetic sequelae), and
  3. post-operative factors.
- Patient factors include a hypercoagulable state – which may be intrinsic due to a known patient coagulopathy, or secondary to major trauma or hypothermia.
- Intraoperative factors include:
  1. vasoconstriction due to any cause – such as hypotension or hypothermia, or
  2. an error in surgical planning and technique such as:
     - choosing a vessel with poor inflow – with failure to perform a 'spurt test',
     - an anastomosis that is under tension, kinked, or twisted,

DOI: 10.1201/9780429399268-42

- rough tissue handling with injury to the intima and exposure of the media,
- thermal injury to the vessels, and
- prolonged use of a vascular clip.
- Post-operative factors such as:
  - prolonged vasospasm in a patient who is cold, in pain, or on vasoconstrictors – including inotropes,
  - hypoperfusion, and
  - external compression from a heavy flap, a drain, or haematoma.

Do you have any contraindications to performing a microvascular procedure?

Yes, these include:
- a patient with a known hypercoagulable state that cannot be corrected and
- a patient who is unfit for relatively prolonged general anaesthesia and the potential need for a subsequent return to theatre.

So, would you perform a microvascular reconstruction in a smoker? Or following irradiation? Or in the extreme elderly?

- Smoking has been shown to only affect the patency of the anastomoses of digital replants. Free tissue transfer has similar patency rates in both smokers and non-smokers.

  However, I would still discourage my patients from smoking as they have a higher rate of other complications (such as poor wound healing or mastectomy skin flap necrosis).
- Irradiation does not affect patency rates, even though the tissue dissection may be more difficult.
- With regard to the elderly, physiological rather than chronological age is what is crucial, as patency rates are equal in all age groups; however, I would be mindful when planning surgery in the extreme elderly as their physiological reserve is decreased compared to their younger counterparts so that complications may cause more serious sequelae than in the young.

How would you manage recipient vessels with severe radiation damage – if no alternatives were available?

- I will first choose the largest possible recipient vessel with high inflow to attempt to counteract the disadvantage at hand.
- In addition, I will:
  - limit dissection of severely damaged vessels to the minimum required,
  - prevent dissection of the intima by passing the needle from 'in to out', whilst ensuring I pass at 90 degrees, as well as
  - reduce the number of required sutures by using a larger suture, if the vessel size allows that.

What is your view on the use of an anticoagulant regime following the anastomosis?

- There is no consensus on an ideal evidence-based anticoagulation protocol for microsurgery.
- My practice includes routine anticoagulation for DVT prophylaxis: I would not routinely start the patient on any anticoagulation specifically for the microvascular anastomosis, to avoid the risk of unnecessary bleeding – except in instances such as:
  - a perforator-to-perforator anastomosis, where I would ask the anaesthetist to give a 5000 U of IV dose of heparin as I start the anastomosis, with a 10-day post-operative course of 75 mg daily aspirin
  - or in the situation of flap salvage, where again, I would give 5000 U of IV heparin after repeating the anastomosis.

How does Aspirin and Heparin work?

- Aspirin inhibits thrombin generation by irreversibly blocking cyclooxygenase, which produces platelet activating factors such as thromboxane.
- Heparin binds to antithrombin III, which in turn, inactivates thrombin.

You are on call and are called by your trainee as the above flap is blue. What would you do?

- I will take this patient back to theatre urgently.
- As the patient is being prepped for theatre, I will review the operative note if I had not performed the operation myself and formulate a plan as follows:
  1. I will first enlist the help of my anaesthetic colleague to correct any hypothermia, hypotension, and vasoconstriction.
  2. I will then lift the flap and check for any causes of obstruction or external pressure such as:
     - a drain,
     - haematoma,
     - anatomical structure, or
     - a particularly heavy flap.
  3. I will then inspect the pedicle to note whether it is:
     - pulsating,
     - in spasm, or
     - whether an obvious thrombus is present.
       Then I will proceed to check the length of the pedicle from the recipient vessel, the anastomosis, to the flap itself looking for kinking or twisting of the pedicle. If present, I will address that-which may require revising the anastomosis if the twist is at the level of the anastomosis.
  4. If the anastomoses are patent but in spasm, I will check again that the patient is warm and apply a topical vasodilator. My first choice is Verapamil – a calcium channel blocker. Other options include 2% or 5% Lignocaine.
  5. If the anastomoses are not patent, I will revise them and take the opportunity to recheck the quality of the recipient vessels, as well as the recipient artery spurt test.
  6. If the anastomoses are flowing but there is still venous insufficiency, then I suspect that the superficial system is not sufficiently drained so I will add another venous anastomosis from the SIEV – which I would have routinely saved at the beginning of the operation, to a recipient vein (such as the retrograde IMV or a preserved DIEP branch in a Type 2 or 3 Moon and Taylor).
  7. If I don't have an SIEV available, then I will debulk the flap and remove the distal zones to decrease the demand on the flap – until flap bleeding is healthy. However, this does mean that flap survival will be at the expense of a smaller reconstructed breast.
  8. If this is not feasible, e.g., due to poor venous flow or severely irradiated veins, then I will use the cephalic vein as a recipient. This may require the use of vein grafts depending on the configuration of the flap, the pedicle, and the position of the SIEV.

How would you handle a size discrepancy between vessels?

- I will manage mild discrepancies by dividing the smaller vessel obliquely to equalize the areas to be sutured.
- With increasing discrepancy, my options include:
  1. a fish mouth incision or spatulation of the smaller vessel,
  2. an end-to-side anastomosis, or
  3. a wedge resection of the larger vessel.
- Lastly, with regards to mild-to-moderate venous mismatches of up to 2 mm, I prefer to use a coupler – by choosing a coupler size in between the ideal size for either vessel, which mildly stretches the smaller vein over the coupler ring and collapses the larger vessel into the other ring. Otherwise, I will hand-sew the anastomosis using the techniques I have discussed.

What is a venous coupler?

This is a device that allows a 'sutureless anastomosis', through the eversion of the vessel ends over two interlocking rigid rings that are 1–4 mm in size – with advantages such as shorter ischaemic times and accommodation of moderate size discrepancy.

- Some studies have shown a lower thrombotic rate compared to hand-sewn anastomoses, although the evidence for this is not strong.

- I am also aware of the development of arterial couplers and those incorporating Doppler flow monitoring, but these have not gained widespread traction yet.

Tell me – how would you monitor the anastomosis?

- I will monitor it clinically if the flap is visible, and the capillary refill is easy to monitor.
- Otherwise, I will use implantable Doppler monitoring in flaps that are either impossible or difficult to monitor visually – such as in buried flaps or in patients who are either very pale or very dark skinned.
- With regards to clinical monitoring, this relies on the flaps':
  - capillary refill-time,
  - temperature (except in intra-oral flaps that will remain warm regardless of perfusion),
  - colour, and
  - turgor.

  If in doubt, I will scratch the skin paddle of the flap – if this is present, with a 25 gauge 'orange' needle to check for both the speed and colour of the return. I find the speed of return a particularly sensitive sign, e.g., in very early congestion where the colour of the return may still be normal.

Let's go back to our scenario, with the patient with a congested flap. What would you do if you find that the whole venous system is filled with thrombus?

- This is a poor indicator for successful salvage, but that is still possible so I will attempt it.
- The flap needs to be thrombolyzed in this instance – with whichever thrombolytic agent is used by my local cardiac unit – most commonly Streptokinase or Urokinase, although others exist.
  1. I will first disconnect the venous anastomosis to prevent systemic thrombolysis. The accompanying drug information sheet will provide advice on how to reconstitute the drug.
  2. I will flush it neat through the flap using one of two ways:
     - If the arterial anastomosis is patent, I prefer to use the arterial pressure to propel the drug through the flap via the largest side branch distal to the anastomosis.
     - If there are no suitable side branches, which is more unusual, then I will take the arterial anastomosis down and flush the drug in the artery, then repeat the arterial anastomosis, and wait 20 minutes for the drug to take effect and for the flap to bleed.
  3. Once that is achieved and the veins are thrombus-free, then I will repeat the venous anastomose(s).

Great, you redo the anastomoses and confirm they are all patent, but the flap does not bleed. What is going on, and how will you manage this?

- This is a 'no-reflow phenomenon', whereby injury to the microcirculation results in failure of flap perfusion despite patent arterial and venous anastomoses.
- The pathophysiology is thought to be due to:
  - ischaemia-induced endothelial cell swelling and membrane disruption, with
  - reperfusion-induced overproduction of reactive oxygen species, and
  - activation of the inflammatory cascade with platelet aggregation.
- This flap is sadly not salvageable, so I will:
  - debride it,
  - dress the wound, and
  - discuss future reconstructive options with the patient when they are awake and ready.

FURTHER READING

1. Cracowski JL, Roustit M. Human skin microcirculation. Compr Physiol. 2020 Jul;10(3):1105–1154.

Case 3.9

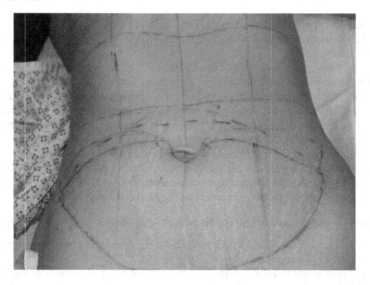

What does this photograph illustrate?

This is a photograph of what appears to be a female patient's abdomen that has been marked for a DIEP flap with perforators marked on the patient's right side, and further vertical lines dividing each side into two sections – illustrating the angiosome concept, with its anatomical, dynamic, and potential territories.

What is an angiosome? Please talk me through the territories you have mentioned.

This is a composite block of tissue supplied by a named artery.

- The anatomical territory of the artery is the area in which vessel branches ramify before anastomosing with adjacent vessels. The vessels that pass between anatomical territories are called choke vessels.
- The dynamic territory is the area into which staining extends after intravascular infusion of fluorescein.
- The potential territory is the area that can be included if the flap is delayed.

What do you mean by a delayed flap?

This refers to the delay phenomenon, which is defined as any preoperative manoeuvre that will result in increased flap survival, such as the elevation of a pedicled flap 2 weeks prior to transfer in order to decrease the chance of distal necrosis.

How does this work?

- It's not completely understood but there are several proposed theories including:
  - improved axiality of blood flow,
  - tolerance to ischaemia after the initial procedure, and
  - altered flap microcirculation.
- In addition, there is evidence of changes in major signalling pathways, such as the mitogen-activated protein kinase (MAPK) and protein kinase C (PKC) pathways, which result in anti-oxidative, anti-inflammatory, and angiogenic effects – such as reduced ischaemia-reperfusion injuries and enhanced tissue regeneration.

DOI: 10.1201/9780429399268-43

How does this alter the microcirculation?

This is not entirely understood and there are numerous proposed theories, such as:

1. the sympathectomy vasodilation theory,
2. the interflap shunting hypothesis, and
3. the hyperadrenergic state.
   - The sympathectomy vasodilation theory proposes that generalized vasodilation occurs following division of sympathetic fibres at the edges of the raised flap.
   - The interflap shunting hypothesis suggests that sympathectomy dilates the arteriovenous anastomoses more than the pre-capillary sphincters, resulting in more blood bypassing the capillary bed. So, during the second operative stage, there is less reduction in flow to the capillary bed than would have occurred had the flap been raised in one stage.
   - The hyperadrenergic state suggests that raising the edges of the flap results in increased vasoconstrictors such as adrenaline and noradrenaline, but at insufficient levels to produce tissue necrosis. The second procedure produces another rise in these substances, but again at a lower level than would have occurred had the flap been raised in one step.

Let us go back to the angiosome concept in this patient – how does it apply to DIEP flaps?

- Zone 1 receives musculocutaneous perforators from the deep inferior epigastric artery (DIEA) and is therefore in its anatomical territory.
- The area of skin lateral to Zone 1 is the anatomical territory of the superficial circumflex iliac artery (SCIA). Blood must travel through a set of choke vessels to reach it from the ipsilateral DIEA. The area of skin on the other side of the linea alba is in the anatomical area of the contralateral DIEA and is within its dynamic territory.
- Zone 4 lies furthest from the pedicle and is in the anatomical territory of the contralateral SCIA. Blood would have to cross two sets of choke vessels to reach it, so is most at risk and frequently discarded – except in very large reconstructions.
- The location of Zones 2 and 3 is dependent on the dominance of the perforators – with medial row dominant flaps having a Zone 2 on the other side of the midline, and the more common lateral row dominant flaps with a Zone 2 lateral to Zone 1.

What would you do if you need to use all flap zones to reconstruct a particularly large breast?

- I will use a bipedicled flap – ideally using the internal mammary vessels for the first set of anastomoses, and the retrograde internal mammary vessels for the second set.
- The alternative is to use the thoracodorsal vessels as the second recipients, if retrograde flow in the internal mammary vessels is insufficient.
- Other options include:
  - the thoracoacromial vessels (but this may have a small vein),
  - the lateral thoracic vessels, or
  - to anastomose one DIEP vessel into the side-branch of the second DIEP vessel, if there is a Type 2 or 3 Moon and Taylor branching pattern.

Why do you prefer the IM vessels?

Their advantages include:

- more superficial vessels – with easier access for microsurgery and better positioning for me as the surgeon, as it avoids working in a relatively deep dark hole, and
- they also allow more medial placement of the flap with less lateral fullness, which is ideal to achieve fullness of the cleavage.

However, I recognize that there is a small chance of a pneumothorax and haemothorax, especially if the area has been severely irradiated.

What would you do if you inadvertently damage the pleura?

- Early detection and management are key to prevent the potential conversion to a tension pneumothorax with continued positive pressure ventilation. This would manifest clinically as increasingly difficult ventilation, progressing to cardiorespiratory decompensation.
- If it is too small to be clinically evident, then I will confirm my suspicion by:
  1. irrigating the suspected area with saline: a pneumothorax will cause bubbling of the air through the saline, as well as
  2. requesting that the anaesthetist performs a Valsalva, which is more sensitive: here, the lung moves away from the surface in a pneumothorax.
- In the case of a confirmed small pneumothorax:
  1. I will simply cover it with a fat graft and place the flap over it to seal the plural breach. I will not attempt to suture it as this may worsen the defect.
  2. I will then obtain a CXR to confirm lung inflation at the end of the procedure: if this is not confirmed, then I will place a chest drain.
- In the event of a larger pneumothorax, or if the anaesthetist notices increasingly difficult ventilation, then I will place the drain more expediently.
- If this is not detected in time, a tension pneumothorax with a patient in extremis will necessitate a needle decompression in the first instance, before insertion of a chest drain.

How would you manage a situation where the IMV is absent?

1. I would perform a cephalic vein turndown: I will first identify the cephalic vein in the Deltopectoral groove and then trace it distally in the arm.
2. Next, I will mark the anterior surface of the vein with Bonnie's blue dye to prevent inadvertent twisting, and
3. Divide it a few centimetres distal to the length required, to ensure the anastomosis is tension-free.

FURTHER READING

1. Wong C, Saint-Cyr M, Mojallal A, Schaub T, Bailey SH, Myers S, Brown S, Rohrich RJ. Perforasomes of the DIEP flap: vascular anatomy of the lateral versus medial row perforators and clinical implications. Plast Reconstr Surg. 2010 Mar;125(3):772–782.

Case 3.10

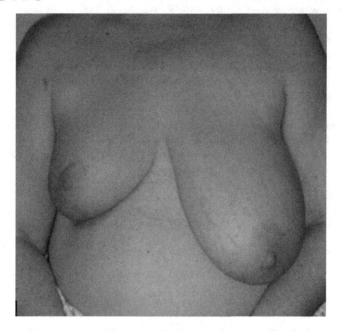

Please describe this photograph.

This is the image of the torso of a lady with a high BMI and marked breast asymmetry – with the left breast significantly larger and more ptotic than the right.

Please describe the anatomy of the breast.

- The breast extends vertically from the second to the seventh rib, and horizontally from the sternocostal junction to the midaxillary line with an axillary extension called the axillary tail of Spence.
- It is composed of multiple lobules – that are interconnected and drained by lactiferous ducts – each of which is composed of hundreds of acini with secretory potential. These are supported by layers of superficial fascia, which are penetrated by Cooper's ligaments that connect the parenchyma to the dermis.
- The IMF is formed by dermal fusion with the superficial and deep fascia.
- The numerous sources of vascular supply to the parenchyma allow numerous pedicles, and consist of:
  - the IMA perforators,
  - the lateral thoracic artery,
  - the thoracodorsal perforators, and
  - the thoracoacromial artery.
- The NAC is supplied by both parenchymal and subdermal vessels.
- Nerve supply to the NAC is from the 4th lateral cutaneous branch in 90% of cases, with additional sources from the 3rd and 5th branches in 10%.
- The rest of the breast skin is supplied by the anteromedial branches of T3–T6 as well as the cervical plexus (C3, C4).

Please describe the embryology of breast development, as well as the stages of breast development.

- Prenatal breast development can be classified into two main processes with:
  1. formation of a primary mammary bud, and
  2. development of a rudimentary mammary gland.

DOI: 10.1201/9780429399268-44

- Bilateral mammary ridges develop from the ectoderm in the 5th week of gestation and extend from the axilla to the groin. Most of these atrophy – except for paired solid epithelial masses in the pectoral region that grow into the mesenchyme to form the primary mammary buds at the end of the first trimester. Failure of this process leads to polythelia in up to 5% of people.
- In the second trimester, secondary epithelial buds appear from indentations on the primary mammary bud, which give rise to lactiferous ducts. These invaginate into the mesenchyme to form a well-defined tubular architecture at 6 months and continue to branch and canalize in the third trimester.
- With regards to the stages of breast development, Tanner described five stages:
  1. stage 1 refers to a prepubertal breast,
  2. stage 2 refers to breast bud formation,
  3. stage 3 refers to further enlargement of the breast and areola,
  4. stage 4 refers to the formation of a secondary mound – due to disproportionate enlargement of the nipple and areola, and
  5. stage 5 being the final adolescent development of a smooth contour with recession of the areola on to the breast.

You mentioned significant ptosis of the left breast. How do you classify breast ptosis?

I use the Regnault classification, which considers the relative positions of the nipple-areola complex (NAC), the breast parenchymal mound and the inframammary fold (IMF) to classify ptosis into four grades: glandular ptosis and Grades I–III.

- Glandular ptosis or pseudoptosis describes a breast with a NAC above the level of the IMF, but with most of the breast parenchyma below the fold.
- Grade I refer to a breast with a NAC at the level of the IMF.
- Grade II refers to a NAC below the level of the IMF, but above the most dependent part of the breast parenchyma.
- Grade III refers to a NAC below the level of the IMF, and at the most dependent part of the breast parenchyma.

She is unhappy with her breast asymmetry and wants a left breast reduction. How do you proceed?

- As with any aesthetic consultation, I will first establish that she is psychologically and medically fit for surgery, before proceeding with a possible surgical plan.
- Assuming her BMI is greater than 30 as the photo would suggest, then I will counsel her strongly to lose weight before we make a final plan, as complications are significantly reduced in those with a BMI less than 30.
- I will arrange to meet with her again when she reaches a safer BMI.
- At this point, I will double check that she is entirely happy with the right breast, as her weight loss may have affected that picture. If so, then I will offer a left-sided reduction with a wise pattern skin excision.
- Regarding the pedicle option:
  - my default choice is the superomedial pedicle, unless the distance of NAC transposition is more than 20 cm – in which case I will suggest a free nipple grafting technique.
  - If the distance of NAC transposition is between 15 and 20 cm, then I will discuss both options – with the understanding that there is a risk of intraoperative conversion to a free nipple graft if she does choose the pedicled option.

Why have you chosen these techniques?

- There is much debate regarding the indications and superiority of different techniques.
- I use a vertical pattern excision in patients requiring smaller reductions and in those with good skin elasticity, which is not the case here, otherwise I will use a Wise pattern.
- I prefer the superomedial pedicle as it allows the creation of better superior pole fullness, and more long-lasting shapes – avoiding the 'bottoming-out' of breasts that occur with inferior pedicle reductions.

- The free nipple grafting technique may 'save' the NAC if an overly long pedicle would otherwise place its vascularity at risk. In addition, the technique would give me more control over the final shape and size of the breast – with the ability to aggressively resect and cone the parenchyma without the risk of distorting the nipple position or compromising pedicle vascularity – which is a particular advantage in patients with gigantomastia. However, its drawbacks include loss of nipple sensation, loss of the ability to breast feed, pigmentary changes to the areola, and the risk of NAC graft loss. So, I will only suggest it if the risk to the nipple is unacceptably high, such as in the case where the NAC will be moved by more than 20 cm or if there is a vascular threat to the NAC that does not respond to more conservative measures.

How will you mark the patient for a wise pattern breast reduction?

- I sit in front of the seated patient.
- I then measure the jugular notch to nipple distance, followed by
- marking the midline, the breast meridian, and the IMF.
- I determine the new nipple position at Pitanguy's point by projecting the IMF onto the breast, check symmetry with the other side and alter it accordingly if needed. I expect the jugular notch to nipple distance to be 21–23 cm.
- Next, I mark the medial limbs to the midline, and
- then ask the patient to lie down to mark the lateral ellipses, as I find this decreases the chance of residual dog ears.
- I finish by double checking all my measurements to ensure symmetry.

How would you define the position of the new nipple, if you find she has significantly asymmetrical IMFs?

I would use landmarks such as the mid-humerus, as well as the jugular notch to nipple distance of 21–23 cm.

Tell me – how would you manage an at-risk nipple? Would you always convert to nipple grafting?

- This is a difficult situation, and the management is somewhat open to debate, as these are very rare cases, with only low volume published case studies, individual case reports, and anecdotal evidence for guidance.
- My management algorithm is based on the timing of the compromise – be it intraoperative or postoperative, and the nature of this – be it arterial or more commonly venous.
- I would have preoperatively counselled the patient regarding this risk, and I will continue to be open and honest – and involve her with regard to the management options, where possible – as I would whilst managing any complication. This will keep her engaged, empowered, and keep her trust.
- If I note an intraoperative ischaemic nipple:
  - I will first check for and reverse factors such as hypotension, hypothermia, or vasoconstriction, then
  - I will try a GTN patch for 30 minutes.
  - If this does not improve matters, then I will proceed with a free nipple graft as this is likely to be due to a non-reversible technical error.
- Intraoperative venous compromise on would closure will prompt me:
  - to check the pedicle is not kinked, or
  - skin closure is not tight: whereby further resection of breast tissue would decrease the pressure.
  - If this improves matters but the problem recurs on skin closure, then I will place tacking sutures and leave them untied, to be progressively tightened and closed in 3–5 days on the ward. This will avoid having to take her back to theatre to achieve wound closure.
  - If it remains blue despite all my measures and I have excluded both kinking of the pedicle, as well as a tight skin closure, then I will place tacking sutures and leave them untied as before – and leech the nipple post operatively – with a plan to progressively close the skin once the congestion resolves.
  - I will discuss this with the patient once she is awake and explain the plan. If she does not accept the risk of nipple loss despite these efforts, then I would convert to a free nipple graft whilst I still can.

- If the patient comes back post-operatively with a blue nipple, then:
  - I will release the periareolar sutures and exclude a hematoma both clinically and on ultrasound – if it is not clinically obvious. If there is a haematoma, then I will take the patient back to theatre for a washout.
  - If there is no haematoma and the nipple improves once the sutures are released, then I will leave the periareolar wound open to heal by secondary intention.
  - If it remains blue, then I will offer the patient the options of conversion to a nipple graft or the attempt to salvage it with leeching, with the understanding that she may end up losing the nipple.
- If the patient returns with a partial or total necrosis of the nipple then I will dress it and let it heal by secondary intention. I will inform her that this may need a nipple reconstruction, in the very rare instance of total loss, once the wound heals entirely.

How does leeching work?

- There are more than 600 leech species, but Hirudo medicinalis is the most frequently applied.
- Their primary effect is to reduce congestion by feeding on blood, with 10–15 ml digested during a 40-minute feed. This is aided by other actions such as:
  - vasodilation: caused by secreted Histamine-like molecules and acetylcholine,
  - an anticoagulant effect: caused by the secretion of hirudin – which is a thrombin inhibitor, and antistasin – which is a factor Xa inhibitor, as well as
  - an antiplatelet effect: caused by various secreted proteins which decrease platelet aggregation and thromboxane production.
- However, it is important to:
  - cover for Aeromonas that is present in their gut and is essential for blood digestion, with broad-spectrum antibiotics such as ciprofloxacin or co-amoxiclav, as well as
  - monitor Hb levels daily.

What are your thoughts on the use of drains in breast reductions? Do you use them?

Despite the evidence that they do not to prevent haematomas, I will still use them in reductions of more than 500 g and in patients older than 50 years of age, as drainage has been shown to be higher in these groups. My rationale is that it would theoretically decrease pressure on the skin and NAC, reduce the recovery time, and possibly decrease scarring – although I recognize there is no strong evidence for this.

Let's consider another scenario: a patient comes for a revision breast reduction as she is upset because her breasts 'are still too big'. This was performed abroad, and the operation note is not available. How would you manage this situation?

This is another difficult situation. If I confirm that she is psychologically and medically fit for revision surgery, then:

- I will encourage her to wait for 1 year before any revision to allow for any swelling and tissues to settle, then
- I will plan for a central mound technique as the previous pedicle is unknown with the understanding that there is a risk of intraoperative conversion to a free graft technique, and I would warn her regarding a higher chance of fat necrosis and nipple loss.

Why do you need to confirm she is psychologically and medically fit? Surely that is already confirmed as she has already had her first breast reduction without any sequelae?

- It is important that I restart a complete assessment of any patient who presents to me – regardless of what procedures they may have had in the past, as we all have different surgical protocols and different levels of accepted risk. Also, the fact that she hasn't had a medical complication the first time may just be down to good luck rather than a good preoperative workup.
- I would also suggest that her current unhappiness with her post-operative result may be due to:
  - poor preoperative workup,
  - an intraoperative error (with the surgeon resecting less tissue than what may have been agreed on), or

– unstable psychology, e.g., if she had requested her current size preoperatively then changed her mind afterwards.

FURTHER READING

1. https://adc.bmj.com/content/archdischild/44/235/291.full.pdf
2. Colen SR. Breast reduction with use of the free nipple graft technique. Aesthet Surg J. 2001 May;21(3):261–271.
3. Sig AK, Guney M, Uskudar Guclu A, Ozmen E. Medicinal leech therapy—an overall perspective. Integr Med Res. 2017;6(4):337–343.

Case 3.11

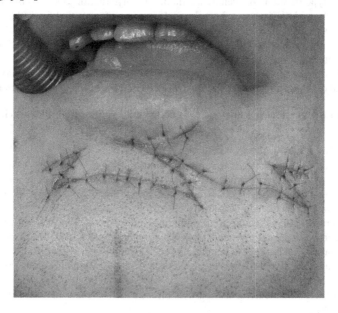

This patient has had Z-plasties performed as part of a scar revision.

What is a Z-plasty? And how would you plan one?

- This is a procedure which involves the transposition of two interdigitating triangular flaps, where the donor site of one becomes the recipient of the other.
- It is used to re-orientate or lengthen a contracted scar – whereby the angle of the Z plasty determines the potential gain in length – with a 25% increase in length for every 15° increase in angle. However, the greater the angle, the more laxity is required to allow transposition. So, 60° angles are most commonly used, giving a 75% increase in length.
- To plan it:
  - I mark the scar – or the portion of it – that needs to be lengthened or re-orientated.
  - Next, I mark the points where I would like the new scar to lie – along the RSTLs, if possible.
  - I then draw a line from the scar to the points, creating triangular flaps that share a common border along it.

Tell me – How will the wound in the photograph heal?

As the skin edges are directly opposed, healing will occur by primary intention and will progress through overlapping phases of haemostasis, inflammation, proliferation, and remodelling – aided by the processes of angiogenesis and wound contraction.

- Haemostasis begins almost instantly after injury, and culminates with the formation of a red thrombus via the intrinsic and extrinsic pathways of the coagulation cascade.
- The inflammatory phase lasts for the first 72 hours and is initiated by factors released by platelets such as PDGF.
  - This attracts neutrophils, and macrophages – which are the key players in this step.
  - Neutrophils debride tissue and phagocytose microorganisms in the first 48 hours.
  - Macrophages attract fibroblasts, by releasing various cytokines such as TGF-ß, PDGF, and Interleukin-1, and promote angiogenesis, by producing VEGF and TNF-α.

DOI: 10.1201/9780429399268-45

- This promotes the start of the proliferative phase that lasts for around 3 weeks. Fibroblasts, which are usually located in perivascular tissue, migrate along networks of fibrin fibres into the wound. They secrete type III and I collagen (in a ratio of 3:1), Glycosaminoglycans (GAGs), and elastin.
- The remodelling phase starts at 3 weeks and continues for up to 18 months, during which equilibrium is reached between collagen breakdown and synthesis:
  - The initially disordered collagen becomes organized with stronger cross-links along the lines of tension, and
  - Type I collagen replaces type III to restore the original 4:1 ratio. The maximum tensile strength of the scar occurs at about 6–8 weeks with 80% of the pre-injury strength.

You've mentioned the processes of angiogenesis and wound contraction. Please tell me more about them.

- Angiogenesis starts with:
  1. migration of endothelial cells towards an angiogenic stimulus (such as VEGF and TNF-a),
  2. followed by proteolytic degradation of the parent vessel basement membrane,
  3. proliferation of endothelial cells behind the leading front of migrating cells, and
  4. finally, maturation of endothelial cells.
- Wound contraction begins soon after wounding and peaks at 2 weeks, with the amount of contraction proportional to the wound depth. This contributes to up to a 40% decrease in the size of full thickness wounds – less so in more superficial wounds, where epithelialization will play a more important role. Myofibroblasts are the key players here, by aligning along skin tension lines to produce contraction along this.
  - They are derived from fibroblasts but contain actin microfilament bundles along their plasma membrane,
  - Hormones, such as vasopressin, bradykinin, and adrenaline, induce myofibroblast pseudopodia to extend.
  - Cytoplasmic actin then binds to extracellular fibronectin, attaches to collagen fibres and retracts-drawing the collagen fibres to the cell, and thereby producing wound contraction.

You've mentioned the coagulation cascade. Please tell me more about that.

- This is a cascade of events that leads to haemostasis.
- The intrinsic pathway begins with the activation of Factor XII after exposure to endothelial collagen in the tunica media and adventitia of damaged vessels.
- The extrinsic pathway is initiated by damaged endothelial cells releasing Tissue Factor, which activates factor VII.
- Both pathways converge via the common pathway whereby prothrombin is converted to thrombin, which in turns activates the conversion of fibrinogen to fibrin.
- The fibrin mesh helps to stabilize the platelet plug, which is initially white if it contains only platelets, but then becomes red when red blood cells are trapped.

So, what is different about foetal wound healing?

- This is characterized by regeneration rather than scarring in the first trimester, with:
  1. absence of inflammation,
  2. rapid deposition of organized collagen – with a normal ratio of type I:III collagen,
  3. a higher concentration of water and hyaluronic acid in foetal extracellular matrix, and
  4. rapid epithelialization.
- Possible pathophysiological theories include:
  1. a lack of TGF-ß1 and TGF-ß2, as well as
  2. the effect of tenascins, which are large extracellular matrix glycoproteins that are present during embryogenesis and then re-expressed at lower concentrations in healing wounds. They are thought to be involved in:
     - the initiation of cell migration during epithelialization,
     - modulation of cell growth and movement, and
     - the deposition and organization of other glycoproteins during tissue repair.

You've mentioned TGF-ß. Please tell me more about that.

- The three mammalian TGF-ß isoforms belong to the TGF-ß cytokine superfamily – members of which regulate wide ranging processes from wound healing to immune function, and cancer progression.
- With regard to wound healing, they are involved in all three stages in addition to angiogenesis, epithelialization, and wound contraction.
- Disordered ratios between the isoforms have been implicated in chronic wounds, as well as excessive scarring, but the full extent of the picture is not yet understood.
- TGF-ß1 is the most prevalent of the three. It is involved in:
  1. the recruitment of neutrophils in the inflammatory phase – along with PDGF,
  2. the stimulation of fibroblasts to produce collagen and VEGF in the proliferative phase,
  3. the inhibition of MMPs during the remodelling phase,
  4. the induction of keratinocyte migration during epithelization, and
  5. the stimulation of myofibroblasts to contract.

What are MMPs?

Matrix metalloproteinases are enzymes that degrade extracellular protein:

- their inhibition is implicated in excessive scarring, and
- their overstimulation is implicated in chronic wounds.

Ok, please continue.

- TGF-ß3 has been shown in some studies to have antagonistic effects to TGF-ß1, with a reversed ratio of TGF-ß3:TGF-ß1 in wounds with minimal scar formation such as mucosa, or scarless wound healing such as in foetal wound healing.
- However, there is evidence to suggest that the reality may be far more complex, with the actual effect of the isoform dependent not just on the presence of the cytokine itself, but also on the ratio of the isoforms, the timing of its release, and the type of tissue it is acting on.

How would this differ from the processes in a wound left to heal by secondary intention?

Wound contraction and ECM deposition will occur to a greater extent – as well as the process of reepithelization, which involves:

1. mobilization of keratinocytes at the periphery (or in appendages in partial thickness wounds) due to loss of contact inhibition,
2. migration of these cells until contact inhibition is re-established, followed by
3. mitosis of basal cells, and finally,
4. differentiation of the cells to re-establish the basement membrane and epithelial layers.

What are the factors that affect the wound healing process that you have described?

These can be local and systemic:

- Local factors include infection and radiation.
  - Infection prolongs the inflammatory phase and activates collagenase.
  - Radiation causes endarteritis obliterans and lymphatic scarring, resulting in local ischaemia and oedema.
- Systemic causes may be inherited or acquired.
  - Inherited causes include:
    - defective collagen – such as in Ehlers Danlos, and
    - abnormal elastin – such as in Cutis laxa and Pseudoxanthoma elasticum.
  - Acquired causes include:
    - malnutrition, such as Hypoalbuminemia and deficiencies in vitamin A, C, D, and Zinc required for collagen synthesis,

- diabetes mellitus that affects white cell activity and local blood supply,
- medication, such as chemotherapy that prevents mitosis of cells, steroids that affect macrophages, and NSAIDs that reduce collagen synthesis,
- lastly, advanced age slows wound healing.

The wound eventually heals but the patient is unhappy with their scar. Please tell me about problematic scars.

- A problematic scar refers to any abnormality of the colour, contour, and texture of the scar manifested as hypo- or hyperpigmentation, keloid, hypertrophic, and depressed scars.
- Hypertrophic and keloid scarring are aberrant forms of wound healing.
     Whilst their absolute causes and pathophysiological processes have not been entirely elucidated, it is accepted that they display continuously localized inflammation, upregulation of fibroblast function, and excessive ECM deposition.
- With regard to hypertrophic scars:
  - Clinically, these are:
    - raised,
    - do not overgrow over the original wound boundaries,
    - can sometimes regress with time, and
    - rarely recur following excision.
  - In addition, they tend to have a predictable cause that results in prolonged inflammation, such as:
    - infection,
    - prolonged epithelialization, and
    - excessive tension.
  - Histologically, they consist of excessive type III collagen arranged parallel with the skin surface.
  - TGF-β1 has been implicated in the pathophysiology, along with other fibrinogenic factors such as IGF-1, by:
    - first delaying the inflammatory phase by inhibiting keratinocyte migration, with
    - a further effect of decreasing the concentration of a cytokine called Stratifin – which is released by differentiated keratinocytes as they signal to the dermis to slow down matrix production by fibroblasts, as well as
    - further promoting collagen deposition by inhibiting MMP action during the remodelling phase.
  - With regard to management of these scars:
    - I would start with non-operative measures, such as silicone-based products, pressure, and massage therapy where applicable, and then
    - progress to offer revisional surgery, if appropriate.
- With regard to keloid scars:
  - Clinically:
    - they extend beyond the edges of the original wound and may cause functional symptoms of pruritus and hyperesthesia in addition to cosmetic concerns,
    - they do not regress and commonly recur following simple excision, and
    - they can occur after the most minor of wounds, and disproportionately affect:
      - darker skinned individuals compared to Caucasian patients, and
      - areas of predilection-such as the sternum, deltoid area, and earlobes, and
      - pregnant patients, and
      - there is some evidence that they may become aggravated in hypertensive patients.
  - The histological features include:
    - 'Keloidal collagen', which consists of whorls and nodules of thick, hyalinized and disorganized type I and type III collagen bundles,
    - a higher concentration of elastin, and
    - tongue-like projections of scar tissue that advance underneath the surrounding normal epidermis.
    - In addition, perivascular chronic inflammatory infiltrates with mast cells are found in the reticular dermis.

- As with hypertrophic scars, the pathophysiology of keloids implicates abnormal TGF-ß1 and MMP signalling pathways. But in addition, keloids have been shown to have:
  - higher Interleukin production in the inflammatory process,
  - higher levels of VEGF,
  - keloid fibroblasts that have an altered phenotype with a higher sensitivity to growth factors and a higher number of growth factor receptors including TGF-ß1, PDGF, and IGF-1 receptors, as well as
  - abnormal mechanosignalling pathways such as the integrin pathway that mediates cell attachment to the ECM.
- With regard to keloid scar management:
  - I would start with non-operative measures such as intralesional steroid injection in combination with pressure therapy where possible, and
  - progress to intralesional excision in combination with steroids. Other alternatives include adjuvant intralesional cryotherapy, interferon injection, 5-FU, Bleomycin, Laser, and radiotherapy.
  - I would also ensure any hypertension is treated, where present.
- With regard to abnormalities in pigmentation:
  - Post inflammatory hyperpigmentation (PIH) of scars results from melanin overproduction or irregular dispersion after cutaneous inflammation and may occur at the level of the epidermis or the dermis.
    - When this is confined to the epidermis, there is an increase in the production and transfer of melanin to surrounding keratinocytes.
    - PIH within the dermis results from inflammation-induced damage to basal keratinocytes, with the release of large amounts of melanin. The free pigment is then phagocytosed by macrophages, now called melanophages, in the upper dermis and produces a blue-grey appearance to the skin at the site of injury.
  - There is limited information about the mechanism and pathogenesis of post inflammatory hypopigmentation.
    - The chromatic tendency of the reaction of melanocytes to trauma is genetically determined and inherited in an autosomal dominant pattern.
    - It is suggested that hypopigmentation may result from inhibition of melanogenesis. However, severe inflammation may lead to melanocyte death with permanent pigmentary changes.

FURTHER READING

1. Mustoe TA, O'Shaughnessy K, Kloeters O. Chronic wound pathogenesis and current treatment strategies: a unifying hypothesis. 2006. Plast Reconstr Surg. 117:35S–41S.
2. Medina A, Scott PG, Ghahary A, Tredget EE. Pathophysiology of chronic nonhealing wounds. J Burn Care Rehabil. 2005 Jul–Aug;26(4):306–319.
3. Li J, Chen J, Kirsner R. Pathophysiology of acute wound healing. Clin Dermatol. 2007;25:9–18.
4. Lichtman MK, Otero-Vinas M, Falanga V. Transforming growth factor beta (TGF-β) isoforms in wound healing and fibrosis. Wound Repair Regen. 2016;24(2):215–222.
5. Wang P-H, Huang B-S, Horng H-C, Yeh C-C, Chen Y-J. Wound healing. J Chin Med Assoc. 2018;81(2):94–101.
6. Whitby DJ, Ferguson MW. Immunohistochemical localization of growth factors in fetal wound healing. Dev Biol. 1991 Sep;147(1):207–215.
7. Chin D, Boyle GM, Parsons PG, Coman WB. What is transforming growth factor-beta (TGF-β)?. Br J Plast Surg. 2004;57(3):215–221.
8. Lichtman MK, Otero-Vinas M, Falanga V. Transforming growth factor beta (TGF-β) isoforms in wound healing and fibrosis. Wound Repair Regen. 2016;24(2):215–222.
9. Pakyari M, Farrokhi A, Maharlooei MK, Ghahary A. Critical role of transforming growth factor beta in different phases of wound healing. Adv Wound Care. 2013;2(5):215–224.
10. Davis EC, Callender VD. Postinflammatory hyperpigmentation: a review of the epidemiology, clinical features, and treatment options in skin of color. J Clin Aesthet Dermatol. 2010;3(7):20–31.

11. Ruiz-Maldonado R, Orozco-Covarrubias ML. Postinflammatory hypopigmentation and hyperpigmentation. Semin Cutan Med Surg. 1997 Mar;16(1):36–43.
12. Ojeh N, Bharatha A, Gaur U, Forde AL. Keloids: current and emerging therapies. Scars Burn Heal. 2020;6:2059513120940499.
13. Rabello FB, Souza CD, Farina Júnior JA. Update on hypertrophic scar treatment. Clinics (Sao Paulo). 2014;69(8):565–573.
14. Huang C, Ogawa R. Keloidal pathophysiology: Current notions. Scars Burn Heal. 2021;7:2059513120980320.

Case 3.12

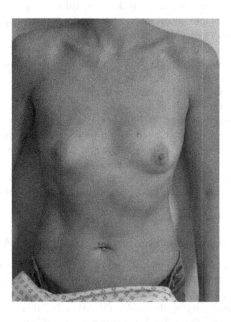

This 17-year-old athletic girl attends your private clinic with her mother asking for bilateral breast implant augmentation. She reports feeling unattractive compared to her peers and is worried the appearance of her breasts may limit her employment prospects in the modelling industry.

How would you proceed?

This is a potentially complex scenario, with several issues to consider including:

1. the medical aspect, with psychological and physical considerations, as well as
2. her age – with consequent legal, and GMC 'Good Medical Practice' implications.
   - From a medical point of view,
     - I will consider her:
       - breast development,
       - chest wall development,
       - psychology, and
       - potential endocrine disorders.
     - The surgical options to anatomically augment her breast include
       - implants,
       - autologous options, or
       - both.
   - From a legal point of view, the 'Family Law Reform Act 1969' in England and Wales, the 'Age Majority Act 1960' in Northern Ireland, and the 'Age of legal capacity act 1991' in Scotland state that the consent of a 16-year-old minor is as effective as that of an adult.
   - However, GMC 'Good Medical Practice' guidance on cosmetic intervention and the BAAPS guidelines suggest a minimum age of more than 18.

In this situation, I would explain that I would refrain from operating until she is 18 years of age, but I will offer to talk her through the general options for her information.

She comes back the following year, with her mother who is very supportive. What now?

- I will re-establish her goals – and explore the reasons for her wanting surgery more carefully – and stress that this procedure may improve her confidence but may not improve her career prospects.

DOI: 10.1201/9780429399268-46

- If her goals are achievable, and she appears to be psychologically healthy, then I will request a psychology assessment to support my decision to treat her, as she is still very young.
- If her goals are not achievable, or I have any doubt regarding her psychological suitability, then I will decline to operate, explain my reasons why, and offer further support with:
  - a referral to a psychologist if she wishes to consider that, and
  - inform her GP, if she consents to that.
- In a patient who is psychologically and medically healthy – with achievable goals, the next step is to establish the mode of breast augmentation. This can be:
  - autologous with lipofilling or flap-based options,
  - non-autologous with implants, or
  - a mixture of both (such as using lipofilling to mask implant edges).

    However, based on the photograph, I would be concerned regarding a lack of adequate autologous donor sites to support a purely autologous option, so I would suggest the latter two options if my examination of her potential donor sites confirms that.

    Also, she would need to be adequately counselled regarding the risks of implants – particularly capsular contracture and the emerging risks of anaplastic large cell lymphoma (ALCL).

What do you mean by psychologically healthy?

How would you assess that, and why don't you just leave it to the psychologist to assess that?

- Judging a patient's psychological health should not be delegated entirely to a psychologist, as I will not perform a purely aesthetic procedure on a patient if I have concerns regarding their psychological suitability – even if a psychologist deems them to be fit.
- As surgeons, we all have varying thresholds for risk – and this is not a medically essential procedure, so I will not take that risk if I do not feel comfortable to go ahead with a patient.
- However, that is not to say that formal psychological assessments are not helpful – they are – particularly in situations where:
  1. I would like confirmation that a patient is healthy and prepared for surgery – even more so in situations such as this, where they are very young, or
  2. for the assessment and treatment of distressed patients whom I have declined to operate on – for either psychological or medical reasons.
- Body dysmorphic disorder (BDD) is a psychiatric condition characterized by a distorted perception of one's body image. I would be concerned by red flags such as:
  - the preoccupation with a minor or perceived defect that disproportionately interferes with their social and interpersonal functioning, and
  - strong or disturbing language when used to describe the defect
- A useful and validated tool is the BDD Questionnaire-Dermatology Version (BDDQ-DV): it is a quick questionnaire, which has been validated in the cosmetic population and has a high sensitivity and specificity.
- Other validated tools include the Dysmorphic Concern Questionnaire, but this has a lower sensitivity.

She is concerned regarding the safety of silicone implants, as she has read several blogs about the Poly Implant Prothese (PIP) scandal and breast implant illness. How do you proceed?

I will inform her of the following:

- With regard to the safety of silicone implants, they are made from medical grade silicone – small quantities of which can be taken up by the body and found in the breast tissue, or in the lymph glands, or elsewhere. This may manifest as inflammatory nodules around silicone deposits called silicone granulomas.
- With regard to the PIP scandal, PIP was a French company that was liquidated in 2010, after the discovery of their fraudulent use of non-medical grade silicone, with a much higher incidence of implant rupture. The implants that are currently used are from reputable companies which are FDA approved.

- However, as we are talking about safety, it is important to mention that there is a very rare form of cancer called ALCL, which has been recognized by the WHO in 2016 to be associated with implants. Rather than a breast cancer, it is a type of cancer of the blood cells that is associated with the capsule around the breast implant.
  - Current evidence is in flux with new information about it being discovered as we speak. To date, cases of breast implant–associated ALCL (BIA-ALCL) have occurred between 2 and 28 years after breast implant insertion with the average time being 8 years.
  - It is most likely to show up as a swelling around the implant causing an increase in the size of the breast, called a seroma.
  - It can usually be successfully treated with an operation to remove the implant and the capsule of tissue surrounding it, but it has also resulted in death in a small number of patients.
  - Because it is so uncommon, international organizations are sharing data and information about this condition.
  - Most of the cases worldwide have occurred in women with textured as opposed to smooth breast implants, with higher numbers in those with implants that have a coarser texture than those with a finer texture.

  However, breast implants continue to have safety approval from Government organizations such as the UK MHRA and the US FDA, and they continue to be used in breast reconstruction following treatment of cancer worldwide.
- Lastly, there have been patient reports of symptoms associated with Breast Implant Illness. This is a term used by some patients who have breast implants and experience a variety of non-specific symptoms that they feel are directly connected.
  - It is important to know that it is not a medical diagnosis, and there is no proven association with breast implants to date; however, ongoing studies are being conducted around the subject.
  - Some patients do report that their symptoms improve if their implants are removed:
    - around half of whom find that the improvement is temporary, and
    - others do not have any improvement at all.

How would you counsel her regarding implant-based augmentations?

I would explain that:

- Early risks include:
  - a haematoma – which would require return to theatre, and
  - infection – which may be require antibiotics if very mild or implant removal-if more severe-with a time gap of 6 months before inserting another one to allow the wound to settle.
- More delayed complications include:
  - implant rotation,
  - capsular contracture,
  - implant rupture (with a 10% risk at 10 years and 50% at 15 years),
  - residual asymmetry,
  - visible ripples and folds,
  - altered sensation to the breasts and nipples, and
  - BIA-ALCL.

  I would also add that there have been patient reports of non-specific symptoms described by some as breast implant illness.

- The chance of requiring a re-operation for any reason is about 1% per year, with capsular contracture being the most common reason. Treated capsular contracture is likely to recur in 50% of cases.
- I will stress that certain features will not improve and may even become more noticeable – such as:
  - cleavage width – which may be especially accentuated by submuscular implants,
  - stretch marks, and
  - visible cutaneous veins
- I will also warn her that her final breast cup size cannot be guaranteed and may vary based on the bra type and shape,

- Sagging may occur with time – although this is unlikely to be a particular concern in this case, and the implant may drop further below the nipple position – which is called 'bottoming out'.
- With regard to future breast feeding – this is not affected in most women, but there is a small risk that she may not be able to breast feed at all, or that her milk is reduced.

She appears to be well informed with reasonable expectations. She would like to have an implant-based augmentation and hopes to go up by about one cup size. How do you plan the procedure?

- This involves:
  - choosing the implant (with the implant size, shape, and surface texture) and
  - choosing the pocket plane.
- With regard to the size of the implant,
  - I will ask her to perform a rice test – the volume of which is converted to a potential implant volume – to test the appropriate sizers. I will warn the patient that the rice volume is not the exact volume that she will eventually have, as it simply provides an indication of the range of implant sizes to be ordered.
- With regards to the shape, my choices are round or anatomical. I prefer to use a round implant to avoid potential complications due to rotation.
- With regards to the surface texture, I will have a careful discussion with her regarding the options of:
  - a smooth implant – with increasingly contested evidence that this increases the risk of subsequent capsular contracture versus textured implants, or
- a textured implant – with emerging evidence that this increases the risk of ALCL – with the approximate risk of 1 in 24,000 women, however the data is continuously changing.
- With regards to the choice of pocket plane:
  - I will assess:
    - her skin quality, nipple to IMF distance, and the upper pole pinch test to see whether the skin pocket will accommodate the desired implant, and
    - any fat donor sites for a potential small volume fat transfer that may be required to disguise implant edges.
  - My choices are subglandular and submuscular planes – which are commonly reproducible and recognized techniques. I am aware of dual and subfascial planes, but I would prefer to avoid these as a new consultant, as they have a higher learning curve and differing definitions in different literature articles.
  - If the upper pole pinch test <2 cm, I will discuss:
    - a submuscular approach or
    - fat transfer to disguise the edges of a subglandular implant.
  - The advantages of the submuscular plane include a reduced risk of:
    - wrinkling, and implant edge visibility, and
    - capsular contracture – although this is increasingly contested, and likely due to the lower chance of a palpable capsule under the muscle layer
  - However, its' disadvantages include:
    - animation,
    - tenderness, and
    - a tugging sensation in the medial aspect – which can be significant, especially in this young athletic girl.

Tell me about capsular contracture.

- This is an excessive version of the foreign body reaction that occurs around any foreign body, including all breast implants, to wall off the implant from the rest of the body.
- It is classified by the Baker system with four stages ranging from stage I with a soft non-palpable implant to stage IV with a painful hard distorted breast.
- Aetiologic theories include:
  - subclinical infection (most commonly by Staphylococcus epidermidis), and
  - a foreign body reaction.

- I would manage symptomatic capsules – i.e., Baker Grades III and IV, with:
  - a subtotal capsulectomy with change of implant and change of plane, if the patient wishes to continue to have an implant, and
  - the alternative is removal, with or without autologous options, with the understanding that she may need to accept a smaller augmentation.

What not perform a capsulotomy?

- I would not advise this procedure as a routine, as it has an up to 90% rate of capsular recurrence and may result in visible ridges.
- However, if the patient does not want a change of implant, or the morbidity of a capsulectomy, then a capsulotomy is an option if she accepts the risks of that.

You proceed with submuscular breast implants, and she comes back with animation and tenderness. This is preventing her from undertaking her daily exercise. Now what?

I would give her the option to:

- simply remove them with no replacement,
- move them to the subglandular plane, with lipofilling to attempt to conceal the implant edges – with the understanding that she may still be left with palpable or visible implants if she doesn't have enough fat, or
- consider autologous options – with the understanding that she may have a smaller augmentation.

FURTHER READING

1. Tebbetts JB, Adams WP. Five critical decisions in breast augmentation using five measurements in 5 minutes: the high five decision support process. Plast Reconstr Surg. 2005;116:2005–2016.
2. BDDQ-DV screening tool: https://practicaldermatology.com/pdfs/pd0215_SF_BDD.pdf
3. https://www.gov.uk/guidance/symptoms-sometimes-referred-to-as-breast-implant-illness
4. https://www.fda.gov/medical-devices/breast-implants/risks-and-complications-breast-implants
5. https://www.legislation.gov.uk/ukpga/1969/46
6. https://www.gmc-uk.org/ethical-guidance/ethical-guidance-for-doctors/cosmetic-interventions
7. https://www.fda.gov/medical-devices/breast-implants/types-breast-implants
8. https://baaps.org.uk/patients/safety_in_surgery/breast_implant_safety.aspx
9. https://www.legislation.gov.uk/ukpga/1991/50/contents
10. https://www.legislation.gov.uk/apni/1969/28/contents

Case 3.13

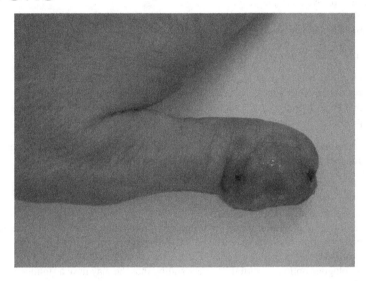

A 50-year-old self-employed roofer presents with a 6-week history of this lesion on their thumb. He initially thought that he may have a type of fungal infection as his nail plate became flaky and came off – revealing this lesion that grew quickly over the next 4 weeks. How would you proceed?

- I am concerned regarding a malignant process, and will proceed with a focused history, examination, and histological confirmation with an urgent biopsy. If this is positive, then I will image him to establish the extent of any local invasion – as well as regional or distant spread, before considering his treatment options within the skin MDT.
- Salient points in the history include establishing:
  - UV exposure,
  - immunosuppression,
  - history of radiotherapy,
  - any personal or family history of skin cancers,
  - medication – particularly immunosuppressants or anticoagulation,
  - hand dominance, and
  - any treatments he may have undergone for the supposed nail infection.
- Next, I will:
  - exclude palpable axillary nodal disease, and
  - perform a full-body exam to assess for any other skin lesions, or intransit disease – in the case of potential melanoma.
- I will then arrange for an urgent biopsy under local anaesthetic.

The biopsy comes back positive for squamous cell cancer, and there are no palpable nodes. How will you manage him now?

- I will image him to establish:
  - the extent of any bony invasion – with a radiograph, and
  - any regional spread – with an ultrasound scan, with fine needle aspiration of suspicious nodes. If this is positive, then he will need a staging CT chest/abdomen/pelvis to exclude more distant spread.
- I will discuss his management options within the skin MDT, with the suggestion that:
  - I excise the lesion and reconstruct the defect with a split skin graft– if there is no bony destruction on the X-ray or

DOI: 10.1201/9780429399268-47

- I amputate the thumb with a 1-cm margin and intraoperative margin control – if bony destruction is evident, with a plan to arrange the reconstruction of his thumb once clear margins are confirmed.
- Radiotherapy is not a primary treatment modality in this case, as it is a relative contraindication in extremities – so is reserved for patients who are not surgical candidates.

Bony destruction is evident on the radiograph, so he agrees to an amputation, but asks about his future reconstructive options. You have a subspecialty interest in hand surgery, so will be performing the thumb reconstruction for him. What are his options?

This question is answered in Case 1.7.

You perform the amputation, but somehow the histological sample is lost in the system. How will you proceed?

- This is a devastating event both for the patient, and for me as the consultant surgeon involved.
  - My first step is to declare this – both to the patient and my organization.
  - I will then work with both the MDT and my patient to decide on the safest management plan.
  - Lastly, I will ensure organizational learning occurs to prevent this happening again.
- As per the GMC's Good Medical Practice:
  - I will fulfil my duty of candour by being open and honest with my patient and record my interaction with them.
  - I will also report this to my hospital's governance system as a major incident to trigger a root cause analysis investigation.
  - Lastly, I will discuss this at the next morbidity and mortality meetings – both at the departmental and skin MDT levels.
- Next, I will suggest to the MDT that we have three possible courses of action – none of which are ideal:
  - Option 1 – would be to simply follow the patient up, as the risk of incomplete excision with a 1-cm margin is low – in the region of 3–5%, according to the BAD guidelines: if this path was chosen, then I would delay any definitive thumb reconstruction for at least 12 months, and possibly up to 3 years to allow for any recurrence to declare itself.
  - Option 2 – would be to sample the stump for histopathological diagnosis of a possible involved margin.
  - Option 3 – would be treat this as the worst-case scenario – with adjuvant radiotherapy, assuming there may have been an incomplete excision, a close margin, or poor prognostic features such as lymphovascular invasion. However, it is important that the patient understands that this would increase morbidity and would also limit their thumb reconstructive options.
- Once an agreement is reached within the skin MDT, I will meet with the patient to discuss their options – along with their next of kin if they wish, and our skin-specialist nurse for additional support. I will also inform them that this will be investigated by the trust as a serious incident, and that they will be updated regarding the outcome of this.
- I will ensure that I organize a personal follow-up consultation for the following week to rediscuss the options, with their risks and benefits, as I recognize that this is difficult information to take in.

You've mentioned a root cause analysis investigation – what is this?

This is the most accepted approach to explore the underlying causes of a serious incident – especially any underlying system and process issues, so that learning points are identified and solutions implemented, to prevent a repeat of the incident.

The patient is thankfully understanding, and grateful for your candour. He agrees to the plan for observation but returns 12 months later with a new palpable node – 4 weeks before he was due to undergo a toe-to-hand reconstruction. What now?

- I will postpone the thumb reconstruction until the patient is fully investigated, and
- arrange a FNA of the palpable node – in clinic if possible, otherwise via an urgent ultrasound scan.

- If the FNA is positive, then this provides a mandate to requesting other investigations such as a staging CT chest/abdomen/pelvis, with discussion of the results in the skin MDT, where I will suggest a level I–III axillary dissection.
- If the FNA is negative, I will arrange an ultrasound-guided true cut biopsy to exclude a false-negative result.

How will you perform the axillary dissection?

- The goal of an axillary dissection – in the context of skin cancer, is to remove all three nodal levels that are located lateral, posterior, and medial to pectoralis minor – with no consensus on its division or resection. I opt to resect it, as:
  - this facilitates the removal of the interval nodes of Rotter, as well as
  - improves the visualization and protection of the lateral pectoral nerve, but I understand that others may simply divide it.
    1. The patient is positioned supine, with a free-draped arm abducted on an arm board, and the incision line infiltrated with adrenaline to aid haemostasis.
    2. I make an incision in a curvilinear fashion 1 cm below the distal hair-bearing area of the axilla.
    3. I then develop the superior flap to the lateral edge of pectoralis major and retract this, followed by
    4. dissection of the inferior flap to the leading edge of LD and retraction of this.
    5. I then follow the LD superiorly to the axillary vein, and
    6. continue along the vein to dissect the axillary contents from distal to proximal – proceeding onto the anterior chest wall – whilst ensuring I ligate all vessels inferiorly, except the thoracodorsal axis that is preserved.
    7. I then identify and ligate the medial pectoral neurovascular bundle-located on the deep surface of the lateral border of pectoralis major and proceed with dissection to the lateral border of pectoralis minor, which I excise.
    8. I then continue with dissection to the subclavian ligament, which is the proximal demarcation of level III.
    9. I ensure I preserve the long thoracic nerve along the lateral thoracic wall.
    10. I then close the skin in layers over a size 15 Blakes suction drain. This is likely to be in for 2–4 weeks, but I remove suction after 5 days, as there is a theory that this reduces the rate of lymphatic drainage into the cavity.

The patient recovers well, and the MDT recommends adjuvant radiotherapy based on the pathology. The patient comes back to clinic 2 months after he completes that, with a dramatic whole arm swelling. There is no sign of erythema or cellulitis. What do you think is going on?

- I suspect he has developed secondary lymphoedema, which I would have pre-warned him about.
  - I will first establish whether the swelling is transient – as I would expect in the early stages of lymphoedema, or persistent. I expect that it would be too early for the development of atrophic skin changes or infections, but I will check that is the case.
  - Whilst there is no acceptable 'gold standard' definition for the presence of lymphedema, many accept a difference of at least 2 cm in circumference at the midpoint of the arm and forearm. This will also serve as an objective reference point to determine future progress.
- Other diagnostic techniques have been described but have not gained traction due to the expense of specialist equipment – such as
  - Perometry, where an infrared optical electronic scanner can demonstrate early changes, and
  - bioimpedance spectroscopy, which assesses the extracellular fluid compartment in the early stages before visible changes occur.
- MRI lymphangiography is useful to determine whether there are lymphatic channels present. However, the gadolinium tracer can enter the venous system making the interpretation of lymphatic channels difficult and can cause an inflammatory reaction and worsen the lymphoedema.
- I will manage this conservatively but aggressively in the first instance – within the skin MDT, and in collaboration with the lymphoedema specialist nurse, or alternatively an occupational

therapist or physiotherapist, if one is not available. They will implement a protocol consisting of decongestive lymphatic therapy (DLT) with four components:
- – compression bandages,
- – skin care to reduce the chances of infection,
- – gentle exercises, and
- – manual lymph drainage to decrease swelling.
- I will not consider surgical options such as liposuction or debulking until the patient develops irreversible static changes much later down the line.
- Other surgical options to re-establish lymph drainage via lymphatic venous anastomosis, a bypass, or a vascularized lymph node are highly controversial in this setting as the theoretical oncological risk is yet to be clarified.

FURTHER READING

1. Cornejo C, Miller CJ. Merkel cell carcinoma. Dermatol Clin. 2019;37:269–277.
2. Kayiran O, De La Cruz C, Tane K, Soran A. Lymphedema: from diagnosis to treatment. Turk J Surg. 2017;33:51–57.
3. https://www.bad.org.uk/library-media/documents/SCC_2009.pdf

Case 3.14

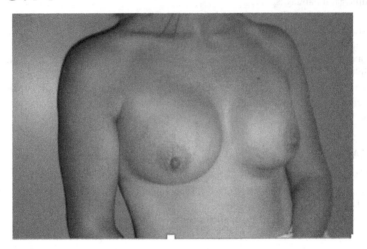

This lady presents to your clinic after undergoing a BBA elsewhere 5 years ago. She complains of hardening of her breasts, with distortion of her breast shape – the right side being worse than the left with deviation of the nipple downwards. She also states that it is uncomfortable at times. How do you proceed? I suspect a capsular contracture. I will seek to find more about:

1. the history of her procedure,
2. any breast cancer history, and
3. any other comorbidities, and
4. her smoking history.

- Salient points with regard to the procedure include:
  1. the reason for the initial operation (to address the size or asymmetry),
  2. confirmation of the time lapse since the operation – which I know is 5 years,
  3. the implant size, type, and pocket, as well as
  4. any post-operative complications that may have led to the capsular contracture.
- I will then proceed with:
  1. examination of her breasts for any visible and palpable signs of capsular contracture, including distortion and tenderness, as well as
  2. palpation of the axillary nodes – which may be reactive, due to a silicone gel bleed or implant rupture.
- If the hardening is palpable but not visible, then it would be classed as a Baker Grade III.
  A painful visible contracture would be classed as a Baker Grade IV.
- I will explain that her symptoms are consistent with capsular contractures, adding that:
  1. this is the commonest post-operative complication following breast augmentation, and
  2. she will require surgery to address this (as medical management has been described, but has a very high rate of recurrence).
- I will request an MRI to:
  1. exclude an implant rupture,
  2. assess the axillae if palpable lymphadenopathy is present, as well as
  3. confirm the implant pocket.
- With regard to the operative management of this, I will determine:
  1. If she is otherwise happy with her current size and shape, and
  2. if she wishes to proceed with another implant-based procedure or would like to consider autologous breast augmentation.

DOI: 10.1201/9780429399268-48

- If she is otherwise fit for a GA:
  - I will counsel her that I will make the intraoperative decision for either a total or anterior capsulectomy:
    - based on the thickness of the capsule, and
    - its adherence to the chest wall, and
  - inform her of the risks of a total capsulectomy – including:
    - bleeding, and
    - a pneumothorax.
- If the capsule is calcified and well formed, then I will proceed with a total capsulectomy, as the planes are well defined to enable safe completion of the procedure. However, I will suggest we limit the procedure to an anterior capsulectomy if it is well adherent to the chest wall.
- If she does not wish to consider another implant-based procedure, then I will suggest augmentation via fat transfer.
- If she does want another implant, then:
  - I will suggest a change of pocket then counsel her regarding the pros and cons of the different options (*as discussed in Case 3.12*).
  - I will also warn her that an implant would also carry a very small risk of BIA-ALCL that is in the region of 1/24,000, but this may change as new evidence is unearthed.

You've mentioned BIA-ALCL, what is that?

- Breast implant-associated anaplastic large cell lymphoma is an uncommon T cell non-Hodgkin lymphoma that was first reported in 1997 in association with breast implants, particularly texturized ones.
- It commonly presents with:
  - an effusion within the peri-implant capsule,
  - less commonly as a capsular tissue mass, and
  - less commonly still, with additional signs such as:
    - erythema,
    - skin lesions, and
    - B symptoms such as unexplained weight loss and night sweats.
- Diagnosis is made by aspiration and cytological evaluation of the peri-implant fluid, with pleomorphic lymphocytes that are negative for anaplastic lymphoma kinase (ALK) and positive for CD30.
  There are numerous proposed theories that are in flux, but which can currently be summarized as:
  - Sustained activation of the immune cascade in chronically overstimulated cells resulting in DNA alteration – via the activation of JAK-STAT signalling pathways. This may be due to:
    1. long-standing biofilm infection – that is associated with implant texturization, and
    2. chronic inflammation – associated with implant-related foreign body reaction,
  - In addition, some patients may have predisposing genetic mutations in JAK-STAT signalling pathways, which becomes relevant with 'second-hit' disease activation from the chronic inflammation or infection.

You mentioned the foreign body reaction. What is this?

- This is a complex immunological cascade that attempts to phagocytose foreign antigens.
- If this is unsuccessful, such as in the case of an implant, then :
  - macrophages and fibroblasts accumulate to lay down collagen and develop a fibrous capsule to wall it off, and
  - neutrophil infiltration and mast cell degradation cause an increase in IL-4 and a T-helper 2 allergy-mediated immune response.
- As I've mentioned before, chronic activation of the immune cascade increases the risk of DNA alteration in overstimulated cells and may lead to activating JAK-STAT mutations in BIA-ALCL.

How would you manage a patient who presents with a unilateral seroma, two years following breast implant insertion?

- This is a very rare presentation that occurs in up to 0.1% of patients.
- My first aim is to exclude BIA-ALCL – which accounts for 10% of patients with late seromas, then manage any other cause of a 'late' seroma – once that is excluded.
- Other causes of 'late' seromas, which occur at least 1 year following insertion, include:
  1. a silicone bleed,
  2. low-grade infection, and
  3. trauma
- Because of this, I will manage her within an NHS breast MDT setting with triple assessment consisting of:
  1. clinical examination,
  2. imaging, and
  3. biopsy
- I will request:
  1. an USS of both breasts and axillae, with an USS-guided FNA of the entire volume of peri-implant fluid for cytology, and ALK and CD30 testing, as well as
  2. a 14-gauge core biopsy of any associated capsular mass or pathological node.
- If the results are positive for ALCL, then:
  - I will manage her within the breast MDT, if I were in a centre with expertise managing this rare disease, or
  - otherwise refer her to one – with the suggestion of implant removal as part of a total en-block capsulectomy, as per the recommendation of current British and American guidelines.
  - I will also record her case in the BCIR, and
  - report this to the MHRA using the 'yellow card' scheme.
- If the result is negative, then I will investigate for the other causes with an MRI – unless the seroma is persistent, in which case I will suggest to the MDT that we repeat the investigation for BIA-ALCL to exclude a false negative result.

Why not simply perform an en-block capsulectomy for all patients in whom you suspect BIA-ALCL – be it in the private or NHS setting? Surely you are comfortable with that procedure from a technical point of view. Why would you consider referring her on?

- I manage all potential cancers within an MDT setting.
- Whilst an en-block capsulectomy is curative in most cases, there are a small number of patients who will need systemic treatment – such as those with loco-regional or distant disease. So, shared management of these patients is essential for optimal outcome with haemato-oncology and breast surgery.
- In addition, an unnecessary en-block capsulectomy would subject the patient to unnecessary morbidity with a risk of a pneumothorax, chronic pain, as well as cosmetic sequelae.

How would you counsel a breast augmentation patient for the risk of this?

I will explain that this is an extremely rare cancer of the blood cells that has been associated with textured breast implants – with a risk of between about 1:300 and 1:30,000 patients, with higher rates in those with a macro-textured surface – with higher surface area and roughness.

Let's change the scenario a little – she has replacement of the implants, then she comes back 2 years later reporting symptoms of brain fog, joint pains, and general fatigue. She believes she has breast implant illness and requests an en-block resection – as is recommended in several patient forums online.

How would you proceed?

- I will examine her and exclude palpable axillary lymph nodes, and any obvious anomalies with her implants.
- I will also request an MRI to exclude a ruptured implant or enlarged lymph nodes.

- If these are normal, I will explain that I want to help her – but that our first course of action should be to exclude other medical reasons for this and request her to see her GP.
- If medical causes are excluded, then I will explain that I would be very happy to remove her implants if she wishes, but that this would not guarantee lasting improvement in her symptoms – if any: as there is evidence to show that half of patients with these symptoms do not notice any improvement after removing the implants. In the other half, some find their improvement is only temporary.
- I will also add that as there is no current evidence for an en-block procedure, and that going ahead with that plan would subject her to unnecessary morbidity, such as a higher risk of bleeding and a pneumothorax.

FURTHER READING

1. DeCoster RC, Clemens MW, Di Napoli A, Lynch EB, Bonaroti AR, Rinker BD, Butterfield TA, Vasconez HC. Cellular and molecular mechanisms of breast Implant–Associated anaplastic large cell lymphoma. Plastic Reconstr Surg. 2021 Jan;147(1):30e–41e.
2. Di Napoli A. Achieving reliable diagnosis in late breast implant seromas: from reactive to anaplastic large cell lymphoma. PRS. 2019; 143(3s):15S–22S.
3. Magnusson MR, Cooter RD, Rakhorst H, McGuire PA, Adams WP, Deva AK. Breast implant illness: a way forward. PRS. 2019; 143(3s):74–81S.
4. Collett DJ, Rakhorst H, Lennox P, Magnusson M, Cooter R, Deva AK. Current risk estimate of breast implant-associated anaplastic large cell lymphoma in textured breast implants. PRS. 2019; 143(3s):30–40s.
5. Rastogi P, Riordan E, Moon D, Deva AK. Theories of etiopathogenesis of breast implant-associated anaplastic large cell lymphoma. PRS. 2019; 143(3s):23–29s.
6. Miranda RN, Medeiros LJ, Ferrufino-Schmidt MC, Keech JA, Brody GS, de Jong D, Dogan A, Clemens MW. Pioneers of breast implant-associated anaplastic large cell lymphoma: history from case report to global recognition. PRS. 2019; 143(3s):7–14S.
7. Turton P et al. UK guidelines on the diagnosis and treatment of breast implant-associated anaplastic large cell lymphoma on behalf of MHRA. Plastic, reconstructive and aesthetic surgery expert advisory group (PRASEAG). JPRAS 2021; 74(1):13–29.
8. Headon H, Kasem A, Mokbel K. Capsular contracture after breast augmentation: an update for clinical practice. Arch Plast Surg. 2015 Sep;42(5):532–543.
9. Clemens N, Horwitz MW SM. How I treat breast implant-associated anaplastic large cell lymphoma. Blood. 2018;132:1889–1898.

Case 3.15

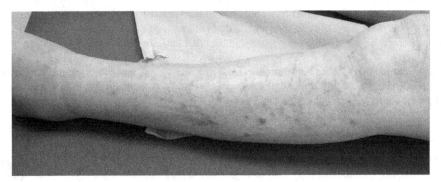

This lady had a lesion excised from the dorsum of the foot 4 years ago whilst abroad, and now presents with pigmented lesions in the lower leg, as you can see in the photograph. She can't recall what type of cancer it was, and she doesn't have any hospital records with her. How do you proceed?

- I suspect intransit melanoma disease. The lack of a known primary makes this a complex situation, as there is:
  - either a true unknown primary – with potentially improved prognosis (as the excised lesion may have been unrelated to this), or
  - the primary was excised, and we just don't have the details, or
  - the primary is currently still present, but unnoticed by the patient or GP.
- I will encourage the patient to explore all options to locate the pathology report of the excised lesion – as this may affect her prognosis, especially if it was indeed, a melanoma.
- I will then examine:
  - the skin of the lower limb for other lesions – especially along the lymphatics that run along the long and short saphenous veins,
  - the lymph nodes in the popliteal fossa and the groin – for palpable disease,
  - the liver edge – for an enlarged liver, and
  - A full-body exam of the skin, as the lifetime risk of a second primary is about 10%.
- I will then plan for a 2-mm margin excision of one of the lesions to confirm the histology, and determine the BRAF status – if positive.

What is intransit disease?

- This is locoregional recurrence that is confined to the superficial lymphatics and occurs in 3–6% of melanoma patients.
- It is defined by the AJCC as clinically evident cutaneous and/or subcutaneous metastases occurring >2 cm from the primary melanoma, in the region between the primary melanoma and the regional lymph node basin.

How is that different from microsatellites and satellite metastases?

- Microsatellites are defined as any microscopic focus of metastatic tumour cells in the skin or subcutis, adjacent or deep to, but discontinuous from the primary tumour.
- Satellite metastases are classically defined as any foci of clinically evident cutaneous and/ or subcutaneous metastases occurring within 5 cm of, but discontinuous from, the primary melanoma.
- In reality, these terms are arbitrary as they have identical survival curves to intransit disease, which suggest this is all the same spectrum of the same process and they are grouped together for staging purposes in the eighth edition of the AJCC.

DOI: 10.1201/9780429399268-49

You go on to excise the lesion, and histology confirms an excised intransit metastasis. How do you proceed?

- This would stage the patient as at least stage IIIB disease – possibly with an unknown primary.
- Treatment of intransit disease depends on several factors:
  1. the volume of intransit disease (whether it is excisable or not),
  2. the location of intransit disease on extremities (for e.g., above or below the knee),
  3. concurrent nodal disease,
  4. concurrent distant disease, and
  5. the overall patient performance status.
- I will:
  1. attempt to find a primary – with a full body exam,
  2. assess for disease burden – by suggesting a total body PET-CT and brain MRI to the skin MDT, to exclude detectable nodal disease and distant metastases, and
  3. request the histological BRAF mutation status of the sample.
- For purely intransit disease that is less than five isolated skin lesions: locoregional treatment routes are considered – such as surgical excision or Laser ablation, with the understanding that they are likely to recur in the near future.
- For purely intransit disease that is more than five isolated skin lesions: I will offer the patient immunotherapy or ILI.
- For nodal metastasis and or stage IV disease: I will suggest referral for systemic therapy with immunotherapy using PD-1 inhibitor or targeted therapy with BRAF and MEK inhibitors.

You have mentioned requesting the BRAF status for this patient: how does that affect clinical management?

- V600E is the most common mutation of the BRAF gene and is involved in the MAP kinase cell signalling pathway that keeps the cell in the mitotic phase.
- Patients with this mutation will respond to targeted therapy with BRAF and MEK inhibitors, which can be used to convert unresectable intransit disease to resectable disease.

The patient has six of these skin lesions with no other disease. How would you counsel them regarding their treatment options?

- Isolated limb infusion is a palliative procedure that can achieve locoregional control but does not change the patient's overall survival. There is a risk of:
  - a lack of response, and
  - impaired limb function.
- Immunotherapy can possibly offer a cure, but carries the risk of:
  - potentially permanent colitis,
  - a perforated colon,
  - permanent endocrine dysfunction – such as hypophysitis, hypothyroidism, or adrenal dysfunction.

So why would you want to attempt to control purely intransit disease?

- Up to 25% of these patients will never develop distant disease, so they will benefit from total control of this stage.
- For the rest, these lesions are very concerning to patients and can be symptomatic – with ulceration and bleeding.

The patient's daughter says she has done some online research, and there have been a few publications suggesting SLNB for intransit disease. What are your thoughts on that? Would you offer this patient this procedure?

No, I wouldn't. I would explain that SLNB is not indicated here, as it is primarily a staging tool, and the patient is already known to have stage IIIB or IIIC disease – which is an immediate indication for systemic therapy.

Let's consider another patient: your dermatology colleague refers a patient with a 2-mm thick MM that they have excised from the leg. There is no palpable lymphadenopathy or sign of intransit disease. How do you manage them?

- I will first examine the orientation of the scar – hoping it is vertical rather than horizontal:
  - If the scar is vertical, and assuming they are fit for further surgery and are N0, then I would offer a SLNB and a 2 cm wider local excision – with reconstruction with a split skin graft or keystone flap, if direct closure is not possible.
  - If the scar is horizontal then a flap will not be possible, as they may eventually require a hemi-circumferential excision of their calf with a 2-cm margin. I will have to reconstruct this with a split skin graft, and counsel the patient regarding their significant risk of distal lymphoedema.

The SLNB comes back as positive. What now?

I will:

1. stage the patient with a PET CT and MRI brain, or whole-body CT,
2. obtain the BRAF status of the primary or nodal deposit, and
3. then discuss this within the skin MDT, and suggest that the patient is offered adjuvant systemic therapy – such as immunotherapy.

Why not proceed with a completion lymph node dissection (CLND)?

Routine CLND is no longer indicated:

- The MSLT-1 study showed that SLNB was the single most important investigation for staging primary melanoma.
- MSLT-2 showed that there is no survival benefit from CLND – despite improved regional control for a small proportion of patients.

As you've mentioned these trials, please tell me about them.

- MSLT-I was the first Multicenter Selective Lymphadenectomy Trial and was designed to address the possible role of sentinel lymph node biopsy in the management of melanoma patients.
  - More than 1300 patients were randomized to either:
    - wide local excision and sentinel lymph node biopsy, with completion lymphadenectomy for those with positive sentinel nodes, or
    - wide local excision alone, and lymph node basin dissection for those with clinical recurrence.
  - This confirmed the prognostic role of SLNB in melanoma, as:
    - there was improved regional disease control and less morbidity in the sentinel node group with early completion lymphadenectomy, compared to those who underwent a lymphadenectomy following clinical recurrence, but
    - there was no change in melanoma-specific survival.
- MSLT-II was designed to establish whether completion lymphadenectomy improves melanoma-specific survival in sentinel node-positive patients versus an observation arm using USS, with a secondary endpoint of disease-free survival:
  - Almost 2000 patients were recruited over 10 years.
  - The results showed a small but significant difference in disease-free survival in favour of the dissection arm that is directly related to reduction of regional node recurrence, with no difference in distant metastasis-free survival.
- So, in conclusion, it appears that careful observation with high-performance ultrasonography of the regional node basins is safe for patients with positive sentinel nodes. Dissection does offer a small improvement in regional nodal control and decreases recurrence slightly overall, as well as providing additional staging information – but this is at the cost of much greater additional morbidity (such as lymphoedema with 24% in the CLND group versus 6% in the SLNB group).

The patient questions the need for 2-cm margins, as she would like to avoid reconstructive surgery if possible. What is the evidence for this?

- The current recommendation for excision margins for 2-mm thick MMs are 2 cm to minimize the risk of locoregional recurrence. This is based on the evidence of at least two phase 3 randomized trials, as well as NICE guidance.
- The UK melanoma study group, along with the British Association of Plastic Surgeons, conducted a large multicentre RCT comparing 1- versus 3-cm margin excision for patients with melanomas that are 2-mm thick. This showed worse outcomes in the 1-cm excision margin group with an increased risk of locoregional recurrence, as well as some evidence on follow-up to say there may even be an increased mortality in this group.
- In addition, a Swedish multicentre RCT compared 2- versus 4-cm margins for melanomas that are more 2-mm thick showing no difference in clinical outcome, but a narrowly increased small risk of local recurrence rate in the 2-cm group.

FURTHER READING

1. Keungand EZ. The eighth edition American joint committee on cancer (AJCC) melanoma staging system: implications for melanoma treatment and care. Expert Rev Anticancer Ther. 2018 Aug;18(8):775–784.
2. Tie EN, Henderson MA. Management of in-transit melanoma metastases: a review. ANZ J Surg. 2019 Jun;89(6):647–652.
3. Leiter U, et al. Complete lymph node dissection versus no dissection in patients with sentinel lymph node biopsy positive melanoma (DeCOG-SLT): a multicentre, randomised, phase 3 trial. Lancet Oncol. 2016;17(6):757–767.
4. Faries MB, Thompson JF, Cochran AJ, et al. Completion dissection or observation for sentinel-node metastasis in melanoma. N Engl J Med. 2017;376(23):2211–2222.
5. Perone JA, Farrow N, Tyler DS, Beasley GM. Contemporary approaches to in-transit melanoma. J Oncol Pract. 2018;14(5):292–300.
6. Gillgren P, Drzewiecki KT, Niin M, Gullestad HP, Hellborg H, Månsson-Brahme E, et al. 2-cm versus 4-cm surgical excision margins for primary cutaneous melanoma thicker than 2 mm: a randomised, multicentre trial. Lancet. 2011;378(9803):1635–1642.
7. Meirion Thomas J, Newton-Bishop J, A'Hern R, Coombes G, Timmons M, Evans J, Cook M, Theaker J, Fallowfield M, O'Neill T, Ruka W, Bliss JM, for the United Kingdom Melanoma Study Group, the British Association of Plastic Surgeons, and the Scottish Cancer Therapy Network. Excision margins in high-risk malignant melanoma. NEJM. 2004 Feb 19;350(8):757–766.

Case 3.16

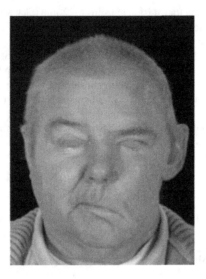

Please describe this photograph.

This is the photograph of a middle-aged man with a left hemifacial weakness. I note left-sided brow ptosis, a lower lid paralytic ectropion, mild alar ptosis, a flaccid left cheek with effacement of the nasolabial fold, and ptosis of the oral commissure. I suspect this is long-standing as I note contralateral deviation of midline structures such as the septum, the tip of the nose and midline of the lips – which occurs with a relatively long-standing unbalanced pull from the right side.

How would you manage a patient with a facial palsy?

- I will take a focused history to establish:
  1. the patient's specific goals – such as achieving:
     - resting symmetry,
     - dynamic symmetry,
     - abolishing any synkinesis, or
     - addressing issues such as oral incontinence or speech difficulties.
  2. the aetiology of the palsy – as this may affect:
     - the patient's general prognosis – and life expectancy if there is a malignancy,
     - the possibility of recovery of nerve function, if it is in continuity – such as a Bell's palsy,
     - potential donor nerves available, and
     - the potential need for adjuvant radiotherapy.
  3. the time elapsed since the palsy – as this will indicate the viability of motor-end plates and the consequent need for muscle transfer – as opposed to neurotization of the native facial muscles with nerve grafts or nerve transfers, and
  4. any patient comorbidities – as this may affect their suitability for general anaesthetic procedures.

How would the patient's prognosis and life expectancy affect your management?

For patients with shortened life expectancies, I will do my best to achieve facial symmetry and movement as soon as possible, such as using a temporalis myoplasty transfer, as opposed to procedures that require time to achieve neurotization.

DOI: 10.1201/9780429399268-50

Please continue

- Regarding my examination:
  1. I will first establish the need for eye protection – as lagophthalmos, if present, is the most pressing issue to address – to prevent the eventual risk of corneal ulceration and blindness in untreated patients.
  2. Next, I will assess their static and dynamic symmetry, as well as for any evidence of synkinesis.
  3. I will then determine their Sunnybrook Facial Grading System (SFGS) score to enable a somewhat objective measure of progress, and
  4. examine for donor nerves such as nerve to Masseter, Hypoglossal, Accessory, as well as Temporalis muscle function.
  5. Lastly, I will establish the impact on the patient using validated facial palsy specific PROMs such as with the Facial Clinometric Evaluation Scale (FaCE). The Facial Disability Index is an equally accepted alternative.
- My management will focus on:
  1. managing the eye,
  2. conservative management – with facial therapy, and chemodenervation – where appropriate,
  3. consideration of surgical symmetrizing options, and
  4. addressing the psychological impact, with a referral for assessment by the MDT psychologist and putting them in touch with 'Facial Palsy UK' for further information and patient support via their local patient support groups.
- In a patient with the possibility of recovery, I will support them with conservative measures to protect their eye as well as facial therapy and observe them for 6 months. If there is no recovery at all during that period, then the chances of them eventually recovering to a functional level are minimal, and I will start to consider surgical options with them.
- Regarding management of the eye:
  - If lagophthalmos is present, then I will assess for a Bells' phenomenon and give him advice regarding eye drops during the day, and nightly chloramphenicol ointment and an eye patch – until I insert an upper eyelid weight – if there is no possibility of recovery.
    Until then, I will also ask the therapists to see him with regard to eyelid stretching to optimize the surgical result – as a short contracted upper eyelid will negate the effect of the weight.
    The alternative is a dynamic option such as neurotization from a cross facial nerve graft – if the timeline is shorter than 12–18 months and the motor end plates are still viable. In addition, there are less commonly used muscle transfer options such as free platysma and pedicled temporalis, but the results of these are very variable – with a much higher failure rate than dynamic options for the smile, so I would avoid them as a new consultant.
  - If he reports epiphora, I will establish from the history if this were:
    - constant – which may be due to defective drainage, and/or irritation of the cornea, or
    - if it is associated with specific movements such as eating, in which case this is hyperlacrimation associated with synkinesis, (termed Crocodile tears or Bogorad's syndrome) and will be responsive to chemodenervation of the lacrimal gland.
    In the case of constant epiphora, I will show him how to correct the paralytic ectropion by repositioning his lower eyelid with tape to see if that resolves matters:
    If it does, then this will indicate to me that surgical correction of the ectropion will resolve that.
    If not, then I will refer him to my ophthalmology colleague in the facial palsy MDT for formal assessment of the ductal drainage system, which may be affected by the lower eyelid malposition.
  - Lastly regarding the lower eyelid paralytic ectropion, I will assess for horizontal laxity:
    - if present, then I will offer a wedge excision to shorten this.
    - If not, then I will offer a lateral tarsal strip advancement, or a static palmaris sling – especially if the medial aspect of the lower lid is affected also.
- Regarding facial therapy, this is vital for both sides of the face and consists of:
  - neuromuscular education of the patient so that they understand the anatomy of their face, and which areas need retraining for improved facial expression and oral competence,

- – stretching of tight, shortened muscles, and
- – the therapeutic management of synkinesis – if present.
- Regarding surgical symmetrizing options, I will consider options for the brow, nasal ala, upper lip, and lower lip.
  - – Regarding the brow, I will offer a direct brow lift if there is no sign of a shortened eyelid (as performing a brow lift in that case will worsen any lagophthalmos).
  - – Regarding the rest of the face:
    - ▪ In a patient who is only interested in/or fit for static options, then I would offer a fascia lata sling with individual slips to symmetrize the ala, and upper and lower lips.
    - ▪ If they are interested in and fit for dynamic options, then I will consider:
      - ○ Neurotization of their facial muscles with a cross facial nerve graft, or nerve transfer if the paralysis is within 12–18 months and the motor end plates are still viable.
      - ○ If the timeline is longer than that, then they will need a muscle transfer as the motor end plates will no longer be viable after 18 months of paralysis. Options include a temporalis myoplasty transfer or a free gracilis transfer.
      - ○ With regard to the lower lip weakness, the asymmetry can be disguised with chemodenervation of the contralateral lower lip depressors in the first instance, and/or consideration of an anterior belly of digastric transfer later on if the patient wishes for a more permanent solution.

How does chemodenervation work, and how would you apply this to facial palsy patients?

- Purified Botulinum toxin causes a neuromuscular blocking effect by binding presynaptically to cholinergic nerve terminals and preventing the release of acetylcholine.
- It can thus be used to improve symmetry by selectively weakening:
  - – contralateral normal muscles, or
  - – ipsilateral muscles affected by hypertonicity and synkinesis – in patients with a post-paralytic picture.

What is synkinesis? And what do you mean by a post-paralytic picture?

A post-paralytic picture describes the clinical sequelae following inflammation and subsequent partial recovery of a facial nerve, with evidence of:
- – hyperactivity and hypoactivity of different facial muscles, as well as
- – synkinesis. This is the involuntary abnormal movement of one muscle when another is activated, such as eye winking when the patient attempts to smile, or abnormal stimulation of the lacrimal gland when they eat (termed 'crocodile tears' or Bogorad syndrome). It is treated with facial therapy and chemodenervation of the muscle affected by the abnormal movement or the abnormally stimulated lacrimal gland.

You mentioned determining the Sunnybrook Facial Grading Score earlier. Why do you use this scoring system in particular?

- There is no perfect scoring system for facial palsy.
- The ideal system would include 3D objective measurement of resting and dynamic symmetry, including spontaneity of movement, as well as synkinesis, and a PROM.
- The SFGS is the most commonly used scoring system by facial palsy surgeons worldwide, due to its relative simplicity and because it includes a score for each of the three most important considerations in facial palsy patients – i.e., resting symmetry, dynamic symmetry, and synkinesis. But its main weaknesses include assessor subjectivity, and a relatively narrow scoring scale (from 1 to 5), which can make it difficult to note subtle differences or progress.
- Alternative systems that also assess the three same three domains include:
  - – the Modified House Brackmann scoring system – more recently modified to include the assessment of synkinesis as well, and
  - – the eFACE scoring system that aims to improve accuracy by offering a wider grading scale than that of SFGS.

    – In addition, to counteract the potential error due to subjectivity, a computerized application has been developed to assess for facial symmetry more objectively, by using facial landmarks. However, the disadvantage is that it is only able to assess resting symmetry, with no dynamic assessment – which is a crucial element.

You mentioned nerve-based options if the motor end plates are still viable: please talk me through these.

- Regarding nerve grafts versus nerve transfers:
  – The advantage of a cross facial nerve graft is spontaneity of movement – when neurotization is successful, however the disadvantages include:
    ▪ failure of neurotization due to axonal drop-off across the graft – which worsens with age. An adequate smile requires about 900 axons to power it, and residual axon numbers in some adult patients with CFNG have been shown to be as low as 100–200 axons.
    ▪ In addition, two stages are required with 6–9 months delay for the axons to grow across the face.
  – In contrast, nerve transfers are one-stage techniques. The most popular option being the nerve to masseter transfer, but others include the hypoglossal and accessory nerves.
  I prefer to use the nerve to masseter transfer as:
    ▪ the descending branch brings 1500 axons so there is minimal risk of failure to neurotize,
    ▪ the nerve is accessible with a short facelift type incision,
    ▪ there is minimal donor morbidity, and
    ▪ there is a quicker period to neurotize as there is a shorter distance for axonal growth to reach their target.
  However, disadvantages include:
    ▪ the need for a period of re-education to produce a voluntary smile without clenching their teeth – as the nerve supplies a muscle of mastication,
    ▪ the eventual absence of spontaneity of movement in most patients, even when a voluntary smile is produced, and
    ▪ post-operative facial resting tone is not as well restored as with a hypoglossal nerve transfer.

How do you locate the descending branch of the nerve to masseter intraoperatively?

- I use a pretragal incision for access, followed by
- dissection through the masseter muscle performed at a point 3 cm anterior to the tragus, and 1 cm inferior to the zygomatic arch.
- The masseter muscle is composed of three leaves: The descending branch of the nerve is located between the most superficial two leaves and the deepest leaf.

Which muscle transfer options would you use to reanimate a smile in a patient with paralysis beyond 18 months?

There is debate in the facial palsy community regarding the ideal muscle transfer option, with the two main camps including a Labbe temporalis myoplasty transfer and free muscle transfers – with a free Gracilis as the most popular choice.

- The advantages of a Labbe procedure include:
  – guaranteed voluntary movement immediately after surgery by clenching their teeth, as there is no need to wait for neurotization of the muscle, which may be worsened with increasing age, or radiotherapy
  – a favourable oblique vector of pull, and
  – it does not transfer any additional tissue bulk in the cheek area, so will not worsen their resting symmetry.
  However, disadvantages include:
  – a variable and mostly moderate excursion of the smile – which tends to be less than that produced by a Gracilis muscle, and

- they will have to undergo several months of rehabilitation to relearn how to activate their temporalis without teeth clenching, and hence convert a 'mandibular' smile – where they must clench their teeth – to a 'voluntary' one.
- There are numerous options for a free muscle transfer. The most popular current option is a gracilis, but alternatives include pectoralis minor, latissimus dorsi, and serratus anterior – amongst others.
- Advantages of a free gracilis transfer include:
  - A greater excursion of smile – if neurotization is successful, and
  - a relatively cheap donor muscle that can be easily raised in the supine position.
  However, disadvantages include:
  - a small risk of flap failure,
  - the need for intraoperative thinning of the muscle – to avoid an excessively bulky cheek and resulting resting asymmetry,
  - the need for a fascia lata sling, as the muscle achieves a dynamic smile but does not correct resting tone.
  - Lastly, it's direction of pull is slightly more horizontal, and consequently considered less favourable than that of the Labbe flap by some surgeons.
  It may be powered by:
    - a cross facial nerve graft, or
    - a nerve to masseter, or
    - by dual innervation – with both a cross facial nerve graft and nerve to masseter to avoid the disadvantages of each.
      The nerve to masseter offers a much higher risk of powerful reinnervation, but with no true spontaneity (as the masseter is a muscle of mastication).
      A CFNG offers the advantage of 'true spontaneity' but does require two stages and carries the risk of a reduced rate of reinnervation compared to the nerve to masseter due to axonal 'drop-off' that occurs along the length of the cross facial nerve graft.
      Dual supply innervation supplements the CFNG with the nerve to masseter: this has the advantage of improving the rates of reinnervation compared to those achieved with a CFNG, but this is at the expense of the loss of some spontaneity.

Let us consider a further scenario: you are referred a patient with a trigeminal and facial nerve palsy. How would that change the potential picture and treatment options that you would offer?

- This has two main consequences:
  1. It places them at particular risk of a neurotrophic keratopathy, and
  2. It results in the loss of the options for a Labbe procedure, as well as the use of the nerve to masseter, and anterior belly of digastric.
- With regard to the neurotrophic keratopathy, I would offer neurotization of the cornea with contralateral supraorbital and supratrochlear nerves as a joint procedure with my ophthalmology colleague.
- Static options such as an eyelid weight, brow lift and fascia lata sling are still available.
- With regard to options for facial reanimation: Nerve-based options include a cross facial nerve graft – if they are young and the contralateral facial nerve is normal. Other nerve sources include the partial hypoglossal nerve or accessory nerve.
- Muscle transfer options will include powering a gracilis muscle with any of the nerve options I have mentioned.

What is neurotrophic keratopathy?

This is a sight-threatening condition – caused by the loss of corneal sensory innervation due to the trigeminal nerve injury – which may result in corneal ulceration and eventual vision loss. This is compounded by a concomitant facial nerve injury with potential lagophthalmos, altered lacrimation, and lower eyelid malposition – resulting in environmental exposure – in addition to the inability to sense damage, if and when it occurs.

FURTHER READING

1. Kasra Z, Thomas S, Weller C, Lighthall JG. Corneal neurotization in the setting of facial paralysis: a comprehensive review of surgical techniques. J Craniofac Surg. 2021;32(6):2210–2214.
2. Banks CA, Bhama PK, Park J, Hadlock CR, Hadlock TA. Clinician-graded electronic facial paralysis assessment: the eFACE. Plast Reconstr Surg. 2015;136:222e–230e.
3. Borschel GH, Kawamura DH, Kasukurthi R, Hunter DA, Zuker RM, Woo AS. The motor nerve to the masseter muscle: an anatomic and histomorphometric study to facilitate its use in facial reanimation. J Plast Reconstr Aesthet Surg. 2012;65(3):363–366.

Case 3.17

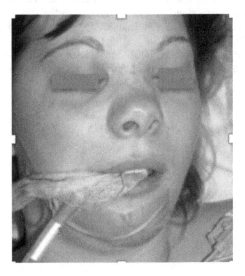

This lady came to see you following a rhinoplasty elsewhere as she was disappointed by the result. Please describe this photograph. What do you think is going on?

- This is an intraoperative photograph of an intubated patient with a saddle deformity of the nose.
- I cannot see a columellar scar, so I expect her primary rhinoplasty was closed.
- I note:
  - skeletal deficiency of the middle third, with
  - an inverted V deformity,
  - interruption of Sheen's aesthetic lines,
  - cephalic rotation of the tip with a prominent infratip lobule, and
  - columellar retrusion.
- In reality, I would request to examine further views, such as:
  - a true lateral view – to assess the position of the radix, the true extent of the deficiency of the dorsum, and consequence on tip projection,
  - a true AP view – to further assess the consequence on the tip such as splaying of the nostrils, and
  - a basal view for further assessment of tip projection.
  The full series would also help assess the nose in relation to the rest of the facial features.

What are the causes of this deformity?

- These may be congenital or acquired:
  - Congenital causes may be
    - an isolated anomaly, or
    - syndromic – such as in Binder's syndrome.
  - Acquired causes may be:
    - traumatic – such as a septal haematoma,
    - iatrogenic – such as over-resection of the dorsum during a rhinoplasty, or
    - infective – such as in syphilis.

How would you prevent this complication during a primary rhinoplasty?

- I use the 'component dorsal hump reduction' technique, which consists of:
  1. separation of the upper lateral cartilage from the septum,
  2. incremental reduction of the septum, followed by

DOI: 10.1201/9780429399268-51

3. incremental dorsal bony reduction using a rasp, whilst continuously using palpation to check the last two steps are adequately performed,
4. this is followed by osteotomies to close an open roof, and
5. the use of spreader grafts/flaps, and suturing techniques – if required.

- I will continuously assess the degree of reduction to ensure that I don't over-reduce.
- I will also ensure that I preserve the transverse aspects of the upper lateral cartilages to maintain the patency of the internal nasal valve, the shape of the dorsal aesthetic lines, and avoid an iatrogenic inverted-V deformity.

How would you assess this patient in clinic?

- I will first establish the patient's specific concerns regarding her nose and her expectations from the revision surgery.
- Salient points in the history include:
  - respiratory symptoms,
  - symptoms of allergic rhinitis or sinusitis,
  - previous nasal trauma,
  - intranasal drug use (which may be prescribed or otherwise), as well
  - time points from the previous surgery, as I would wait at least 1 year before undertaking revision surgery.
- My examination will involve:
  - analysing the anatomical characteristics of this patient from the frontal, lateral and basal view,
  - assessing for any physiological consequences, and
  - marrying this information with the patient's specific concerns and their history.
  Specifically,
- From the frontal view:
  1. I will assess for any midline deviation, which may be bony or septal.
  2. I will then follow Sheen's dorsal aesthetic lines, which start from the medial superciliary ridge to the tip-defining points.
  3. Next, I will assess for the nose in thirds:
     i. In the superior third: the bony vault width should be 80% of the ideal alar base.
     ii. In the middle third: I will evaluate for any contour deformity, such as a V deformity.
     iii. In the lower third:
        - I will evaluate for the width of the alar base, which should be equal to the intercanthal distance.
        - I will then assess the tip for:
          ○ two symmetrical tip-defining points,
          ○ a supratip point,
          ○ the junction between the infratip lobule and columella, and
          ○ a diamond shape ideally formed by these four points, with a horizontal line bisecting both tip-defining points and dividing the diamond into two equilateral triangles

Please tell me – what do these four points represent anatomically?

- The tip-defining points represent the light reflecting points of the domal segment of the middle crus of the lower lateral cartilage.
- The supratip point represents the junction between the middle and lateral crus.
- The junction between the infratip lobule and columella represents the junction between the middle and medial crus.

Okay, please continue

- From the lateral view:
  1. I will start with the length of the nose (from the radix to the nasal tip), with the ideal length in a Caucasian patient equal to 0.67 of the midface.

2. Again, I will evaluate the nose in thirds:
    i. In the upper third, I will evaluate the position and depth of the radix: this should be at the level of the upper lash line.
    ii. In the middle third, I will assess the dorsal line.
    iii. In the lower third, I will assess the tip for:
        - any supratip breaks,
        - alar retraction,
        - excessive columellar show,
        - tip projection – which is measured from the alar cheek junction to the nasal tip, and ideally equal to 0.67 of the nasal length, and
        - tip rotation – with an ideal nasolabial angle of 90–95 degrees in males, and 95–110 degrees in females.
3. Next, I will evaluate the position of the forehead and chin.
- From the basal view, I will assess:
1. the columellar contour,
2. columellar length, which should be one half of tip length,
3. any septal deviation, and
4. the shape of the nostrils – which should be tear drop shaped, with the apex medial to the base.
- Next, I will examine for any respiratory obstruction with the Cottle manoeuvre and inspect for septal deviation, as I would expect that both the internal and external nasal valves are affected in all but minimal deformities.
- I will finish my examination by assessing the soft tissue envelope – as skin thickness can affect post-operative swelling, and skin retraction would affect my choice of surgical approach.
- Lastly, I will evaluate her photographs prior to her primary rhinoplasty to establish what might be a congenital anomaly (e.g., cephalic rotation of the tip), and what was a result of the procedure.

In what way would skin retraction affect your approach?

I would choose an endonasal approach in those with moderate retraction, and a gingivobuccal sulcus approach in cases of severe soft tissue retraction – as an open rhinoplasty approach in a tight envelope will risk dehiscence of the columellar incision, and even possibly vascular compromise.

As you've mentioned vascular compromise, please tell me about the normal vascular supply to the nose.

- This is from the facial and ophthalmic arteries:
    - The most important source artery is the facial artery – with its superior labial artery, and angular artery branches.
        The superior labial artery gives off a columellar branch in 2/3 of people, which is sacrificed in an open tip rhinoplasty, leaving the lateral nasal artery, which is a branch of the angular artery to supply the tip. This may be unilateral or bilateral, and lies 2 mm above the alar groove, so injury from an alar base resection during a concomitant open rhinoplasty may lead to tip necrosis.
    - The ophthalmic artery supplies the upper third – with branches such as the anterior ethmoidal artery, dorsal nasal artery, and external nasal artery.

So, in that case, would you avoid an open technique?

My default position is to use an open technique unless contraindicated, as I believe this allows me better analysis, and the ability to precisely correct deformities – although I am aware that many more experienced surgeons may prefer the closed approach as there is less consequent morbidity from disruption of the soft tissue envelope, but it does require more experience as there is less visibility of structures.

You mentioned the internal and external nasal valves: what are they? And what is the Cottle manoeuvre?

- These are formed by the relationship between the upper and lower lateral cartilages with the nasal septum.

- They are involved in the regulation of airflow, as their configuration creates collapsible tubes that are affected by inspiratory negative pressure – akin to the Starling resistor model of the upper airway, where the increased airflow velocity causes an increase in transmural pressure and leads to subsequent airway collapse.
- The internal valve:
  - is formed by the junction of the lower border of the upper lateral cartilage and the nasal septum, and is normally 10–15 degrees.
  - It regulates airflow resistance, as it is the narrowest point of the nasal airway. A narrower angle creates airway obstruction and is assessed with the Cottle manoeuvre, whereby the patient is asked to inspire, then they are asked to pull their cheek laterally and repeat. Any improvement in airflow is a positive sign and indicates that the patient would benefit from a spreader graft.
- The external valve is formed by the lower edge of the lateral crus and nasal septum, as well as contributions from the alar soft tissue. External valve collapse is seen if the nostrils collapse on inspiration.

How would you correct a saddle nose deformity?

This is based on the severity of the deformity:

- Patients with minimal deformities have:
  - a depression above the supratip,
  - with normal tip projection and rotation.
      As the deformity is minor with sufficient septal cartilage, I will manage this with a dorsal septal onlay graft to restore septal height, and spreader grafts to correct the internal nasal valve.
- Patients with moderate deformities have:
  - a recessed dorsum,
  - with decreased tip projection, and even cephalic rotation, with
  - more inferior position of the radix, and
  - separation of the nasal bones from the upper lateral cartilages, resulting in an inverted V deformity of the middle third and interruption of Sheen's lines.
      As the septum is deficient, I will use conchal or rib cartilage for dorsal septal onlay grafts, columellar strut grafts and dorsal septal grafts to support and improve tip projection and derotation, as well as spreader grafts to address the middle third V deformity.
- Those with major deformities have:
  - an absent middle third and even superior third in some cases, resulting in a short nose appearance,
  - with major retraction of the mucosa, and
  - a flattened and broad tip.
      I will use the costal cartilage of the 7th rib to reconstruct the dorsum, as well as the same tip grafts as I've mentioned before. I will use the endonasal or sublabial approach to address the soft tissue retraction, as I have mentioned earlier.

What would you do if the conchal cartilage is of poor quality, in a patient with moderate deformity?

I would use diced cartilage wrapped in deep temporal fascia, or rib cartilage.

What problem would you foresee with costal cartilage, and how would you manage that?

- It tends to resorb and warp, with a greater risk in those with a particularly tight soft tissue envelope.
- I will cross that bridge if and when I came to it, and use other donor sites, such as:
  - diced cartilage with fascia if the defect is small, or
  - split calvarial, iliac crest, or costal bone for larger defects.
- The disadvantage of bone is that it provides an unnaturally rigid feel, despite the advantage of a rigid structure.
- Lastly, I am aware of commercial costal cartilage allografts which would avoid another donor site.

How would you counsel the patient?

- As well as discussing the proposed surgery itself, I will discuss the recovery as well as the complications.
- With regard to the post-operative recovery:
  - I will explain that a nasal splint is worn for 1 week, and that they may have nasal packs.
  - If an open approach has been undertaken, they will have sutures to remove at 1 week.
  - I will advise the patient to elevate the head as much as possible, avoid bending and stooping, and avoid blowing their nose.
  - A saline nasal spray can be used for comfort as needed, and there may be light oozing from the nostril in the first week.
- With regard to complications:
  - Early complications include bleeding, swelling, infection, CSF rhinorrhea, and DVT/PE.
  - Intermediate complications include wound healing problems, open roof deformity, asymmetry, irregularities, and respiratory obstruction. In addition, tip numbness, and changes in the colour, and texture of the skin may occur. Lastly, skin necrosis is a possibility – especially in secondary cases.
  - Late complications include an altered or loss of sense of smell, excessive callus formation, pollybeak deformity, a saddle nose deformity, and persistent nasal obstruction. Septal damage includes perforation or collapse. In addition, a poor external scar is a risk if an open approach is used. Lastly, I would prepare them for dissatisfaction with their result, as there is a significant revision rate.

How would you manage a septal perforation?

- My management algorithm is based on:
  - its size, and
  - whether it is symptomatic.
- Small perforations:
  - if asymptomatic, can be managed conservatively.
  - If symptomatic, e.g., producing a whistling noise, then I would offer a silicone nasal plug or a mucosal local flap repair. In this patient who has had two rhinoplasties, I would veer towards a silicone nasal plug as I would be more concerned about scarring and vascularity of the septal mucosa.
- In a patient with a larger perforation that is symptomatic, a flap repair would be necessary as a silicone plug would not be suitable. My flap choice is based on the quality of the nasal mucosa:
  - If it is of good quality, then I would use a local advancement flap from the residual septum and nasal vestibule.
  - If this is not suitable, as I suspect may be the case in this patient, then I will use regional flaps such as a FAAM flap or nasolabial flap.

How would you proceed if the patient is to be treated with a silicone plug?

The first aspect is sizing to ensure it is comfortable and does not cause adjacent tissue necrosis. It is important that the patient understands that the plug will need to be intermittently cleaned and changed for hygiene reasons.

FURTHER READING

1. Rohrich RJ, Muzaffar AR, Janis JE. Component dorsal hump reduction: the importance of maintaining dorsal aesthetic lines in rhinoplasty. Plast Reconstr Surg. 2004;114(5):1298–1308; discussion 1309–1312.
2. Durbec M, Disant F. Saddle nose: classification and therapeutic management. Eur Ann Otorhinolaryngol Head Neck Dis. 2014;131(2):99–106.

Summary of Topics Covered

TRAUMA/BURNS/ADULT UPPER LIMB

Burns

- Indications for transfer to a burns centre and transfer protocol
- Clinical assessment of burns
- LASER Doppler assessment
- Escharotomy
- Inhalation injuries
- Pathophysiology of thermal burn
- Physiological response to burns
- Physiology of burns healing
- Fluid resuscitation
- Fluid creep
- Nutrition in a burn patient
- Burns dressings
- Early burns surgery
- Burns contractures
- Toxic shock syndrome
- Toxic epidermal necrolysis
- Electrical injury

Upper Limb

Management of a fight bite:

- Management of joint destruction
- Infection of the deep spaces of the hand
- Compartment syndrome of the upper limb
- Volkmann's ischaemic contracture

Scaphoid fracture:

- Scaphoid anatomy
- Scaphoid non-union advanced collapse
- Scaphoid lunate advanced collapse
- Wrist ligaments

Digital amputation:

- Factors affecting outcome
- Management of patient
- Indications and contraindications for replantation
- Post-operative anticoagulation regime
- Management of missing amputates in hand with multiple digital amputations
- Delayed reconstruction
- Thumb reconstruction algorithm
- Outcome measures
- Scoring systems
- Power and precision grips

Management of a mangled hand:
- Concept of the 'acceptable hand'
- Importance of hand aesthetics
- Timing of reconstruction
- Principles of tendon transfer
- Patient rehabilitation regime
- Management of joint contractures
- Intrinsic muscle weakness

Two-stage tendon repairs:
- Indication
- Surgical technique
- Complications of tendon reconstructions
- Lumbrical plus finger
- Quadriga effect
- Leddy and Packer injuries
- Alternatives to tendon reconstruction
- Tendon graft donor sites
- Rehabilitation
- Outcome measures

Brachial plexus injury:
- Anatomy
- General approach
- Indications for surgery
- Reconstructive goals in pan-plexus injury
- Timing of exploration and repair
- Signs of preganglionic injuries
- Management of patient with acute injury
- Management of patient with old injury
- Obstetric injuries

Dupuytren's disease:
- Pathophysiology
- Management
- Non-surgical options
- General surgical options
- Skin incision options
- Management of residual PIPJ contracture
- Management of white finger on tourniquet release
- Management of exposed flexor tendon
- Management of iatrogenic nerve injury
- Management of skin flap necrosis

Facial/Lower Limb Trauma

Lower limb trauma:
- Emergency room assessment of open lower limb injury
- Evidence for antibiotics
- Gustilo and Anderson classification
- Signs of a high energy injury

- Management of a transferred patient
- Principles of planning a lower limb reconstruction
- Preoperative imaging
- Timing of surgery
- Primary wound excision of lower limb injuries
- Zone of injury
- Management of the acutely ischaemic limb
- Reconstruction of venous injuries
- Management of the physiologically unstable patient
- Indications for primary amputation
- Management of a patient with absent plantar sensation
- Management of a patient with segmental muscle loss
- Management of bone loss
- Open foot injuries
- Below-knee amputation – technique
- Stump complications
- Compartment syndrome of the lower limb
- Management of an unconscious patient with potential compartment syndrome
- Contraindication to surgical release of compartment syndrome
- Management of rhabdomyolysis
- Osteomyelitis
- Management of degloving injuries

Craniofacial trauma:
- Drawing of LeFort fractures
- Assessment of patient with a possible pan-facial fracture
- Surgical airway
- Definitive airway
- Surgical cricothyroidotomy
- Secondary survey
- Management of retrobulbar haemorrhage
- Lateral canthotomy and cantholysis
- Principles of LeFort fracture management
- Management of suspected rhinorrhoea

Diabetic foot ulcers:
- Management
- Pathophysiology of diabetic foot ulcers
- Pathophysiology of diabetic neuropathy
- Charcot foot collapse
- Management option for osteomyelitis in the infirm
- Management in the fit patient

ACUTE HEAD AND NECK TUMOURS/CONGENITAL ANOMALIES/ TRUNK AND PERINEAL RECONSTRUCTION

Head and Neck

Management of patient with preauricular swelling:
- Management of negative or equivocal FNA/core biopsy in suspected malignancy
- Management of facial nerve
- Nerve-sparing parotidectomy

- Use of nerve stimulators
- Frey's syndrome
- Management of nerve infiltration
- Recipient vessel choice
- Venous anastomosis
- Management of short facial artery stump
- Safe pedicle transport into neck
- Neck dissections – indications, types, risk, technique, and management of complications
- Management of palpable neck node
- HPV status and head and neck SCC
- Risk factors for oral SCC
- SLNB and oral SCC
- Management of unknown primary of the head and neck

Reconstruction of patient with hemi-maxillectomy and orbital exenteration defect:
- Reconstructive goals
- Management of patient unfit for a free flap
- Prosthetic option
- Indications for adjuvant radiotherapy

Osteoradionecrosis:
- Indications for surgical management
- Planning of reconstruction
- Airway management
- Preoperative indications for elective tracheostomy
- Description of surgical tracheostomy
- Post-operative management of tracheostomy patient
- Safe decannulation protocol
- Management of intra-oral dehiscence
- HBO therapy

Laryngopharyngeal reconstruction:
- Flap selection and design
- Considerations with regard to concomitant reconstruction of external skin defect
- Management of primary pharyngeal closure in radio-recurrent patient
- Management of a patient with low BMI
- Nutritional assessment
- Refeeding syndrome
- Frailty assessment
- Management of a pharyngeal leak/fistula
- Management of a suspected chyle leak
- Physiology of normal voice production
- Options to re-establish voice in laryngectomy patients
- Long-term sequalae of largyngectomy

Paediatric Plastic Surgery

Congenital melanocytic naevus:
- General management plan
- Risk stratification

- Indications for routine screening for neurocutaneous melanosis
- Pathophysiological theories for increased risk of melanoma
- Laser management
- Tissue expansion
- Routine monitoring of patients with congenital melanocytic nevi
- Management of suspected malignant transformation
- Dermoscopy features of CMN
- Management of child with seizures

Prominent ears:

- Timing of surgery
- Preoperative assessment
- Goals of surgery
- Surgical techniques
- Description of personal technique and rationale
- Non-surgical options
- Preoperative counselling
- Post-operative management

Trunk

Management approach in delayed breast reconstruction:

- Effect of oncological factors on operative plan
- Effect of chemotherapy and predicted survival on operative plan
- BMI cut off and management of a patient with a high BMI
- Management of a patient with a previous laparotomy
- Management of a patient with a failed DIEP following radiotherapy
- Recipient vessel choice
- Technique to maximize use of all flap zones
- Management of pneumothorax
- Management of absent IMV
- Use of preoperative imaging
- Reconstruction of quandrantectomy defect

Perineal reconstruction:

- Approach to reconstruction
- Rationale for flap reconstruction in radio-recurrent patient
- Flap of choice
- Description of VRAM flap reconstruction
- Options to decrease abdominal donor site morbidity
- Component separation
- Vaginal reconstruction

Chest wall reconstruction:

- Aims of sternal reconstruction
- Management of patient with mediastinitis
- Workhorse reconstructive flaps
- Management of patient with osteomyelitis
- Reconstruction of a sternectomy

Abdominal wall reconstruction:
- Management options including component separation

Hypospadias:
- Draw a cross-section of the penile shaft
- Pathophysiology
- Chordee
- Embryology of male genitalia and hypospadias
- Management of a baby with hypospadias
- Surgical algorithm
- Description of technique for one and two stage repairs
- Horton's test
- Release of curvature
- Timing of surgery
- Risks of surgery
- Management of a fistula
- Management of a urethral stricture

Pressure sores:
- Management of a patient with pressure sores
- Staging
- Extrinsic and intrinsic causal factors
- Non-surgical management
- Management of pressure sores in spinal injury patient
- Planning of buttock rotation flap
- Management of pressure sore in head injury patient

Cleft and Craniofacial

Cleft lip and palate:
- Embryology
- Theories for initiation of elevation of palatal shelves
- Treatment timeline
- Risk of future children being affected
- Treatment controversies
- Anatomy of a cleft palate deformity
- Management of a palatal fistula
- Alveolar bone grafting
- Cleft lip repair
- Management of whistle deformity
- Management of the nose
- Management of child with hypernasal speech
- Pharyngeal closure patterns

Craniosynostosis:
- Aims of treatment of a patient with a non-syndromic synostosis
- Management of patient
- Management of potentially raised ICP
- Positional plagiocephaly

Pfeiffer syndrome:

- Contribution of FGFR mutation
- Management of patient
- Chiari malformations
- LeFort III advancement
- Monobloc procedure

Treacher Collins syndrome:

- Facial clefts
- Embryology of facial development
- Phenotypes of cleft numbers 6–8
- Treatment timeline
- Options for hearing restoration
- BAHA
- Middle ear implants
- Classification of microtia
- Embryology of inner ear formation
- Management of a patient with microtia
- Autologous reconstruction
- Positioning of ear reconstruction
- Complications
- Management of maxillary hypoplasia

Congenital Hands

Polydactyly:

- Embryology of the hand and embryological insult in synpolydactyly
- Management of patient

Syndactyly:

- Embryological insult
- Management of patient
- Contraindications to surgical release
- Rationale and algorithm for timing of surgery
- Management of bilateral symmetrical syndactylies
- Principles of release
- Draw the incision lines and discuss
- Options to avoid skin grafting
- Disadvantages of skin grafts
- Classification of congenital hand malformations
- Syndromic associations
- Principles of management of an Apert hand
- radial deficiency
- Pollicization

GENERIC TECHNIQUES, COMPLEX WOUNDS, VASCULAR ANOMALIES, AND AESTHETICS/SKIN CANCER/GENERAL PROFESSIONAL CAPABILITY

Hidradenitis Suppurativa

- Scoring system
- Patient management
- Reconstructive options

Necrotizing Fasciitis
- Initial management
- Finger sweep test
- Scoring systems
- Description of intra-operative management
- Excisional techniques
- Reconstructive options

Facial Palsy
- Assessment of a patient with facial weakness
- Flaccid and post-paralytic facial palsy
- Facial palsy management algorithm
- Scoring systems
- Nerve to masseter – location
- Cross facial nerve grafting
- Labbe temporalis myoplasty
- Free muscle transfer
- Neurotrophic keratopathy
- Selective chemodenervation

Aesthetic

Facial rejuvenation:
- Effects of facial ageing
- Assessment of facial ageing
- Treatment options
- Facelift types
- Management of post-operative facial weakness
- Management of recurrence of jowling
- Reduction of haematoma risk
- Management of post-operative cheek swelling
- Neck lift assessment
- treatment algorithm to address the neck

Breast asymmetry:
- Breast ptosis – classification
- Management of breast asymmetry
- Breast reduction techniques
- Marking of breast reduction
- Management of asymmetrical IMFs
- Management of an at-risk nipple
- Drains and breast reduction
- Revision breast reduction
- Psychological assessment

Breast augmentation:
- Preoperative assessment for breast augmentation
- PIP scandal
- Breast implant illness
- Safety of breast implants

- Counselling a patient for breast augmentation
- Alternatives to implant-based augmentation
- Planning an implant-based augmentation
- Dual plane augmentations
- Capsular contracture and management
- Management of post-operative animation and tenderness

Implant capsular contracture:

- Management of a patient with a capsular contracture
- BIA-ALCL
- Management of a delayed unilateral seroma
- Management of a patient requesting en block resection for self-reported breast implant illness

Rhinoplasty:

- Saddle deformity of the nose
- Prevention of saddle deformity
- Assessment of rhinoplasty patient
- Management of a saddle deformity
- Open vs closed technique
- Internal and external nasal valves
- Graft donor sites
- Management of septal perforation

Generic Techniques/Basic Science

Flap classification:

- Flap circulation
- Flap conditioning
- Pathophysiology of delay phenomenon
- Anastomotic healing
- Risk factors for anastomotic thrombosis
- Microsurgery with severe radiation damage
- Contraindications to microsurgery
- Post-operative anticoagulation regime following microsurgery
- Mechanism of action of aspirin and heparin
- Management of blue flap
- Management of vessel size discrepancy
- Venous coupler
- Monitoring of anastomosis
- Flap salvage
- No reflow phenomenon
- Causes of free flap failure
- Ischaemia-reperfusion injury

Wound healing:

- Z-plasty
- Process of wound healing
- Angiogenesis
- Wound contraction
- Coagulation cascade

- Foetal wound healing
- TFG-beta
- MMPs
- Secondary intention wound healing
- Factors affecting wound healing
- Keloid scars
- Hypertrophic scars
- Hyper and hypo pigmented scars

Skin Cancer

SCC:
- Assessment for a possible subungual skin cancer
- Management of biopsy proven SCC of the thumb
- Indications for adjuvant radiotherapy
- Management of lost histological sample
- Management of possible regional spread
- Axillary dissection
- Lymphedema
- Management of patient with distant metastatic spread
- Inguinal dissection
- Pelvic node dissection

Melanoma:
- Intransit disease
- Management
- BRAF status
- Management of a patient with a primary MM
- Management of a positive SLNB
- Resection margins for melanoma

BCC:
- Mohs surgery
- Dermoscopy
- Recipient vessels in reconstruction
- Management of patient unfit for a free flap
- Management of close deep margin
- Gorlin syndrome

Ethical/medicolegal issues:
- Safeguarding
- Consent
- Critical incident management
- Root cause analysis
- Duty of candour
- GMC's good medical practice
- Legal capacity
- GMC good medical practice guidance cosmetic intervention
- Management of an underage patient seeking a cosmetic procedure

General Basic Science Questions Interspersed in the Book

- Nerve injury types
- Nerve healing
- Anatomy of peripheral nerve
- Physiology of nerve conduction
- Bone healing, membrane induction
- Distraction osteogenesis
- Microscopic injury to vessels
- Zone of trauma/injury
- Osteomyelitis-Pathophysiology of and imaging
- Microcirculation of the skin and regulation
- Angiosome concept
- Perforating pattern of DIEA
- MRI mechanism of action
- Tendon anatomy
- Tendon healing
- Flexor pulley system
- Negative pressure therapy
- Radiotherapy – mechanism of action and pathophysiology of complications
- LASERS
- Tissue expansion – pathophysiology, planning and surgical technique
- Dermoscopy
- Pathophysiology of osseointegration
- Mathes and Nahai classification
- Structure of the skin
- Function of the skin
- Normal palmar fascial anatomy
- Embryology of ear formation
- Flap raising surgical technique (Fibula, ALT, Radial Forearm)
- Cross-section of the leg and location of fasciotomy incisions
- Breast anatomy
- Embryology of breast development
- Stages of breast development
- Mechanism of action of leeching
- Foreign body reaction
- SIRS
- ARDS
- DIC
- CRPS

Abbreviations

3D – 3 Dimensional
ADH – AntiDiuretic Hormone
AER – Apical Ectodermal Ridge
AJCC – American Joint Committee on Cancer
ALT – Anterolateral thigh flap
AP – AnteroPosterior
APB – Abductor Pollicis Brevis
APL – Abductor Pollicis Longus
ATLS – Advanced Trauma Life Support
ATP – Adenosine Triphosphate
AV – Arteriovenous
AVA – Arteriovenous Anastomosis
AVN – Avascular Necrosis
BAD – British Association of Dermatologists
BAHA – Bone Anchored Hearing Aid
BCC – Basal Cell Carcinoma
BCIR – Breast and Cosmetic Implant Registry
BIA-ALCL – Breast Implant Associated Anaplastic Large Cell Lymphoma
BMI – Body Mass Index
BMP – Bone Morphogenetic Protein
CABG – Coronary Artery Bypass Graft
CCG – Clinical Commissioning Group
CK – Creatine Kinase
CLND – Completion Lymphadenectomy
CMCJ – Carpometacarpal Joint
CNS – Central Nervous System
CPAP – Continuous Positive Airway Pressure
CRP – C Reactive Protein
CRPS – Complex Regional Pain Syndrome
CT – Computed Tomography
CTA – Computed Tomography Angiography
DAO – Depressor Anguli Oris
DCIA – Deep Circumflex Iliac Artery
DIEP – Deep Inferior Epigastric Perforator flap
DLI – Depressor Labii Inferioris
DM – Diabetes Mellitus
DVT – Deep Vein Thrombosis
ECM – Extracellular Matrix
ECRB – Extensor Carpi Radialis Brevis
ECRL – Extensor Carpi Radialis Longus
EDC – Extensor Digitorum Communis
EDC – Extensor Digitorum Communis
EIP – Extensor Indicis Proprius
EMSB – Emergency Management of Severe Burns
ENT – Ear Nose and Throat
EPL – Extensor Pollicis Longus
ER – Emergency Room
FAMM – Facial Artery Musculomucosal flap
FCU – Flexor Carpi Ulnaris
FDA – Food and Drug Administration
FDP – Flexor Digitorum Profundus

FDS – Flexor Digitorum Superficialis
FGF – Fibroblast Growth Factor
FNA – Fine Needle Aspiration
FNAC – Fine Needle Aspiration Cytology
FPL – Flexor Pollicis Longus
FRCS – Fellowship of the Royal College of Surgeons
FTSG – Full Thickness Skin Graft
GA – General Anaesthetic
GCS – Glasgow Coma Scale
GP – General Practioner
GTN – Glyceryl Trinitrate
HPV – Human Papillomavirus
ICP – Intracranial Pressure
ICSRA – Intercompartmental Supraretinacular Artery
IGAP – Inferior Gluteal Artery Perforator flap
IGF – Insulin like Growth Factor
IJV – Internal Jugular Vein
IMA – Internal Mammary Artery
IMF – Infra-mammary fold
IPJ – Interphalangeal joint
IV – IntraVenous
LA – Local Anaesthetic
LASER – Light Amplification by the Stimulated Emission of Radiation
LD – Latissimus Dorsi
LD – Latissimus Dorsi flap
MACS – Minimal Access Cranial Suspension
MCPJ – Metacarpophalangeal Joint
MDT – MultiDisciplinary Team
MHRA – Medicines and Healthcare products Regulatory Agency
MMP – Matrix Metalloproteinase
MRC – Medical Research Council
MRI – Magnetic Resonance Imaging
MT – Metatarsal
MTPJ – Metatarsophalangeal Joint
NAC – Nipple Areolar Complex
NICE – National Institute for Health and Care Excellence
NL – Nasolabial
NO – Nitric Oxide
NPA – Nasopharyngeal Artery
NV – Neurovascular
NSAID – NonSteroidal Anti-Inflammatory Drug
OMT classification – Oberg Manske Tonkin classification
OPG – Orthopantomogram
ORN – Osteoradionecrosis
ORIF – Open Reduction Internal Fixation
PAP – Profunda Artery Perforator flap
PCOS – Polycystic Ovary Syndrome
PDGF – Platelet Derived Growth Factor
PDS – Polydioxanone Suture
PE – Pulmonary Embolus
PET – Positron Emission Tomography
PIA – Posterior Interosseus Artery
PIPJ – Proximal Interphalangeal Joint
PMH – Past Medical History
PMH – Past Medical History

PROMs – Patient Reported Outcome Measures
RBC – Red Blood Cell
RCT – Randomized Controlled Trial
RFFF – Radial Forearm Free Flap
RIG – Radiologically Inserted Gastrostomy
ROM – Range of Movement
RSTL – Relaxed Skin Tension Line
RTA – Road Traffic Accident
SALT – Speech and Language Therapist
SCC – Squamous Cell Carcinoma
SCIA – Superficial Circumflex Iliac Artery
SCM – Sternocleidomastoid
SGAP – Superior Gluteal Artery Perforator flap
SIEV – Superficial Inferior Epigastric Vein
SLNB – Sentinel Lymph Node Biopsy
SMAS – Superficial Musculoaponeurotic System
SPECT – Single Photon Emission Computed Tomography
SSG – Split Skin Graft
TAP flap – Thoracodorsal Artery Perforator flap
TBSA – Total Body Surface Area
TFL – Tensor Fascia Lata
TGF beta – Transforming Growth Factor beta
TNF alpha – Tumour necrosis Factor alpha
TNM – Tumour Node Metastasis
TPN – Total Parenteral Nutrition
TSST – Toxic Shock Syndrome Toxin
TUG – Transverse Upper Gracilis flap
UOP – Urine Output
USS – Ultrasound Scan
UVB – Ultraviolet B
VEGF – Vascular Endothelial Growth Factor
VRAM – Vertical Rectus Abdominis Myocutaneous flap
WHO – World Health Organization
WNT – Wingless Type Signalling Centre
ZM – Zygomatic Maxillary
ZPA – Zone of Polarizing Activity

Index

Printed in the United States
by Baker & Taylor Publisher Services